MW01156682

HYDROTHERAPY
for Health and Wellness

THEORY, PROGRAMS & TREATMENTS

RICHARD EIDSON

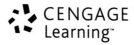

CENGAGE
Learning™

Australia • Brazil • Japan • Korea • Mexico • Singapore • Spain • United Kingdom • United States

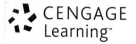
CENGAGE
Learning™

Hydrotherapy for Health and Wellness:
Theory, Programs, and Treatments
Richard Eidson

Vice President, Milady: Dawn Gerrain

Publisher: Erin O'Connor

Acquisitions Editor: Martine Edwards

Product Manager: Jessica Burns

Editorial Assistant: Mike Spring

Director of Beauty Industry Relations:
Sandra Bruce

Marketing Manager: Gerard McAvey

Production Director: Wendy Troeger

Content Project Manager: Angela Iula

Art Director: Joy Kocsis

Technology Project Manager: Sandy Charette

For product information and technology assistance, contact us at
Career Professional & Group Customer Support, 1-800-648-7450

For permission to use material from this text or product,
submit all requests online at **www.cengage.com/permissions**
Further permissions questions can be e-mailed to
permissionrequest@cengage.com

Library of Congress Control Number: 2007941007

ISBN-13: 978-1-4180-4929-4
ISBN-10: 1-4180-4929-8

Milady
5 Maxwell Drive
Clifton Park, NY 12065-2919
USA

Cengage Learning products are represented in Canada by Nelson Education, Ltd.

For your lifelong learning solutions, visit **milady.cengage.com**

Visit our corporate website at **www.cengage.com**

Notice to the Reader
Publisher does not warrant or guarantee any of the products described herein or perform any independent analysis in connection with any of the product information contained herein. Publisher does not assume, and expressly disclaims, any obligation to obtain and include information other than that provided to it by the manufacturer. The reader is expressly warned to consider and adopt all safety precautions that might be indicated by the activities described herein and to avoid all potential hazards. By following the instructions contained herein, the reader willingly assumes all risks in connection with such instructions. The publisher makes no representations or warranties of any kind, including but not limited to, the warranties of fitness for particular purpose or merchantability, nor are any such representations implied with respect to the material set forth herein, and the publisher takes no responsibility with respect to such material. The publisher shall not be liable for any special, consequential, or exemplary damages resulting, in whole or part, from the readers' use of, or reliance upon, this material.

1 2 3 4 5 XXX 11 10 09 08

Contents

CHAPTER 4

CHAPTER 5

CHAPTER 6

CHAPTER 9

About the Author

Richard Eidson is a hydrotherapist and hydrotherapy educator. He has also invented and holds three patents on hydrotherapy equipment. Richard has an undergraduate degree in social psychology, which has provided him with a deeper understanding of the mental and emotional benefits of hydrotherapy treatments. He also has an MBA, which has been helpful in understanding the marketing and financial management aspects of hydrotherapy programs. Richard is a licensed massage therapist as well, with special training in shiatsu.

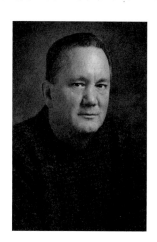

Richard's experiences not only as a therapist, educator, and inventor, but also from operating a wellness facility, have provided him with the knowledge and experiences for writing this textbook. In addition, he has done extensive research on hydrotherapy, especially into the behavior of water found in natural settings, in the human body, and in its use in hydrotherapy treatments. During his research, he has visited and researched some of the most important hydrotherapy sites of current and historical significance in North America, including Hot Springs, Arkansas, and Saratoga Springs, New York, as well as the main hot springs facilities in California, Colorado, and western Canada. His international research includes trips to Germany (including Baden-Baden and Bad Worishofen, the home of Kneipp therapy), as well as Vichy, France. Other research projects have included trips to Greece, India, Japan, Thailand, Oman, and Bali (Indonesia). He has been able to personally visit all of the locations in various parts of the world that are described in Chapter 8: History of Hydrotherapy.

Several of the photographs in this textbook were taken by Richard during his travels and during the photo shoot for the textbook. These photographs are intended to give visual expression to the special and unique experiences of the many aspects of hydrotherapy.

Richard resides in Fairfield, Iowa, where he runs a wellness center and a company for inventing hydrotherapy equipment. He provides consulting, education, and training in hydrotherapy and continues his research into hydrotherapy through travels both nationally and internationally. His personal Web site detailing his teaching and research in hydrotherapy is www.studyhydrotherapy.com.

Acknowledgments

Support from many people, educational resources, and health and wellness hydrotherapy facilities have been fundamental in developing this textbook. First, I would like to thank Sandra Moren—a friend and a fellow Milady author—for her inspiration and creative ideas. Monica Brown, a respected spa consultant who helped develop the spa and wellness industry we see today, has also contributed creative suggestions and inspiration. Jessica Burns, my developmental editor at Milady, helped me at every step along the way. Other people who have helped with their support and inspiration are Grace Jull, Susan Gove, and Ken West.

I would also like to recognize the resources of knowledge in various fields and the authors who created them. The *Textbook of Medical Physiology* by Arthur Guyton and John Hall was of great value in helping me understand the dynamic, fluid, cellular nature of the human body. Rod Nave, of the department of physics and astronomy at Georgia State University, created the HyperPhysics Web site, which provides a comprehensive explanation of the scientific behavior of water in an easy-to-understand format.

Finally, I would like to acknowledge some of the wellness facilities that offer hydrotherapy treatments. People at the following facilities provided me with invaluable education and experiences in hydrotherapy: Friedrichsbad and Caracalla in Baden-Baden, Germany; the Edelweiss Kneipp Kur Wellness Hotel, in Bad Worishofen, Germany, and German M. Schleinkofer, Kneipp hydrotherapy educator and author of several textbooks on hydrotherapy; and the Centre Thermal des Domes in Vichy, France, for education in the French tradition of hydrotherapy.

The author and publisher would like to acknowledge the following reviewers, who supported us through the development of this text. We are grateful for your input and appreciate your insightful suggestions:

Monica Tuma Brown, Spa Development Consultant, Minnesota

Cathy Fournier, Massage Therapist and Hydrotherapy Instructor, Canada

Susan Gove, Massage Therapist, Hydrotherapy Instructor, Spa Trainer, and Guest Speaker, Georgia

Sharon Howerton, Hydrotherapy Instructor and President of Oceanus: The Ocean Therapy Institute, North Carolina

Grace Jull, Kripalu Center for Yoga and Health, Massachusetts

Rachel Rowen Karlsberg, Medical Aesthetician Practitioner and Educator, California

Patricia Lyons, Registered Nurse, Indiana

Carol Mae, Massage Therapist and Hydrotherapy Instructor, Washington

Sandra Alexcae Moren, Kyron Spa and Salon Consulting, Author, and Educator, Canada

Julie Onofrio, Massage Practitioner and Writer/Web Developer, Washington

Tonya Payne, Educator, Spa Owner, Therapist, and Nutritional Expert, Illinois

Introduction

The hydrotherapy education presented in this textbook will allow therapists to develop a new set of therapy skills to help clients attain all of their health and wellness goals. This textbook, which has been created for students and therapists, is intended to provide hydrotherapy education for use in various professional settings, including private practices, health and wellness centers, fitness centers, spas, skin care centers, and schools.

Hydrotherapy education can be easy, enjoyable, and creative and can enhance the skills of any therapist. It is not just learning how to perform a few hydrotherapy treatments, it is also about gaining comprehensive knowledge, skills, and experience to use the full potential of hydrotherapy as a therapeutic modality. Hydrotherapy education can also help therapists develop a greater appreciation and relationship with water that can enhance their ability to work with it as a therapeutic tool. This textbook teaches about the behavior of water in the natural environment, inside the human body, and as it is used in hydrotherapy treatments. A key point is that the basic principles of the behavior of water in each of these three areas are the same—the measurable, predictable way in which water behaves is the same wherever it is found. Thus, there is a natural synergy between water inside the body and water used in hydrotherapy to transform the body. It is this synergy that a therapist learns to work with to produce profound health and wellness transformations in a client.

Human beings have always had a natural relationship with water. We were born in a total water environment, the surface of the Earth is 70% water, and each of us is 60% water. Hydrotherapy education is simply the process of taking this natural relationship with water and transforming it into a remarkable relationship between water, the therapist, the client, and the client's health and wellness goals.

This relationship is not new. Hydrotherapy has been an essential element of all great health and wellness traditions for thousands of years. This tradition continues to the present day because it works in multiple and profound ways. And it will continue to develop in the future, offering even greater applications in the art and science of health and wellness, as well as unfolding a much greater appreciation of this incredible substance that we simply know as "water."

In this textbook, each chapter provides education on a key element of hydrotherapy. All the chapters, taken together, develop a more complete, holistic knowledge of hydrotherapy, as well as basic treatment skills and training in a wide range of hydrotherapy treatments (see Figure 1).

This textbook follows the standard teaching format of text explanations, related tables, illustrations, and photographs. Some chapters also provide teaching exercises. There is also an on-line companion Web site that provides additional information for each chapter, including color photographs, links to educational Web sites, scientific research, and teaching demonstrations. These resources are available for use by both teachers and students in a classroom setting and for home study. This textbook can also be used by professional

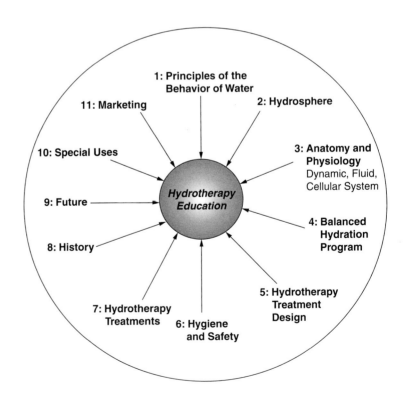

therapists who want to learn more about hydrotherapy and its practical application as a therapeutic modality.

The following is a brief introduction to each of the 11 chapters.

Chapter 1: Principles of the Natural Behavior of Water

This chapter introduces the principle ways in which water behaves. It is the natural behavior of water that allows for all the complex physiological activities in the human body, for the beautiful expressions of water in the natural environment and for its use as a therapeutic tool in hydrotherapy. Each of the principle behaviors of water are measurable and predictable, which allows them to be used with greater precision. The following are the principle behaviors of water that are presented in this chapter:

- Heat capacity
- Solvent
- pH levels
- Suspension
- Gravity
- Pressure
- Osmosis
- Evaporation
- Buoyancy

Teaching exercises are given for each principle, providing students with hands-on experience.

Chapter 2: Hydrosphere: One Dynamic Water System

In Chapter 2, we learn that all water that we use for hydrotherapy (and all other uses) has its source in the hydrosphere—the Earth's one dynamic water system. The total amount of water on Earth remains relatively constant and is found in beautiful natural dynamic expressions, including the oceans, lakes, rivers, waterfalls, rain, snow, ice, glaciers, and hot springs. This one dynamic, integrated water system is continually purifying itself and distributing this "fresh" water to all areas of the planet. The hydrosphere is not only the source of water used for hydrotherapy treatments, but also much of the understanding of the principles of hydrotherapy has been gained over time from people's experiences with water in natural settings—for example, at hot springs or the ocean. Greater knowledge of the hydrosphere connects us to the "source" of water as well as providing greater insights into the natural behavior of water as it is used in hydrotherapy.

Chapter 3: Dynamic Fluid Anatomy and Physiology and Hydrotherapy

The study of water also provides a greater understanding of the anatomy and physiology of the human body. The human body is approximately 60% (10 gal) water, and all this water is in a continual state of dynamic circulation. Water in the body is an essential part of every one of our 100 trillion cells and of every physiological process that takes place in our bodies. The fact that the body is mainly water provides insight into why hydrotherapy is such a powerful therapeutic tool. In hydrotherapy, water is brought into contact with the body to transform the fluid dynamics of water inside the body. Hydrotherapy can be used to work on localized areas of the body or the body as one integrated system. This chapter presents insights into working with the body at the structural level and also at the dynamic fluid, cellular level.

Chapter 4: The Balanced Hydration Program: A Key to Health and Wellness

Chapter 4 discusses why proper hydration is so essential for our health and wellness and why when the body's hydration level falls below a certain level, problems begin to develop and become greater with increasing levels of dehydration. Today, we have a better understanding of how much water the body naturally loses each day and how much water intake is needed to stay properly hydrated. This chapter presents the Balanced Hydration Program, which allows you to consult with your clients to help them improve their daily hydration behaviors. This program provides recommendations not only about the optimal amount of water but also about the percentage of drinking water relative to water from beverages, the timing of water intake throughout the day, and the source and quality of water intake. By making improvements in these key areas, a client can make significant, positive changes in his or her total daily hydration behavior. The benefits of this program can be very significant, not only for improved hydration, but also for weight management as well as decreasing the level of intake of potentially harmful (toxic)chemicals.

Chapter 5: Understanding the Key Elements of Hydrotherapy Treatments

Certain key elements are common to all the hydrotherapy treatments taught in Chapter 7. Chapter 5 discusses each element in detail. A greater knowledge of each key element helps in the understanding the significance of each element and how they function together to produce desired therapeutic outcomes. The following are the key elements of a hydrotherapy treatment that are discussed in this chapter:

- Client
- Therapist
- Hydrotherapy equipment
- Products, including herbs, seaweed, algae, mineral salts, clay, essential oils, and hydrosols
- Water: The role of water in each hydrotherapy treatment
- Steps of the treatment: The step-by-step instructions for each treatment
- Facility: Includes the hydrotherapy treatment room and other rooms used in the hydrotherapy program

An understanding of these different elements is helpful in being able to design specific hydrotherapy treatments and programs to be used as part of ongoing health and wellness programs.

Chapter 6: Hygiene and Safety

The use of water in hydrotherapy treatments creates certain unique conditions that require special hygiene and safety procedures. Water used in hydrotherapy treatments can come into contact with all or part of the client's body. This water can then come into contact with the hydrotherapy equipment, floor, and other surfaces in the treatment room. Because a large number of germs can be contained in just one drop of water, all equipment and surfaces that have come into contact with water used during the treatment must be cleaned and *disinfected*. Proper disinfection procedures are necessary to kill germs and thereby eliminate possible infection of the client or the therapist.

There are also special safety issues associated with the use of water in hydrotherapy treatments, including protection against scalding or slipping. In addition, some hydrotherapy treatments, especially heating treatments, can make c lients dizzy, causing them to have difficulty when moving. Therapists must take added measures to ensure each client's safety.

Chapter 7: Hydrotherapy Treatments

In this chapter, students learn the general principles of performing treatments in a specific category of hydrotherapy, for example,
steam therapy. Students also learn how to perform a variety of treatments in that category, for example, steam treatments for relaxation,
detoxification, skin care, preparation for massage, and inhalation
therapy. This provides both the knowledge and skills to work with
any treatments in all of the categories. It also provides the knowledge and skills to design new treatments in each category. The key
categories of hydrotherapy treatments covered are hydrotub (bath),
underwater hydromassage, steam, shower, hydromassage table, hot
and cold compresses, cryotherapy, and misting.

Chapter 8: History of Hydrotherapy—
Ancient to Present

The study of the historical use of hydrotherapy shows that it has
been a major component of the great health and wellness traditions
throughout time. We find the use of hydrotherapy in Ayurveda from
India and in the traditional health and wellness programs of Japan,
both of which are more than a thousand years old. Both of these traditions have also been used continuously until the present day and are
now popular at wellness centers and spas around the world. The great
hydrotherapy traditions of the Greeks and Romans have had a major
influence on modern hydrotherapy. In addition, the use of hydrotherapy, including medical hydrotherapy, by many European countries
has been used continually for several hundred years. The history of
hydrotherapy teaches us that it has worked for thousands of years and
can be applied in similar ways today to help clients achieve the same
health and wellness goals that clients have always valued.

Chapter 9: The Future of Hydrotherapy

This chapter discusses ways in which hydrotherapy is continuing to
develop insights into the further development of hydrotherapy in the
future. The areas discussed in this chapter include the following:

- Water: Continuing scientific developments in understanding the behavior of water, especially at the molecular level
  and its behavior in the human body.
- Natural products: More natural products are becoming
  available from around the world as well as a greater understanding of their use in hydrotherapy.
- Hydrotherapy equipment: Improvements in design
  features, such as greater comfort, better control over

water temperature and pressure, and more multipurpose equipment.

- Wisdom from the past: Greater research and understanding into the historical uses of hydrotherapy can provide deeper insights into the development of hydrotherapy in the future.

- Shared knowledge: Through the Internet and other modern forms of communication, greater sharing of information about hydrotherapy among therapists from around the world will lead to a greater global team approach in the further development of treatments and programs.

- Hydrosphere: A greater understanding of the behavior of the hydrosphere in the future, can lead to a greater understanding of the natural behavior of water as well as our connection to the planet's one global water system. and the total concept of nature leading to better insights into the further development of hydrotherapy.

- Nature Paradigm: We are gaining a greater understanding of the total concept of what we mean by nature and what is natural, including alternative health approaches such as hydrotherapy. This will continue to provide insights into the use of hydrotherapy and a greater appreciation of how all natural systems are intimately connected.

Chapter 10: Unique Uses of Water for Health and Wellness

This chapter discusses some of the "unique" uses of water for healing and wellness. Much is known about water—both scientifically and from the use of water in traditional hydrotherapy treatments. However, much remains to be learned about the full potential of the use of water as a therapeutic modality. A better understanding of the role of water in healing and wellness may come from insights gained through many of the unique uses described in this chapter.

One area of the special use of water for healing and wellness involves water in natural settings. Nothing is done to the water, it just seems to have special qualities that produces unique effects. Some of the examples discussed include:

- Healing baths
- Sacred bath
- Special hot springs, waterfalls, lakes
- Natural water settings for meditation and contemplation

- Water from some remote locations know for its special power for producing greater health and longevity
- The beneficial effects from the recreational use of water in natural settings

Another area of the unique use of water includes normal water that has been modified by some form of technology or human intention that then transforms the people it comes in contact with, such as the following:

- Crystals or gemstones
- Color light therapy
- Natural and primordial sounds
- Transforming water through intention (e.g., blessing water)
- Enhanced drinking water for greater health and wellness
- Principles of feng shui and Sthapatya Veda for enhancing the "chi" or "prana" (life force) of the water

In each of these example, the question is, "What is it about these waters that gives them special healing and wellness properties and how can this understanding allow us to use more of its full potential for health and wellness?"

Chapter 11: Marketing Hydrotherapy Programs

This chapter provides education on how to market and promote hydrotherapy treatments and programs. Clients are often not as familiar with hydrotherapy as they are with more traditional programs such as massage and skin care. Therefore, it is necessary to find creative ways to educate and interest clients in a facility's hydrotherapy programs. The following are some of the suggestions for promoting these programs:

- Engaging brochures, DVD presentations, and Web sites
- Personal client interview to provide education and recommendations about all programs, including hydrotherapy
- Water themes as part of a facility's atmosphere and décor—for example, small fountains, natural sounds of water, or beautiful photographs of natural water settings

In summary, this textbook has been designed to provide students and therapists with the knowledge and skills to:

- Perform treatments in a wide range of hydrotherapy categories, including hydrotub (bath), underwater hydromassage, steam, shower, hydromassage table, hot and cold compresses, cyrotherapy, and misting.

- Have comprehensive knowledge and skills of the general principles of each of these categories.
- Design hydrotherapy treatments and programs for use in specific health and wellness programs.
- Understand the complex health and wellness goals of clients and be able to recommend treatments and programs to allow clients to achieve their personal goals.
- Maintain high standards of hygiene and safety during (and after) hydrotherapy treatments.
- Communicate and successfully market hydrotherapy treatments and programs to current and potential clients.

This edition features an Online Companion™ that is a useful supplement for instructors and interested readers that provides instrumental resources and activities, in addition to what the book provides. For the instructors such resources and activities include:

- Sample lesson plans
- Additional discussion questions
- Answers to the Chapter Review Questions featured in the core text

The Online Companion also includes a section devoted to readers who are seeking additional information. Sections are made up of the following components:

- Links to relevant and up-to-date information on Hydrotherapy
- Scientific Research on Hydrotherapy
- Teaching examples and case studies
- Forms to be printed for your own use or in a classroom setting, such as client interview form and hydration forms
- Frequently Asked Questions and Helpful Hints
- Bibliography of related titles and scientific research

The Online Companion™ icon appears at the end of specific chapters to prompt you to go online and take advantage of the many features provided.

You can find the Online Companion™ web site at http://www.milady.cengage.com.

Principles of the Natural Behavior of Water

KEY TERMS

hydrotherapy	solvent	negative ions
hydrosphere	diffusion	pumping
mole	solute	osmosis
hydrogen bond	hydrophilic	evaporation
cohesion	hydrophobic	humidity
surface tension	pH level	buoyancy
adhesion	suspension	specific gravity
kinetic energy	blood plasma	
heat capacity	gravity	

INTRODUCTION

Hydrotherapy is the use of water as a therapeutic modality to help clients attain and maintain all their health and wellness goals. To better appreciate how water is used in hydrotherapy as a therapeutic modality, it is helpful to understand some basic principles of water's natural behavior. Water behaves in several well-known and predictable ways. Knowing these principles helps us understand how water behaves inside the human body, in the natural environment, and in hydrotherapy treatments. From a scientific understanding of the behavior of water, researchers are able to develop mathematical formulas that can be used to accurately predict the precise behavior of water according to each basic behavioral principle of water. This knowledge also provides precise ways to measure the behavior of water in terms of temperature, flow rate, and other variables.

Hydrotherapy
The use of water as a therapeutic modality to help clients attain and maintain all their health and wellness goals.

Additional knowledge about the behavior of water, especially for its use in hydrotherapy, is also gained through direct experience with the different ways in which water behaves, whether it be from teaching exercises, during hydrotherapy treatments, or in the natural environment. This chapter includes a simple teaching exercise for each of the different ways in which water behaves. By experiencing these different natural behaviors of water, including buoyancy and heat exchange, therapists can better understand the nature of water. Every hydrotherapy treatment involves at least one principle of the behavior of water; thus, it is possible to continue to learn about the behavior of water while performing hydrotherapy treatments. For example, in a flotation treatment, buoyancy is the main principle that produces the therapeutic effects. In a steam treatment, the principle of heat exchange is the main dynamic principle. One can also learn about the principles of water's behavior from experiences in natural settings, such as a waterfall, the ocean, or hot springs. The **hydrosphere** refers to the one water system on Earth, which has a fixed volume of approximately 332 million cubic miles (mi^3). All of this water in the hydrosphere is in a state of constant circulation and is found in different dynamic formations, such as the ocean, clouds, rivers, rain, snow, and glaciers (see Figure 1–1).

Understanding the basic principles of the behavior of water, both intellectually and from direct experience, will give a therapist greater knowledge and skills in using water as a tool for therapeutic transformations. It also allows a therapist to develop a deeper personal connection with water that can then be used in therapeutic settings to enhance the outcome of hydrotherapy wellness treatments. This chapter discusses the elements that are fundamental in understanding the behavior of water: water molecules, heat capacity, movement, solvent, suspension, and buoyancy.

Hydrosphere
Earth's entire water system.

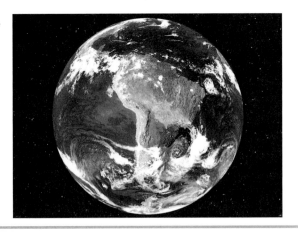

Figure 1–1 Hydrosphere of South America *(courtesy of NASA).*

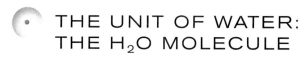

THE UNIT OF WATER: THE H₂O MOLECULE

The various ways in which water behaves are based on the structure and behavior of water molecules—the basic unit of water—and how those water molecules interact not only with each other but also with other types of molecules. Any amount of water is made up of a certain, measurable number of water molecules. The molecular weight of water is 1 mole (mol), which is equivalent to 18.02 g, or 18.02 mL (see Teaching Exercise 1–1). A **mole** of any substance is a combination of the atomic weights of the atoms that make up that substance (see Table 1–1). One mole of any substance,

Mole

A combination of the atomic weights of the atoms that make up a substance.

1–1 TEACHING EXERCISE

1 mol of water = 18.02 mL

- The molecular weight of water (H_2O) is 18.02 g. This is equivalent to a volume of 18.02 mL.
- 1 mol of any substance, including water, contains 6,023,000,000,000,000,000,000,000 molecules (6.023×10^{23}).
- Any amount of water in any state—solid, liquid, or vapor—represents a specific amount of water molecules. Even the total estimated amount of water on Earth, which is 332,500,000 mi^3, is made up of a specific number of water molecules.
- Fill a small measuring glass with 18.02 mL (18.02 g) of water. This is 1 mol of H_2O.

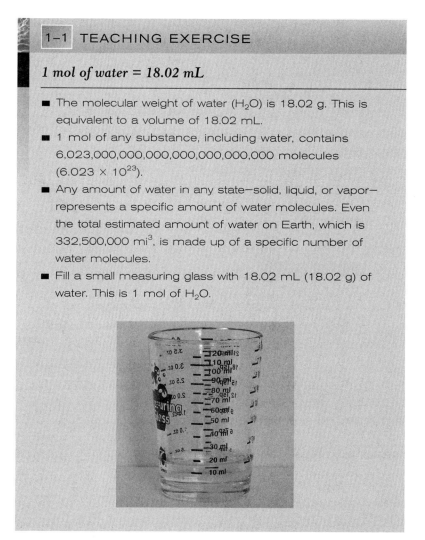

Table 1–1   Atomic Structure of Water

1 mol is the amount of any substance that has a mass in grams equal to the sum of the atomic masses of all its atoms. 1 mol of any molecule always has the same number of molecules–6.023×10^{23}.

Atomic mass of hydrogen	1.01
Atomic mass of oxygen	16.00
Atomic mass of H_2O	18.02
1 mol of H_2O (weight in grams)	18.02
Number of water molecules in 1 mol of H_2O	6.023×10^{23}
$6.023 \times 10^{23} =$ 6,023,000,000,000,000,000,000,000	6.023×10^{23}

including water, contains 6,023,000,000,000,000,000,000,000 molecules (6.023×10^{23}). Therefore, 1 mol of water, which consists of two hydrogen atoms and one oxygen atom (H_2O), weighs 18.02 g and contains 6.023×10^{23} water molecules (see Figure 1–2 and Plate 4).

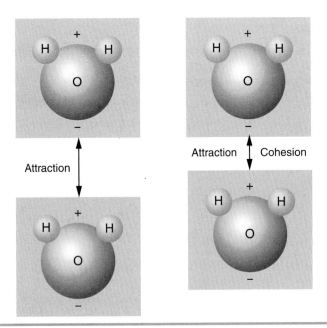

Figure 1–2 H_2O molecule: Hydrogen bond.

Behavior of Water at the Molecular Level

Cohesion

Water molecules have a slightly positive electrical charge on the hydrogen side of the molecule and a slightly negative electrical charge on the oxygen side. According to the law of attraction, the negative end of one water molecule (the oxygen side) is attracted to the positive end (the hydrogen side) of another water molecule, creating a cohesive force of attraction between the water molecules. **Hydrogen bond** is the term used to describe this cohesive attraction between water molecules. This **cohesion** between water molecules allows water to behave as a liquid between temperatures of 32°F (0°C) and 212°F (100°C). In other words, the water molecules have an attraction strong enough to each other to stay connected in the liquid form. At temperatures below 32°F (0°C), water molecules will freeze into a solid crystal, hexagonal structure. At temperatures above 212°F (100°C), water will boil; the heat from this boiling will produce evaporation of liquid water to the vapor state. Even at temperatures below boiling, some water molecules are always evaporating from the surface of the water. For example, solar heating of the ocean increases the temperature of the water, which, in turn, increases the rate of evaporation of water molecules from the ocean's surface. (See Teaching Exercise 1–2.)

Hydrogen bond
The term used to describe the cohesive attraction between water molecules.

Cohesion
The attraction between water molecules that allows water to behave as a liquid between temperatures of 32°F (0°C) and 212°F (100°C).

Surface Tension

Cohesion of water molecules also produces the phenomena known as surface tension. **Surface tension** occurs because water molecules on the surface of water have a greater attraction to each other than to the water molecules below the surface. This principle of water can be seen in the behavior of water drops: Surface tension keeps the water molecules in the drops from spreading out in a thin film. It is what gives raindrops and dew drops their shape. Surface tension also creates a greater resistance to objects entering the water—for example, the resistance that is experienced when diving into water. (See Teaching Exercise 1–2.)

Surface tension
Water molecules on the surface of water have a greater attraction to each other than to the water molecules below the surface.

Adhesion

Adhesion is the behavior of water that allows water molecules to be attracted to the molecules on the surface of other substances. For example, small drops of water can stick (attach) to the side of a glass cup, a leaf, or a flower. Adhesion of water molecules to the

Adhesion
The behavior of water that allows water molecules to be attracted to the molecules on the surface of other substances.

1–2 TEACHING EXERCISE

Cohesion, Surface Tension, and Adhesion

Use an eye dropper to create several drops of water on a nonabsorbent surface. The photograph shows water drops on a leaf. The water drops on the surface illustrate the following ways that water behaves.

- **COHESION:** The attraction between molecules of water allows water to remain in the liquid state in a certain temperature range.
- **SURFACE TENSION:** The water molecules on the surface of a water drop have greater attraction to each other than to the water molecules below the surface. This allows water to form drops, instead of spreading out into a thin layer.
- **ADHESION:** Water molecules are attracted to other molecules on the surface of other objects. This gives water drops the ability to stick to other surfaces without running off, as shown in the photograph.

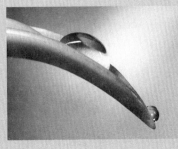

glass molecules, as an example, keeps the drops of water attached to the side of the glass. When the water drop becomes large enough, the force of gravity will cause it to flow down the side of the glass. This property of adhesion also creates some resistance to the flow of water through water pipes in homes or through the blood vessels (in the form of blood plasma) of the circulatory system. As water flows through these pipes or vessels, the water molecules that come in contact with the surface of these structures are attracted to them, which creates some resistance to the flow of the fluid. (See Teaching Exercise 1–2.)

Kinetic Energy

Water molecules have a high level of **kinetic energy,** as they are constantly in a state of random motion. Because of the small size of water molecules, it is not possible to see them moving in a glass of water, but this does not mean they are not in a state of constant motion (see Teaching Exercise 1–3). Because of their kinetic energy, water

kinetic energy
The extra energy an object possesses due to its motion.

1–3 TEACHING EXERCISE

Kinetic Energy and Diffusion

Water molecules are in constant motion, even though we do not see them moving in a glass filled with water.

1. Place 5 drops of food color into a large glass of water at room temperature. The kinetic energy of the water molecules influences the rate at which the food color molecules diffuse in the water. Note how much time it takes for the food color molecules to dissolve.

2. Repeat Step 1, but this time with hot tap water. How long does it take? The greater the water temperature, the greater will be the kinetic activity (speed of the water molecules), and the force of collision between water molecules, which increases the rate of diffusion (mixing) of the food color molecules.

During hydrotherapy treatments, when we increase the temperature of water inside the human body, we increase the rate of diffusion as well as the metabolic rate of the cells. This increase occurs as the kinetic energy of the water and other molecules within our body increases.

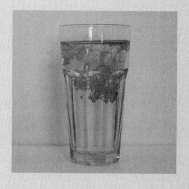

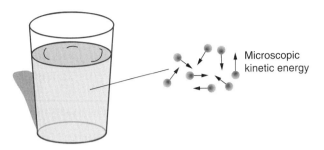

In a glass of water, water molecules are moving at high speeds, constantly colliding with other water molecules. As the temperature of water increases, the speed and force of the collisions of water molecules increases. In the human body, a water temperature of 98.6°F/37°C creates the ideal rate of movement of water molecules for the metabolic functions of the cells.

Figure 1–3 Movement of water molecules: Kinetic energy.

molecules move at high speeds of hundreds of meters per second (see Figure 1–3). The greater the water's temperature, the greater will be the speed and the force of collision of the water molecules.

This natural movement of water at the molecular level influences the metabolic activity that takes place in every cell of our body. In the body, a constant core temperature of approximately 98.6°F (37°C) is necessary to produce a speed and energy of water molecules that is optimal for normal cellular metabolic activity. Even a slight increase or decrease in this core temperature can alter normal cellular functioning. Different hydrotherapy treatments use different water temperatures to increase or decrease the core or surface temperature of the body, producing different therapeutic benefits.

 ## BEHAVIORS OF WATER

Heat Capacity

Heat capacity
The behavior of water by which it absorbs heat (increases in temperature) or releases heat (decreases in temperature).

Heat capacity is the behavior of water by which it absorbs heat (increases in temperature) or releases heat (decreases in temperature). Although all substances absorb and release heat, water has some unique features. First, water has a high heat capacity, which means it can absorb a large amount of heat without a significant rise in temperature. For water in the liquid form, it takes 1 calorie (cal) of heat to increase the temperature of 1 g of water 1°C. Substances

Table 1–2   Heat Capacity

Substance	Amount of Heat (in cal)
Water	1
Copper	0.023
Copper	0.023
Aluminum	0.023
Ethanol	2.44

such as copper have a low heat capacity, which means it takes much less heat to increase their temperature (see Table 1–2).

Water is the only substance that exists naturally in all three states: solid (frozen), liquid, and gas (vapor). (See Teaching Exercise 1–4.) The temperature of water determines in which state it will be. As frozen water is heated, it becomes liquid. As the temperature continues to increase, there is greater evaporation of water molecules. When water reaches a temperature of 212°F (100°C), the water boils, and all additional heat produces evaporation of water molecules. When water cools and condenses back to the liquid state, it releases the same amount of heat to the environment that it gained when it was heated. This phase transition of water from solid to liquid to gas is shown in Figure 1–4.

As will be discussed in Chapter 2, there is a fixed amount of water on Earth. Of this total amount, 97.99% is in the liquid state (mainly the ocean), 2% is in the frozen state (ice packs and glaciers), and less than 0.001% is in the atmosphere in the form of water vapor. Water cannot heat itself; it must be heated by some external heat source. For water on Earth's surface, the main source of heat is solar heat (energy) from the sun (see Figure 1–5). Solar heating of the ocean and other surfaces of water increases the water temperature, thus increasing the rate of evaporation. The ocean's ability to absorb large amounts of solar heat is what keeps Earth's surface temperature within a normal range. Water is also heated and cooled by people using electricity, gas, and solar technologies for such activities as bathing, cooking, and cleaning, as well as for many industrial, agricultural, and commercial activities.

For use in hydrotherapy treatments, water may be heated or cooled, depending on the type of treatment. Some hydrotherapy treatments use heated or cooled water to increase or decrease the client's surface and/or core body temperature. The core temperature of water in the body is maintained at a constant temperature

1–4 TEACHING EXERCISE

Water in Three States: Solid, Liquid, and Gas

1. Add 18 mL of water into a measuring cup (1 mL of water = 1 g of water). Remember that 18.02 g of water equals 1 mol of water and that 1 mol of water contains 6.023×10^{23} water molecules.

2. Place the measuring cup in a freezer. Once the water is frozen, remove it from the freezer. Lowering the temperature of the water molecules caused a change in state from liquid to frozen water. The volume of the water also increased. When water freezes, the volume increases by 4%.

3. Place the measuring cup on a table, preferably where it will come in direct contact with sunlight for solar heating. Water molecules will evaporate from the surface of the water. Note how long it takes for all the water molecules to evaporate. (The rate of evaporation will be greater with increased heat.)

Water is the only natural substance that exists naturally in all three states. The total amount of water in the hydrosphere is in a continual process of transformation between liquid, gas, and solid states.

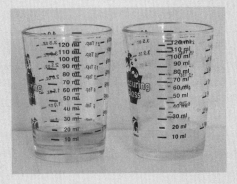

of approximately 98.6°F (37°C). However, when a therapist places a client in a hydrotub that has a water temperature of 104°F (40°C), the client's core body temperature will increase due to heat exchange between the hotter water in the hydrotub and the cooler water in the client's body (see Teaching Exercise 1–5). The use of steam therapy,

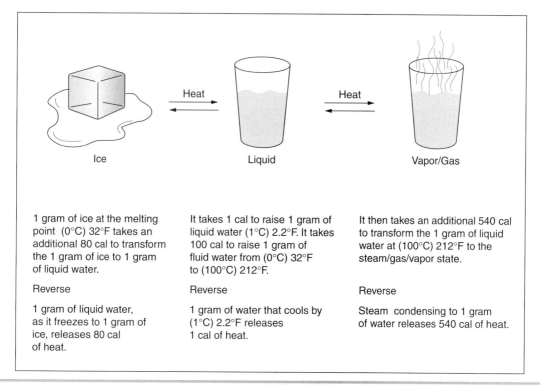

Ice · Liquid · Vapor/Gas

1 gram of ice at the melting point (0°C) 32°F takes an additional 80 cal to transform the 1 gram of ice to 1 gram of liquid water.

Reverse

1 gram of liquid water, as it freezes to 1 gram of ice, releases 80 cal of heat.

It takes 1 cal to raise 1 gram of liquid water (1°C) 2.2°F. It takes 100 cal to raise 1 gram of fluid water from (0°C) 32°F to (100°C) 212°F.

Reverse

1 gram of water that cools by (1°C) 2.2°F releases 1 cal of heat.

It then takes an additional 540 cal to transform the 1 gram of liquid water at (100°C) 212°F to the steam/gas/vapor state.

Reverse

Steam condensing to 1 gram of water releases 540 cal of heat.

Figure 1–4 States of water: Ice, liquid, gas.

Figure 1–5 Solar heating of water: Sun and ocean *(image copyright Nat Ulrich, 2008. Used under license from Shutterstock.com).*

1-5 TEACHING EXERCISE

Heat Exchange

Water will exchange heat with whatever it comes into contact. For example, if warm water comes into contact with cool air, then the water will lose heat to the air, which will heat the air. If the air temperature is hotter than the water, then water absorbs the heat—the water becomes hotter and air becomes cooler.

1. Fill a gallon container with warm water from a sink. Try to get the water temperature as close to 98.6°F as possible by adding warm or cooler water (use a temperature gauge).

2. After 4 or 5 hours, check the water temperature again. During this time, there will have been heat exchange between the warmer water and the cooler room temperature of about 70°F. Note the change in temperature.

The human body maintains a constant core temperature of about 98.6°F. The main heating source that keeps the body warm is the heat generated by the metabolic activity of each of the 100 trillion cells of the body! To experience the principle of heat exchange used during hydrotherapy, perform the following steps.

1. Place your hand in water that is no hotter than 104°F (40°C) to 108°F (44°C). (You should be able to use a sink filled with water for this exercise.) Heat from the water will flow to the lower temperature of your hand, increasing the surface and core temperature of your hand, as well as the temperature of the blood flowing through your hand.

2. Place your hand in cold tap water in a sink. Heat from your hand will flow to the colder water, decreasing the surface and core temperature of your hand as well as the blood flowing through your hand.

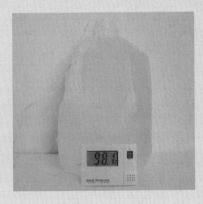

showers, and other techniques can also raise or lower the body's surface and core temperatures. Likewise, hot or cold compresses can produce changes in temperature in more localized areas of the body.

The human body gains and loses heat from and to the environment in four ways: conduction, convection, radiation, and evaporation.

1. Conduction is the heat exchange that takes place when the human body is in direct contact with another object. For example, the body gains heat when sitting in a hot tub at 104°F by being in direct contact with water. Water in contact with the body conducts heat 20 times greater than air at the same temperature. This is the main reason immersion in water that is warmer or cooler than the body can rapidly increase or decrease the skin and core temperature.

2. Convection is the heating or cooling of the body by flowing water or air at a different temperature across the body. Air, blowing from a fan, will have a greater cooling effect on the body. Water in a hot tub that is circulating will heat the body more quickly than when the water is still.

3. Radiation is the transfer of heat from objects in the form of infrared rays. Normally, the body is hotter than objects in a room at 70°F, and heat will radiate to the cooler objects in a room. At room temperatures of around 70°F, the amount of heat being produced by the body and being lost is about equal, so generally we feel comfortable. If a person is in a hot tub, surrounded by water that is at 104°F, the radiant heat of water will flow to the cooler temperature of the body (98.6°F), increasing the body temperature.

4. Evaporation of water plays a significant role in cooling the human body in order to maintain a constant core temperature of approximately 98.6°F (34°C). When the body's core temperature increases—for example, due to exercise—sweat, which is mostly water, is produced by the skin's sweat glands. Heat from the body is absorbed by the sweat on the skin, causing the sweat to evaporate. As the water in sweat evaporates from the skin, heat is removed from the body, thereby cooling the body. The evaporation of 1 g (1 mL) of sweat will remove 580 cal of heat from the body. Sweating is essential for cooling the body whenever there is an increase in the core temperature. (See Chapter 3.)

Solvent

An important behavior of water is that it acts as a **solvent,** or a substance within which other substances can dissolve. Water is sometimes referred to as a universal solvent, because so many substances dissolve in it. When a certain substance, such as salt or sugar, is placed in water, it completely dissolves until the molecules are equally present throughout the water. If you place 100 g of sugar in a measuring cup and add enough distilled water to make 1 L of solution, you will create a 10% sugar solution.

Gases such as oxygen and carbon dioxide will also dissolve in water. Water from any source, including the ocean, lakes, rivers, groundwater, or rain, will contain some dissolved minerals and gases in solution. When flowing water comes in contact with rocks, soil, oxygen, and carbon dioxide, the minerals and gases from those items dissolve in the water.

Likewise, different fluids found in the body are composed mostly of water and have precise amounts of dissolved minerals (electrolytes), glucose, oxygen, and carbon dioxide. Examples of some of the main fluids in the body are blood, interstitial fluid, cellular fluid, lymphatic fluid, and cerebral spinal fluid.

The rate (speed) of **diffusion** of various substances (**solutes**) dissolving in water depends on the temperature of the water, the amount (concentration) of the substance dissolving, and the distance the solute has to travel. Thus, the greater the concentration of the substance dissolving, the greater the temperature of the water, and the shorter the distance the dissolving substance needs to travel, the greater the rate of diffusion will be. In the body, diffusion is the primary way that nutrients, oxygen, hormones, and other substances move between blood plasma, interstitial fluid, and fluids within the cells.

Therapists use water's solvent property to dissolve various products in water to produce different beneficial effects during a hydrotherapy treatment. For example, certain bath salts, such as products from the Dead Sea or natural sea salt, can be dissolved in different concentrations in water used for a hydrotub treatment. Substances that dissolve naturally in water are said to be **hydrophilic** (*hydro* means "water," *phyllic* means "love"). Substances that do not dissolve in water, such as oils, are said to be **hydrophobic** (*phobic* means "fear").

Because water is such a powerful solvent, all water in the liquid form found in the hydrosphere—for example, the ocean—has minerals, gases (e.g., oxygen and carbon dioxide), and other substances dissolved in it. To produce water that is free from dissolved substances, technology is required to distill the water and remove any dissolved molecules. Distilled water, which is pure water with all minerals and other dissolved substances removed, is created by boiling water, condensing the steam from the boiled water back into water in its liquid form, and then collecting the liquid water. Because water is such a powerful solvent, however, a small number of molecules from the container, the air, or a filter may dissolve in the distilled water after it is created. Distilled water is used for various industrial, medical, and personal uses, as well as in some hydrotherapy treatments that require mineral-free water.

Acidity, Alkalinity, and the pH Scale

The **pH level** is a measure of how acidic or alkaline a specific solution is (see Figure 1–6). The technical definition of an acid is any substance that yields more hydrogen ions (H^+) when dissolved in water. An alkaline substance is any substance that yields more hydroxide ions (OH^-) when dissolved in water. When a substance dissolved in water contributes more H^+, it makes the solution more acidic. For example, when lemon juice or vinegar is dissolved in water, it makes the water more acidic, because both of these substances are very acidic. When a substance dissolved in water contributes OH^-, this makes the solution more alkaline. See Teaching Exercise 1–6. Pure (distilled) water has a pH of 7, which means it has an equal number of H^+ and OH^- and is thus considered neutral. Table 1–3 shows the pH of some common fluids (solutions), including fluids found in the human body. The surface of the skin is more acidic and has a pH of approximately 5.5. Therapists, especially estheticians, are trained to understand how different solutions, each with their own pH level, will produce different effects when they come into contact with the surface of the skin.

pH level
A measure of the acidity or alkalinity of a specific solution.

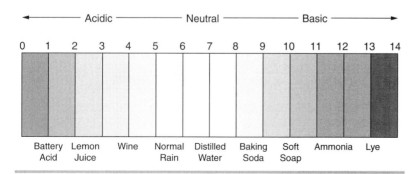

Figure 1–6 pH scale: Acids and bases.

1–6 TEACHING EXERCISE

Changes in pH of Water Solutions

Any solution of water, such as blood, orange juice, or mineral water, has a specific pH level. Any solution that is added to distilled water will change the water's pH from neutral (7) to more acidic or alkaline.

1. Use a simple pH measuring kit. Place distilled water in the kit's container, and then add the testing drops. The color will be in the neutral range—a very light orange. Note: Test strips used for measuring pH could be used for this demonstration instead of the pH kit.
2. Add about 5 drops of lemon juice, which is very acidic. The color of the water will turn very yellow, which indicates the water is very acidic.
3. Remove the water in the kit and rinse the container with water. Add distilled water and the drops of the testing liquid. The water should once again be in the neutral range.
4. Add 5 drops of milk of magnesia, which is very alkaline. Shake the container a bit. The color will turn deep purple, which means the water is now very alkaline.

During hydrotherapy treatments, whatever we place in water will change the pH of the water, even if it is only a small amount.

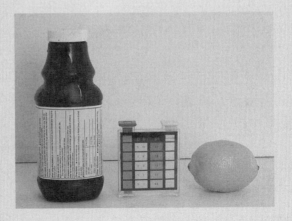

Table 1–3   pH Values of Common Substances

Substance	pH Value
Lemon juice	2.3
Carbonated soft drink	3.0–3.5
Coffee	4.8
Pure water (distilled)	7.0
Milk of magnesia	7.45
Urine	4.6–8.0
Blood	7.5–7.45
Cerebral spinal fluid	7.4
Bile	7.6–8.6

Suspension

Some substances, such as sand or essential oils, can be mixed with water but will not dissolve in the water. Substances that mix with water but do not dissolve in it are said to be in **suspension.** Such substances will separate to the top or bottom of the water when there is no longer activity causing the substances to mix with the water. For example, sediment in a stream is kept mixed (suspended) by the movement of the flowing water. When this movement stops or decreases, the sediment will settle to the bottom of the stream. Water that will be used for drinking water must have any sediment removed. This is done with filters and gravity, the latter of which allows heavy particles to settle out. Similarly, substances that are lighter than water and that are suspended in water will float to the top when the mixing ceases. Thus, because oils are lighter than water, they will quickly move to the top of the water.

The red and white blood cells and the platelets in human blood are in suspension (not dissolved) in the blood. The constant movement of blood through the circulatory system keeps these cells mixed in the blood. When blood is removed from the body for testing, these blood cells will eventually settle out by gravity. After red and white blood cells and platelets have separated from the blood, the fluid portion that remains is **blood plasma,** which is 55% of the total volume of the blood. Blood plasma, which contains various dissolved substances such as electrolytes, glucose, and proteins, is 91.5% water. The remaining 45% of the blood volume consists of

Suspension
Substances that mix with water (but do not dissolve) and will separate when the mixing action ceases.

Blood plasma
The liquid that remains after red and white blood cells and platelets have been separated from the blood.

red and white blood cells and platelets suspended (not dissolved) in the blood plasma.

In hydrotherapy, substances, such as mud, clays, or oils, may be mixed with the water for use during a treatment (see Teaching Exercise 1–7). These substances will not dissolve in the water;

1–7 TEACHING EXERCISE

Suspension

1. Fill a 1 gal or $\frac{1}{2}$ gal container with water so the container is 75% full.

2. Add a $\frac{1}{2}$ cup of sand or fine gravel and shake the container to mix the sand. Note how the sand quickly settles to the bottom of the container when the mixing ceases. Sand is heavier than water, so it sinks in water.

3. Empty and then use the same container. Again, fill the container with water so that it is about 75% full. Then add about 100 mL of oil, such as olive, corn, or vegetable oil. Shake the container to mix the oil and water. Note how the oil quickly settles to the top of the container when the mixing ceases. Oil is lighter than water, so it will float. Also, oil does not dissolve in water and is therefore said to be hydrophobic, "water-fearing."

During hydrotherapy treatments, we normally add products to the water. Many products, such as salts, dissolve in water. Others, such as oils or clays and mud, must be mixed into the water before it comes into contact with the client's skin. These substances will settle to the top or bottom soon after the mixing ceases.

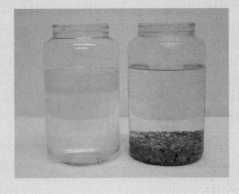

instead they must be mixed with the water being used. Once the mixing stops, the substances will eventually settle to the bottom of the water, in the case of mud or clay, or rise to the top, in the case of oils.

Movement

For water to flow (move), some force (energy) must be applied to it. For example, the force of gravity produces the movement of water in a river. Movement of blood plasma, which is 91.5% water, through the circulatory system is created mainly by the pumping of the heart. The main forces that produce movement (flow) of water are gravity, pressure, osmosis, and evaporation.

Gravity

Gravity, a force that causes water to flow from a higher elevation to a lower elevation, plays a major role in the movement of water in the hydrosphere (see Chapter 2). Some examples of the effects of gravity are the flowing of streams and rivers and the falling of rain and snow. The ability of water to flow into our homes is often produced by the force of gravity of water coming from a water tower. Likewise, water that drains from our homes does so by the force of gravity. Water flowing by gravity has considerable energy and can create significant force, depending on the amount of water and the angle of the water's flow. An example of this force of gravity can be seen in a waterfall (see Figure 1–7 and Plate 15) or the generation of hydroelectric power.

Gravity
The force that causes water to move (flow) from a higher elevation to a lower elevation.

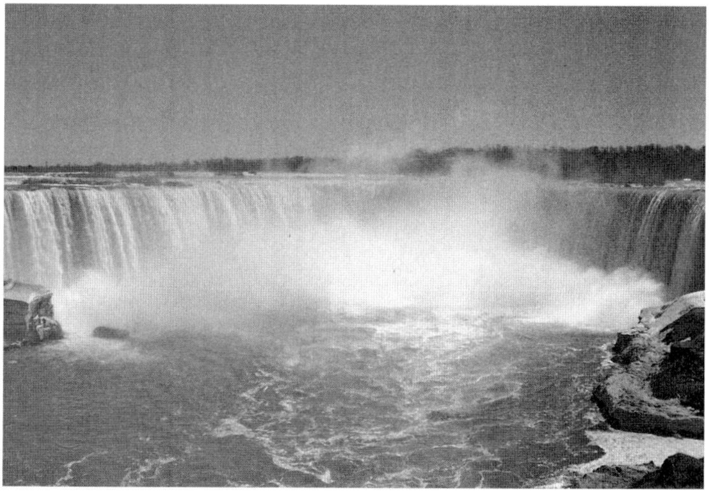

Figure 1–7 Niagara Falls: Flowing water is energy.

In hydrotherapy, water flowing under the force of gravity can be used to create the water pressure of a shower or of a handheld hose. This water pressure can be controlled and varied in intensity, depending on the goal of the treatment. For example, water pressure of a handheld shower used to remove a product from the body, such as clay, can be relatively light. However, the water pressure from the same handheld shower applied to the back or shoulders can be made much stronger to create a hydromassage effect (see Chapter 7). The teaching exercise for gravity is to just observe this principle functioning in our everyday experiences of water, for example, water draining from a bathtub or flowing in a river.

Under certain conditions, an increased number of negative ions are produced by water flowing due to the force of gravity. **Negative ions** are molecules that have gained an extra electron. The greater the turbulence and force generated by the force of gravity, the greater the number of negative ions that are produced. This effect can be found around waterfalls or around streams and rivers with a turbulent flow (see Figure 1–7). An increase in the number of negative ions in an environment has been associated with an increased sense of well being and other health benefits.[1] In hydrotherapy, an increased number of negative ions are created by the turbulent effect of showers and from the production of steam. For example, in a Vichy shower hydrotherapy treatment (see Chapter 7), the client lies on a wet table and is showered by as many as seven showerheads at once. This produces not only a hydromassaging effect but also a significant number of negative ions in the treatment room (which also benefits the therapist).

Negative ions
Molecules that have gained an extra electron.

Pressure

Applying pressure to water through a **pumping** action (force) will cause water to flow. The amount of pressure created depends on the power of the pump, the diameter (size) of the pipes, and the distance the water is pumped. Whereas forces of evaporation, condensation, and gravity are the main forces that produce movement of water in the hydrosphere, in living systems, including human beings, blood (which is mainly water) is pumped by the heart (see Teaching Exercise 1–8). This pumping action creates a certain flow (volume) and pressure (e.g., blood pressure). The human heart pumps about 3,600 gal of blood a day; the blood pressure created in the arteries and capillary system from this pumping is essential to the body's health. Normal blood pressure in the arteries is 120/80 mmHg; in the capillaries of the kidneys, it is 55 mmHg; and in the general capillary system, it is 35 mmHg (see Chapter 3). Blood, which is

Pumping
Applying pressure, or force, to water to cause water flow.

1–8 TEACHING EXERCISE

Pumping and How the Heart Pumps

In the hydrosphere, water usually moves by the processes of gravity and evaporation. In living systems, however, blood (which mainly water), is pumped by muscle contractions of the heart.

1. Place one end of a simple siphon pump in a 1 gal container filled with water. (Simple siphon pumps are normally used for siphoning gas and be purchased at stores like Wal-Mart.)

2. Squeeze the bulb with one hand while you press the tube closed with your other hand. Release the pressure on the bulb and the tube at the same time. Continue this process for 1 min. Feel how much effort it takes.

This simple procedure is a similar principle to the way your heart pumps blood. It is amazing to think your heart pumps 3,600 gal of blood each day!

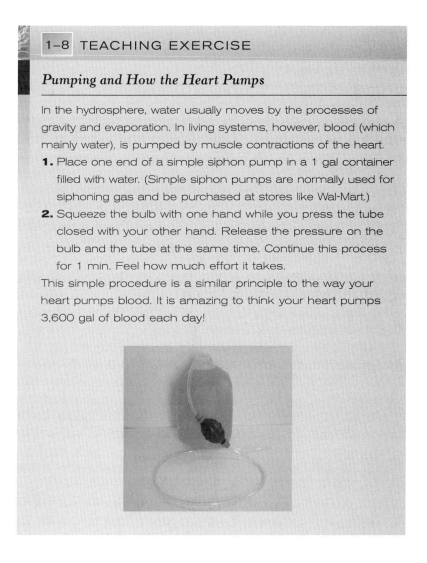

mainly water, flows through a blood vessel system that is greater than 60,000 miles long, and the natural alignment of this system is important for maintaining proper blood flow and pressure.

Modern technology has allowed the development of mechanical water pumps, which are powered mainly by electrical motors. Water pumps are often used in hydrotherapy to generate water pressure. This water pressure is usually used to generate streams (jets) of water in hydrotubs, hot tubs, footbaths, and aquatic pools. These streams of water create a powerful hydromassaging effect on the body. A handheld hydrowand is sometimes used, which allows a therapist to direct water pressure (usually underwater) to specific, localized areas of the client's body. Some hydrotubs and baths force compressed air into the water, which creates water movement as well as water pressure on the client's body, producing a hydromassaging effect.

Osmosis

Osmosis is the movement of a solvent through a selectively permeable membrane. In living systems, when the solvent is water and the selectively permeable membrane is the cell plasma membrane, there will be movement of water from an area of higher water concentration through the membrane to an area of lower water concentration. Selectively permeable means that only water molecules are allowed passage through the cellular membrane and not solutes like sodium ions (Na^+). Thus, when the solution on one side of a cellular membrane has a higher concentration of water molecules than the solution on the other side, the water molecules will flow from the area of higher concentration to the area of lower concentration. Increasing the water temperature also increases the osmotic pressure of the water. During a hydrotherapy treatment, if the temperature of the skin or the core body is increased, the osmotic pressure (rate of osmosis) will increase resulting in an increased flow of water and pressure (see Teaching Exercise 1–9). Osmosis produces a flow (movement and pressure) of water that is essential to the healthy fluid dynamics and circulation in all living systems. Osmosis is the main force that creates the flow of water between the interstitial fluid and the fluid inside the cells of the body and from interstitial fluid back to the blood capillaries (see Figure 1–8). If the balance of osmotic pressure increases or decreases beyond normal levels, cells in the body can swell or shrink in volume producing negative effects and even death in some circumstances. The pumping action of the heart and osmotic pressure are the two main forces responsible for dynamic circulation in the human body.

Osmosis
The movement of water from a higher concentration of water molecules to a lower concentration through semipermeable membranes, or membranes that allow the passage of the water molecules but nothing else.

Evaporation

Evaporation is the transition of water from the liquid (and the frozen state by sublimation) to the gas (vapor) state. Water molecules that evaporate move into the air (atmosphere) and become part of the mixture of gases in the atmosphere (see Table 1–4). An example of evaporation in the hydrosphere is solar heating of the ocean, which increases the temperature of water on the ocean's surface. This added heat causes a greater amount of water molecules to evaporate from the surface of the ocean into the atmosphere in the gas state; the greater the amount of heat, the greater the amount of evaporation. Because there is greater solar

Evaporation
The transition of water from the liquid (and the frozen state by sublimation) to the gas (vapor) state.

1–9 TEACHING EXERCISE

Osmosis

1. Use a medium-sized egg. Weigh the egg and then place the egg in a cup of vinegar for about 24 hours, until the shell dissolves. A medium-sized egg will usually weigh about 50 g. (The weight of the shell is less than 2 g, and is not important in our calculation.)

2. Then place the egg in a cup filled with corn syrup.

3. Water will flow by osmosis through the membrane of the egg, going from an area of higher concentration inside the egg to an area of lower concentration in the corn syrup. After about 5 hours, weigh the egg again to find out how much water was lost. (Remember that 1 g of water = 1 mL of water.) The egg should weigh approximately 25 g, which means that about 25 mL of water moved by osmosis out of the egg.

4. Now, place the egg in a bowl of distilled water for about 5 hours. Water will flow by the force of osmosis from the distilled water, which has a higher concentration of water molecules, to the area of lower concentration inside. The egg should now weigh about 70 g, which means about 50 mL of water moved into the egg by osmosis.

In the human body, pressure produced by the pumping action of the heart and by osmosis are the main forces that create most of the circulation of water in the body.

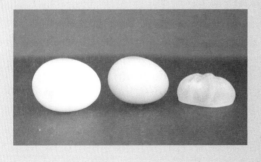

heating of water in tropical regions, there is much greater evaporation and **humidity,** a measure of the amount of water vapor in the air.

Solar heating of oceans, lakes, rivers, and other surface water produces evaporation and movement of water molecules to higher

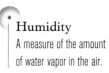

Humidity
A measure of the amount of water vapor in the air.

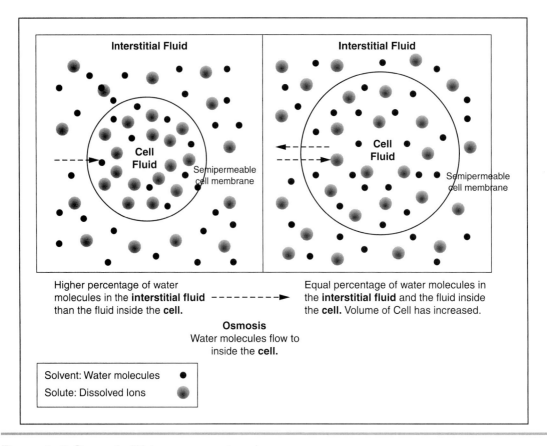

Figure 1-8 Osmosis: Water movement and pressure.

elevations in the atmosphere (see Figure 1–9). This is the dynamic process by which water flows from lower to higher elevations, bringing water from ocean and surface water sources to the highest mountain elevations, including the top of Mount Everest.

In hydrotherapy, evaporation can be used to move water from the source of the steam (the steam generator) to the client's body,

Table 1–4	Percentage of Atmospheric Gases
Nitrogen (N_2)	78.084%
Oxygen (O_2)	20.946%
Carbon dioxide (CO_2)	0.0349%
Water (H_2O)	0.01–4% (variable)
Other	< 0.003%

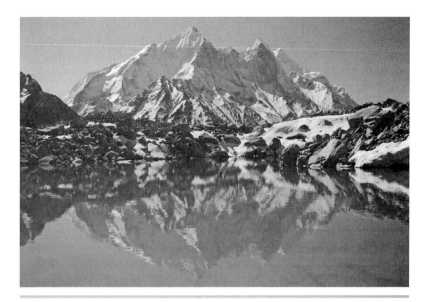

Figure 1-9 Upward movement of water: Evaporation *(image copyright Galyna Andrushko, 2008. Used under license from Shutterstock.com).*

as in a steam room. During steam therapy, as water is boiled, a large amount of steam (gas/vapor) is generated. The steam immediately rises (movement) and expands (movement) to fill the entire steam room, cabinet, or canopy, significantly increasing the amount of water molecules in the air (humidity) and raising the temperature. The movement of water molecules by evaporation is also used for inhalation therapy. When inhaled, steam will fill the lungs with water molecules in the gas state—especially the 300 million alveoli, which is where the exchange of oxygen and carbon dioxide takes place within the lungs. Products such as essential oils and herbs can be added to water used for steam inhalation. These products will also evaporate and enter the lungs. Therapists often use this method to introduce natural products into the bloodstream through capillary exchange in the lungs. There is also greater evaporation of water molecules during heated showers or baths. The level of humidity will increase in showers or baths, especially in a small, closed area, though not at the same rate as created by the generation of steam.

Buoyancy

Buoyancy is another important behavior of water that is used during many hydrotherapy treatments. The force of **buoyancy** reduces the weight of an object placed in water. If the total volume of an object placed in water is lighter than the same volume of water, then the

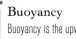

Buoyancy
Buoyancy is the upward force on an object produced by the surrounding liquid.

Specific gravity
The weight in grams of 1 cubic centimeter of a substance.

object will float. If the total volume of an object is heavier than the same volume of water, then the object will sink. For example, a cork floats, and a rock sinks. The total volume of the human body (approximately 17 gal) is about 5% heavier than the same volume of water. Therefore, the human body will sink in water. However, the body will weigh only about 5% of what it normally weighs. (See Teaching Exercise 1–10.)

Any object's level of buoyancy can be measured. The weight of water is used as a standard of measure to compare the weight of other objects: 1 cubic centimeter (cm^3) of water has been given a weight of 1 g. This amount is known as the **specific gravity** of water. As a comparison, the same volume (1 cm^3) of aluminum has a specific gravity of 2.5. Because aluminum's specific gravity is higher than water's, aluminum will sink in water. However, because a cork of the same volume has a specific gravity of 0.05, it will float in water. (See Table 1–5.)

In hydrotherapy, the principle of buoyancy can be applied in many ways. When a client is in a hydrotub, flotation tank, or aquatic pool, the effects of buoyancy can produce deep relaxation, reduction of pain, and an increased sense of well-being. Buoyancy, by reducing the force of gravity on the body, makes it possible for clients with injuries, disabilities, weight issues, and other problems to float, move, and exercise in water. Buoyancy also decreases vascular resistance to the pumping of blood, making it easier for the heart to pump blood. Special hydrotubs and pools allow a therapist to work directly with a client for various therapeutic purposes in an almost-gravity-free environment. Modern therapies have been developed that allow for special therapist–client interaction by using hydrotubs and pools with special design features. One of

Table 1–5   Specific Gravity of Various Substances

Weight of a volume of a substance compared with the same volume of water. The volume normally used is 1 cm^3.

Substance	Specific Gravity
Water	1.000
Mercury	13.600 (sink)
Gold	19.300 (sink)
Oils/Lipids (fat)	0.970 (float)
Human body	1.035–1.075* (sink)

* This range is for normal weight individuals.

1–10 TEACHING EXERCISE

Buoyancy

1. Use an empty 1 gal plastic container with a lid.

2. With your hands, submerge the container in water, perhaps in a bathtub, large sink, or tub.

3. Notice how much effort it takes and how much the water pushes against the container.

4. Because 1 gal of water weighs 8.345 lb, the empty container is displacing 8.345 lb of water (i.e., the container is pushing up with a force of 8.345 lb).

An average-sized human body has a volume of about 17 gal. Imagine you have an empty 17 gal container and you need to push it completely under water. The force would be 17 times greater than the force used for the 1 gal container. This teaching exercise gives an idea of the force of buoyancy pushing up against an object.

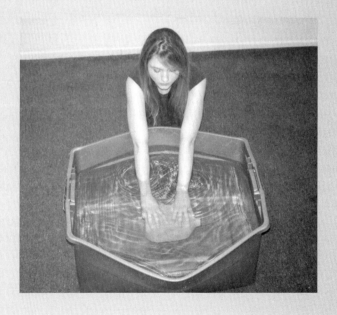

most successful forms of modern hydrotherapy has been the development of WATSU®, a specific therapeutic approach in which the therapist is in the pool with the client, moving the client passively through a series of flowing movements. A more detailed description of WATSU is given in Chapter 5.

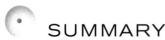

SUMMARY

To develop comprehensive hydrotherapy knowledge and skills, it is important to understand the basic ways in which water behaves (see Figure 1–10). This knowledge will also help in understanding the relation between water in the hydrosphere, water in the human body (60%), and water used in hydrotherapy treatments. Scientific information about the way water behaves allows us to create measurable, predictable ways for the use of water in hydrotherapy. It also gives many profound insights into the complex relationship between water used for hydrotherapy and the therapeutic changes produced inside the fluid dynamic system of the human body, which is mostly water. In addition, as we give hydrotherapy treatments, we directly experience these basic principles of the behavior of water as the fundamental dynamic elements at the basis of the wellness transformations being produced.

The basic unit of water is the water molecule (H_2O), which consists of two hydrogen atoms and one oxygen atom. The behavior of a water molecule interacting with other water molecules, as well as with molecules of other substances, is at the basis of all the principle behaviors of water. Any amount of water consists of a specific number of water molecules: 1 mol of water (18.02 g) contains 6.023×10^{23} water molecules. A water molecule has a slight positive charge on the hydrogen side and a slight negative charge on the oxygen side. The opposite charge causes water molecules to be attracted to each other through the force of cohesion, creating what is known as a hydrogen bond. Surface tension is produced because water molecules on the surface of water are more attracted to each other than they are to water molecules below the water's surface. Water molecules are also attracted to the molecules on the surface of some other substances, such as glass, which is what allows water to adhere to these surfaces.

Water has a high heat capacity because it can absorb and release a large amount of heat with a minimal change in its temperature. This behavior of water is essential to maintaining normal temperatures in the hydrosphere and in the human body. Changes in water temperature are responsible for the transition of water from solid to liquid to gas. Hydrotherapy uses this property of water to absorb and release heat to increase or decrease the temperature of the body's surface and core.

Water is a powerful solvent, and most bodies of waters in the hydrosphere are solutions of various minerals and gases found in the soil. Likewise, different fluids in the human body are mainly water with dissolved minerals (electrolytes), gases, and other substances. In hydrotherapy, certain products are dissolved in water that then

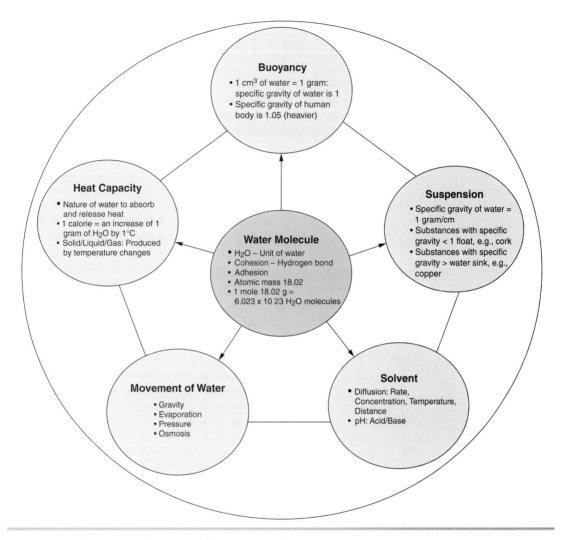

Figure 1–10 Behavior of water – Basic principles.

comes into contact with the client's body, producing different types of therapeutic effects.

Substances that dissolve in water (solutes) change the pH level of the solution, making it either more acidic (lower pH level) or more alkaline (higher pH level). Certain solutions—for example blood plasma in living systems—require a constant pH level (in this example, about 7.35–7.45) that must be maintained at all times for the normal functioning of the system.

Some substances can be mixed in water but do not dissolve in it. When the force that is creating the mixing ceases, the substances will separate from the water. Substances that are heavier than water will settle to the bottom, whereas substances that are lighter than water will float to the surface. During hydrotherapy treatments, products that do not dissolve in water, including mud, clay, and essential oils, must be mixed with the water.

For water to move, there must be some force applied to it. Movement of water is created mainly by the forces of gravity, evaporation, osmosis, and pressure by pumping. Gravity produces movement of water from higher elevations to lower elevations. Water flowing under the force of gravity can produce considerable pressure. When water evaporates from the liquid (or frozen) state, it goes into the gas state, becomes part of the atmosphere, and rises and expands. In the hydrosphere, water is mainly heated by solar energy and moves from the lowest elevations (sea level) to the higher elevations, where it condenses into rain, snow, or ice.

Water inside living systems moves mainly by the pumping action of the heart or by osmosis. Osmosis is the movement of water though cellular membranes that allows water molecules to pass through but restricts the movement of other molecules. Water moves from an area of higher concentration of water molecules through the membrane to an area of lower concentration (i.e., water follows solute). Movement of water by pumping is found mainly in living systems and is produced by contractions of muscles—mainly, the heart. This action pumps more than 3,600 gallons per day and is essential for moving blood through the more than 60,000 miles of blood vessels. Some hydrotherapy treatments use mechanical pumps to move water and to create water pressure, as in the hydrojets of a hydrotub.

Buoyancy is a behavior of water that reduces the weight of an object placed in water. Objects with a heavier volume than the same volume of water have a higher specific gravity and will sink; objects with a lighter volume than the same volume of water have a lower specific gravity will float. Because the total volume of the human body is slightly heavier than the same volume of water, the human body will slowly sink in water. In hydrotherapy, buoyancy has many useful applications, including reducing the effects of gravity on the body and creating a deep sense of relaxation.

REFERENCE

(1)   Howard, P. J. (1998). *The Owner's Manual for the Brain: Everyday Applications from Mind Brain Research*. Boston: Boston Press.

REVIEW QUESTIONS

1. What is the basic unit of water?

2. Describe the force of attraction between water molecules.

3. Give an example of surface tension and adhesion of water.

4. Which causes greater transfer of heat, when the body is in contact with cold air or cold water?

5. If a person is sitting in a hot tub with water temperature of about 104°F, will there be greater heating of the body if the water in the hot tub is also circulating?

6. Explain the way the evaporation of water in sweat on the skin reduces the temperature of the body.

7. What is the behavior of water that allows it to moves from lower elevations to higher elevations (uphill)?

8. What is the principle behavior of water that causes water to moves from higher to lower elevations?

9. How many gallons of blood does the heart pump each day and how long is the blood vessel system in the body?

10. What are the two main forces responsible for circulation of the main fluids (blood, interstitial, cellular, lymphatic, and cerebral spinal fluids) in the body?

11. Describe the principle of buoyancy.

12. Describe principles of the behavior of water functioning in a session in a hot tub.

13. How can understanding the principles of the behavior of water help a therapist develop greater skills in the use of water for hydrotherapy treatments?

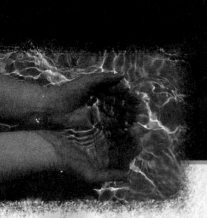

Hydrosphere: One Dynamic Water System

KEY TERMS

hydrology   infiltration
hydrologic cycle   balneotherapy

THE HYDROSPHERE

The Earth is one planet with one water system. *Hydrosphere* refers to all the water systems on our planet that behave as one dynamic, interconnected system; it includes for example, the atmosphere, oceans, lakes, rivers, glaciers, and groundwater and mineral springs (see Table 2–1). Scientists calculate that there is a total of 332 million mi^3 of water on Earth, that this amount remains relatively constant, and that all the various water systems of our planet combine to form one, total, dynamic, and interconnected system (see Figure 2–1 and Plate 1). The general understanding is that 70% of the Earth is covered with water. However, this is only water in the liquid and frozen states. When we also consider water in the vapor state in the atmosphere, the we see that 100% of the surface of Earth is covered by water and that we are in constant contact with this water. In fact, our comfort is greatly influenced by the various levels of humidity in our environment.

Knowledge of hydrotherapy is intimately connected with knowledge of the hydrosphere. Water that we use for hydrotherapy treatment, as well as water we use for hydration and other purposes, comes from various sources and locations in the hydrosphere. Much of what has been learned about the therapeutic use of water for hydrotherapy has come from experiencing the behavior of water in such natural settings as hot springs, oceans, lakes, and waterfalls.

Table 2–1   Percentage of Water on Earth

Total (fixed) amount of water on earth	332 million mi^3
Percentage of water in ocean (salt water)	97.200%
Percentage of water in ice caps and glaciers	2.014%
Percentage of water in groundwater (shallow and deep)	0.680%
Percentage of water in surface water (lakes, rivers, snowpack)	0.009%
Percentage of water in atmosphere	0.001%

Hydrology, the science that deals with the behavior of water on our planet, describes the properties, distribution, and total circulation of water on and below Earth's surface, as well as in the atmosphere. The **hydrologic cycle** refers to the dynamic sequence of conditions through which water passes—from vapor in the atmosphere to precipitation on land or water surfaces, returning to the atmosphere as a result of evaporation and transpiration (see Figure 2–2 and Plate 2). The total amount of water on our planet remains basically the same but is constantly circulating and changing between liquid, solid, and gas states (see Chapter 1) as it is being purified and recycled. All living systems, including human beings, depend on this continual cycle of purification, renewal, and distribution.

Hydrology
The science that deals with the behavior of water on our planet.

Hydrologic cycle
The sequence of conditions through which water passes, from vapor in the atmosphere to precipitation on land or water surfaces, returning to the atmosphere as a result of evaporation and transpiration.

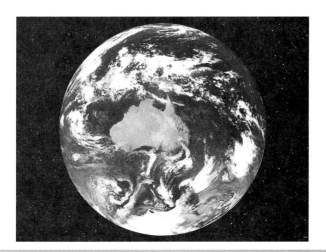

Figure 2–1 Hydrosphere of Australia *(courtesy of NASA).*

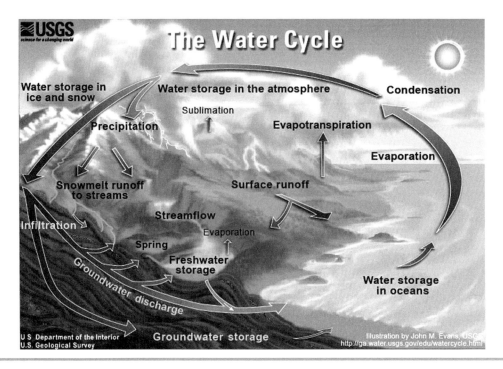

Figure 2–2 The hydrologic cycle *(courtesy of U.S. Department of the Interior/U.S. Geological Survey <http:// ga.water.usgs.gov/edu/watercycle.html>).*

Satellite photos of Earth reveal that even though we give various names to different geographic locations of the ocean, they are all just different regions of one interconnected water system. The various rivers and groundwater systems on the planet, though separate from each other, eventually flow back to the same ocean system. The dynamic, hydrologic cycle begins when heat from the sun is absorbed by water on the surface of the ocean (or other water sources), causing water to transform from a liquid state to gas molecules by evaporation. During evaporation, water molecules rise into the atmosphere and remain there until cooler temperatures cause them to condense back into the liquid state. These smaller water droplets combine to form larger droplets and eventually return to the land or ocean by the force of gravity in the form of rain, snow, and ice crystals.

Water that falls on land in the form of rain, snow, or ice will eventually begin to flow, under the force of gravity, from higher to lower elevations. Surface water, mainly in the form of lakes and rivers, will naturally flow back to the ocean, though some of it will evaporate back into the atmosphere before reaching the ocean. Even water contained in glaciers and snowpacks will eventually melt and return to the ocean or evaporate back to the atmosphere

Table 2–2   Average Residence Time of Water

Glaciers	20–100 years
Seasonal snow cover	2–6 months
Soil moisture	1–2 months
Groundwater, shallow	100–200 years
Groundwater, deep	10,000 years
Lakes	50–100 years
Rivers	2–6 months

(see Table 2–2). Some evaporation can occur directly from water in the frozen state to the gas state, which is a process known as sublimation. Some of the water that falls on land will be absorbed by the soil through the process of **infiltration** and will form groundwater under the surface. As this water flows over rocks and through the soil, minerals as well some oxygen and carbon dioxide, will dissolve in the water. All surface water and groundwater contain some combination of dissolved minerals and gases from this process (see Table 2–3). Groundwater, both deep and shallow, is one of the main sources for drinking water and other daily uses. It is this continual,

Infiltration
The process by which some of the water that falls on land is absorbed by the soil to become groundwater.

Table 2–3   Water Analysis: Hot Springs, Arkansas

Constituents	Milligrams per Liter (mg/L)
Calcium	71.00
Magnesium	7.50
Sodium	2.70
Potassium	1.00
Fluoride	0.20
Iron	0.01
Zinc	0.01
Total dissolved solids (TDS)	221
Alkalinity ($CaCO_3$)	190
pH	7.7

Table 2–4   Hydrosphere: Principles of Behavior of Water

Water Principle	Interaction/Experience
Heat exchange and heat capacity	Solar heating of ocean, lakes, and rivers
Solvent	Minerals, oxygen, and carbon dioxide dissolve in water as it comes in contact with air, soil, and rocks
Gravity	Movement of water from higher to lower elevations
Evaporation	Movement of water from lower to higher elevations
Buoyancy (suspension)	Soil and organic matter mixed (suspended) in water

natural circulation (hydrologic cycle), that brings water in different amounts and at different times to all regions of the planet and that is fundamental to the growth and health of all living systems.

It is interesting to note that the principles that govern the behavior of water described in Chapter 1 are the same principles that govern the behavior of water in the hydrosphere and the hydrologic cycle (see Table 2–4). We see the principle of heat exchange in the solar heating of the ocean, lakes, and rivers. The solvent property of water allows the diffusion of minerals, oxygen, and carbon dioxide in water as the water comes into contact with the atmosphere, rocks, and soil. The dynamic movement of water in the hydrologic cycle is due mainly to evaporation, which brings water to higher elevations, and to the flow of water by gravity, which brings water to lower elevations. Soil, organic matter, and other substances that are suspended (mixed, but not dissolved) in water are moved by flowing water from one region to another and play an important role in many ecosystems. See Teaching Exercise 2–1.

Living systems are also a natural part of the hydrologic cycle. Water evaporating from the leaves of plants and trees returns to the atmosphere, increasing the amount of water (humidity) in the atmosphere. Most of this moisture will eventually return in the form of rain. In general, regions on the planet that receive more rainfall (e.g., the tropics) will have more growth and biodiversity.

2-1 TEACHING EXERCISE

Hydrologic Cycle

1. You will need a 2 to 2.5 gal clear plastic container with a lid.

2. Place 35 g of sea salt in a measuring cup; then add enough distilled water make to 1 L of salt water. This will make a 3.5% saltwater solution, which is the same salinity as water in the ocean. Then add about 5 drops of blue food color.

3. Place some aquarium stones, pebbles, or small stones to one side in the plastic container. This represents land. Then add the 1 L of salt water from the plastic container; this represents the water in the ocean. Place the lid on the container (see photo).

4. If possible, take the temperature inside the container by using a temperature gauge that has an outdoor probe.

5. If possible, place the container in direct sunlight for direct solar heating.

Model of Hydrologic Cycle

1. Heat from the room (or from direct sunlight) will transfer heat to the water. Water molecules will begin to evaporate from the surface of the water. The greater the heat, the greater the rate of evaporation. The humidity will increase inside the container.

2. As the humidity level increases, condensation of water from a gas to a liquid begins, and small water droplets will form on the inside sides and top of the container. These water droplets are pure water, with no salt or food color molecules. This water would be pure enough to drink.

3. When the condensed water drops get large enough, gravity will cause the drops on the sides of the container to slide down back to the salt water. Water drops on the top of the container will drop back to the salt water, similar to raindrops.

2-1 **TEACHING EXERCISE** *(Continued)*

This exercise illustrates how the total amount of water in the hydrosphere does not increase or decrease, but simply recirculates. The model includes all the basic elements of the hydrologic cycle, including heat (solar heat), evaporation (purification), condensation, and precipitation.

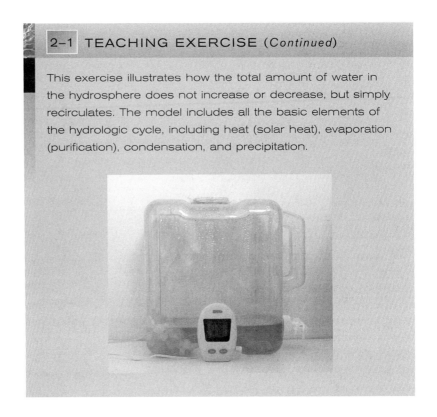

We (human beings) are also a natural part of the hydrosphere and hydrologic cycle (see Figure 2–3). The total population of people on the planet is about 6.6 billion. Because each person is, on average, 60% water (about 10 gal of water per person), this means that at any time, about 66 billion gallons of water in the hydrosphere is found inside human beings. Each day, every person naturally loses about 2.5 qt (2.5 L) of water in the form of urine and evaporation of moisture from the skin and lungs. This means that on a global scale, the total population of human beings each day has a water intake of about 4 billion gallons of water and naturally loses about 4 billion gallons of water. This creates a continual flow rate of about 4 million gallons per minute, the size of a small river.

All water consumed by the world population comes from water sources in the hydrosphere, returns to the hydrosphere, and is part of the hydrosphere. The hydrosphere is a unifying natural system for all forms of life, including human beings, as all living systems get water, which is essential for life, from this same system. Through the hydrosphere—through the Earth's one dynamic water system—we are all connected.

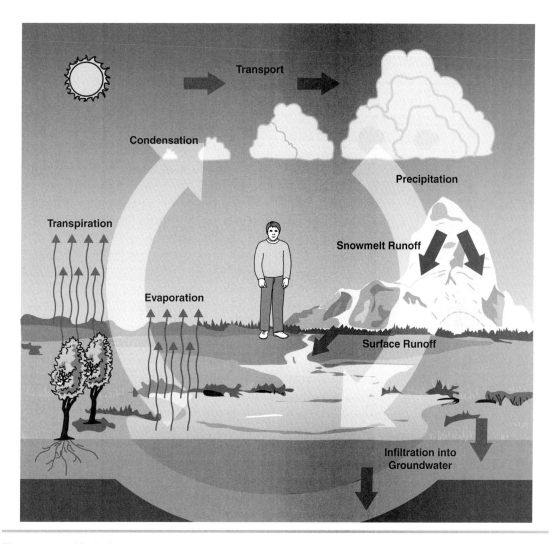

Figure 2–3 Hydrologic cycle and human beings.

EXPRESSION OF WATER IN THE NATURAL ENVIRONMENT: BEAUTY, BALANCE, AND HEALING

During a hydrotherapy treatment, a therapist uses water in some form to produce specific therapeutic transformations. Another form of hydrotherapy occurs when people come into contact with water in one of its expressions in the natural environment.

Water creates much of the beautiful landscapes of our environment, and interacting with water in one of these natural settings is a form of hydrotherapy. For example, spending time at the ocean, a mountain lake, a waterfall, or a hot spring can have a profoundly calming, balancing, and restorative benefit. This is why many health and wellness resorts are located in natural settings where water is a major theme.

Today's world has many forms of modern stress. There are increasing levels of air, water, noise, and other types of pollution, which produce physical, emotional, and mental stress. Overcrowded cities and increased traffic are another growing source of strain. The constant use of computers, televisions, cell phones, and other electronic devices can have negative effects on our health. The increasingly rapid pace of life, social conflicts, and problems on a global scale are producing greater levels anxiety. Together, these modern stresses are contributing to—and even causing—many of our physical, mental, and emotional problems. People deal with these negative influences in different ways. One way is to spend time in natural settings, especially water settings, away from our more artificial, man-made environments. Doing so can have significant healing and balancing benefits. Most people enjoy taking time to be in nature for rest and renewal, recreation, healing, simply to enjoy the beauty of nature. Some individuals and communities incorporate the beauty of water in their homes and communities by building fountains or landscaping with pools and lakes (see Figure 2–4).

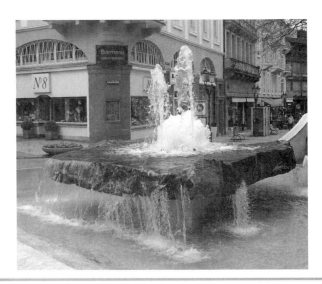

Figure 2–4 City water fountain in Germany.

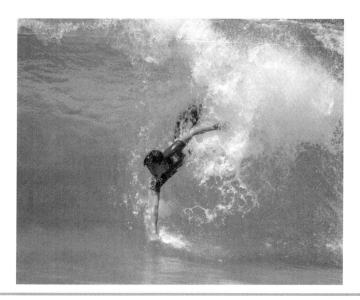

Figure 2–5 Body surfing *(compliments of Greg Rice, www.GregRImagery.com <http://www.gregrimagery.com/>, Sandy Beach, Ohau, Hawaii).*

Some people enjoy a more calming, meditative time in nature, while others prefer a more dynamic interaction with water, such as swimming in the ocean, riding a wave, bathing in a hot springs, skiing down a mountain, or skating on a frozen lake (see Figure 2–5 and Plate 3). In fact, much of our recreational and sports activities are based on interacting with water in some form in the hydrosphere (see Figure 2–6). The Winter Olympics is founded entirely on interacting with water in the frozen state, and much of the Summer Olympics involves activities in water in the liquid state, including swimming, diving, and rowing. The therapeutic value of the experience of water in these natural and man-made settings can be very beneficial.

THE HYDROSPHERE AS A SOURCE OF KNOWLEDGE OF HYDROTHERAPY

The behavior of water in natural settings and the positive healing effects that come from these experiences have taught us much about many of the uses of water for hydrotherapy. Many of the principles used in hydrotherapy originated from experiences of individuals who were aware of and studied the healing properties of water. There is a centuries-old tradition of the use of hydrotherapy use in the great

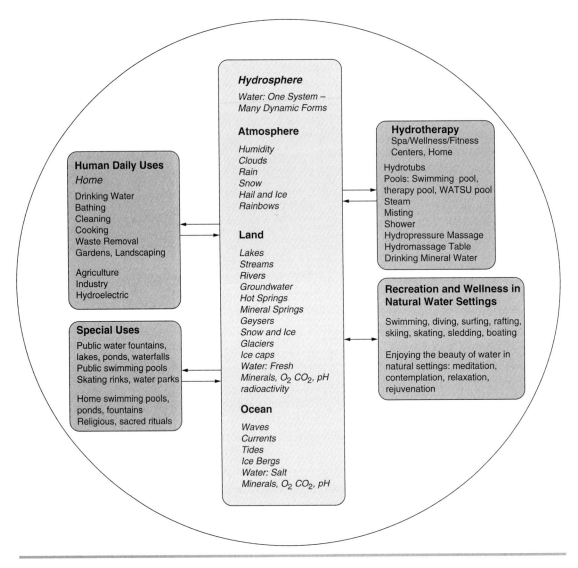

Hydrosphere

Water: One System – Many Dynamic Forms

Atmosphere

Humidity
Clouds
Rain
Snow
Hail and Ice
Rainbows

Land

Lakes
Streams
Rivers
Groundwater
Hot Springs
Mineral Springs
Geysers
Snow and Ice
Glaciers
Ice caps
Water: Fresh
Minerals, O_2 CO_2, pH
radioactivity

Ocean

Waves
Currents
Tides
Ice Bergs
Water: Salt
Minerals, O_2 CO_2, pH

Human Daily Uses

Home

Drinking Water
Bathing
Cleaning
Cooking
Waste Removal
Gardens, Landscaping

Agriculture
Industry
Hydroelectric

Special Uses

Public water fountains, lakes, ponds, waterfalls
Public swimming pools
Skating rinks, water parks

Home swimming pools, ponds, fountains
Religious, sacred rituals

Hydrotherapy
Spa/Wellness/Fitness Centers, Home

Hydrotubs
Pools: Swimming pool, therapy pool, WATSU pool
Steam
Misting
Shower
Hydropressure Massage
Hydromassage Table
Drinking Mineral Water

Recreation and Wellness in Natural Water Settings

Swimming, diving, surfing, rafting, skiing, skating, sledding, boating

Enjoying the beauty of water in natural settings: meditation, contemplation, relaxation, rejuvenation

Figure 2–6 Hydrosphere and people.

holistic health and wellness traditions, including Japanese, Greek, Roman, and European traditions, as well as Ayurveda from India. This use of hydrotherapy continues today as part of modern health and wellness programs (see Chapter 8).

Balneotherapy
The study and use of natural mineral water for improving health and wellness.

Balneotherapy is the study and use of natural mineral water for improving health and wellness. The use of natural mineral water, both internally and externally, has been found to be effective in treating specific medical conditions and maintaining general health and wellness. Many European countries, including Germany and France, have long traditions of balneotherapy as well as the use of the natural mineral waters during "health vacations," where the emphasis is on relaxation, rejuvenation, and prevention. There has been a considerable amount deal of scientific research done on effectiveness of such approaches, especially in Europe and Japan.[1]

HARMING THE HYDROSPHERE

Human activity is having a profound impact on the hydrosphere. These activities, including toxic pollution, destruction of the natural environment, and global warming, are having a harmful effect on both local and global water systems.

One source of water pollution is from toxic chemicals that are finding their way into community water supplies and global water systems (see Figure 2–7 and Plate 8). Recent water analysis has found a vast array of trace levels of pharmaceutical drugs in the drinking water of at least 41 million Americans. Harmful micro-organisms from sewage and septic systems, as well as from farm animals and wild animals, can also get into our water systems. Toxic substances, such as chlorine, are added to the water supply to kill disease-causing microbes, though these are added at levels that are currently considered safe by the EPA for public health. In addition, some forms of air pollution are increasing the acidity of moisture in

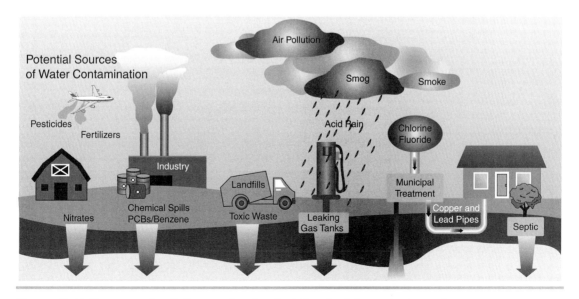

Figure 2–7 Sources of pollution and water *(evolution of pollution, waterwise.com).*

the atmosphere, which then returns to land in the form of acid rain. Acid rain can be especially harmful to living systems that depend on a constant pH level for water in their natural environment.

Another harmful behavior for the hydrosphere is the dumping of various forms of garbage into the different water systems, especially ocean, lakes, and rivers. Normal trash and larger items are being dumped in water systems, often without any regulation, especially into the oceans. This can not only prove harmful for marine life, but can also impact the local water system for countless years.

Another behavior is the overuse of water supplies from different groundwater and surface water sources. Many groundwater systems are being depleted much faster than they can be recharged. Likewise, surface water sources are also being overused, especially for agricultural irrigation.

The destruction of wetlands, deforestation, and diversion of water created by dams and irrigation is also damaging the hydrosphere. These systems are a part of the hydrosphere, and their destruction is creating related problems for the human populations that are connected to these systems. Global warming—depending on the effect it is having on the hydrosphere in terms of melting ice caps, changing rain patterns (droughts), and increasing destructive weather patterns (hurricanes)—can also have a major negative impact on the normal, balanced functioning of the hydrosphere.

HYDROTHERAPY FOR THE HYDROSPHERE

The activities of the hydrosphere's water systems are very dynamic, balanced, and precise. For example, the ocean temperatures remain relatively constant in different regions. Normal rainfall patterns can be predicted within specific ranges for different geographic areas. However, the effects of toxic pollution, destruction of the environment, and global warming are exceeding the balancing and purify ability of these water systems. Up to a point, these systems can reestablish balance from these destructive influences—but there are limits. To protect the hydrosphere, it is necessary to reduce, and potentially eliminate, as many of the causes of these problems as is possible. Hydrotherapy for the planet essentially means stopping behavior that is producing the toxic problems previously mentioned.

Comprehensive education about protecting our water systems is essential for solving these problems. This requires more effective education not only for everyone connected with business, industry, agriculture, and government but also for every individual—every person is part of the hydrosphere, and every individual's actions can protect or harm the Earth's one water system.

There is a growing understanding through science and education about the need to immediately address these problems. Sometimes, change is forced by the obvious negative consequences of destructive human behavior. For example, in the 1960s, toxic pollution from multiple sources severely damaged the Hudson River in New York State and the area came to be known as "an open sewer." A similar situation occurred on Lake Erie around the same time. Disasters like these motivated the creation of the Clean Water Act of 1972. This act established regulations to control industrial and other sources of pollution. The Clean Water Act, combined with activity by environmental groups and other concerned individuals, produced a significant improvement in the health of these waters. It also illustrated one very positive feature of the hydrosphere: Once behavior that is damaging a specific area, region, or location of the hydrosphere stops, as it did in Lake Erie, natural dynamics can restore various degrees of health and balance to the system. This ability to maintain and restore balance is common to all living systems, including the human body and is also true of the hydrosphere. However, there are limits to this ability, and these limits are a serious concern today regarding the hydrosphere. The most important thing that can be done to protect the hydrosphere is to stop doing the things that are harming it. Legislation and the enforcement of laws that limit these harmful activities are often necessary. International cooperation between nations to reduce pollution is essential, as the activities of any one country can harm the entire global water system.

Conservation is another way to protect the available water supply. Most of the water (95%) that we use is for industrial and agricultural activities, and much can be done by industry and agriculture to reduce this amount. Some of the same efforts that are being made to control water pollution by industry and agriculture are also being made to control their excessive water use. In addition, we, as individuals, can do more to conserve the amount of water that we each use. The U.S. Environmental Protection Agency (EPA) estimates that the average home wastes 14% of its water due to leaks in faucets, toilets, and other water-related fixtures. There are many simple, practical ways to reduce unnecessary water use. For example, installing more efficient toilets, washing machines, and showerheads can reduce daily water use. A significant amount of water is also used for maintaining lawns, which could be reduced by different landscaping designs.

The following are a few of the ways that hydrotherapists (therapists trained in the use of water as a therapeutic modality) can play a greater role in protecting the waters of the hydrosphere:

- Educate clients on the importance of water for their health and wellness (see Chapters 3 and 4).
- Provide education about the behavior of the hydrosphere, our relationship with the hydrosphere and how our health, both short-term and long-term, is connected with the normal functioning (health) of the hydrosphere.
- Participate in and support programs of any kind that educate the general public about the importance of protecting our planet's water systems.
- Support any programs that help stop existing activities that are harming our planet's natural water supply, including toxic pollution, destruction of the natural environment, and global warming.

 ## THE HYDROSPHERE: NATURE'S DRINKING FOUNTAIN

All water that is used for our daily hydration needs comes from various sources in the hydrosphere. The main sources of water for hydration and home uses come from groundwater, springs, and surface water such as lakes and rivers.

In most communities, a municipal water treatment plant purifies water for use by the public. Organic and inorganic contaminants are removed, along with any sediment. Disinfectants, such as chlorine, are added to kill disease-causing microbes. Sometimes, fluorine is added to promote dental health. The quality of the water produced by these treatment plants is analyzed at regular intervals and must meet government standards for acceptable levels of various contaminants.

The Maximum Contaminant Level Goal (MCLG) is the acceptable level of a contaminant in drinking water below which there is no known or expected risk to health. Maximum Contaminant Level (MCL) is the highest level of a contaminant that is allowed in drinking water. MCLs, which are enforceable standards, are set as close to MCLGs as feasible, using the best available treatment technology and taking cost into consideration. An example of a toxic substance that is often found in a water supply is chlorine, which is added as a disinfectant. The MCL for chlorine is 4.0 mg/L, which means that amounts below that level are considered safe. (Units are in milligrams per liter, which are equivalent to parts per million [ppm].) Eye and nose irritation and stomach discomfort can be produced by chlorine in the water at levels above the MCL. Another example of an MCL for a toxic substance is that for copper—1.3 mg/L. At levels above 1.3 mg/L, copper can cause short-term gastrointestinal distress, and long-term exposure to an elevated copper level can cause kidney and liver damage. The EPA has published a comprehensive listing of known water contaminants that can potentially be found in water sources (see Table 2–5).[2]

Ideally, our water supplies should be completely free from any contaminants, either natural or man-made. Because this ideal is not currently a practical reality, the question becomes, what are safe levels of potentially harmful substances in water? There is considerable controversy about acceptable levels of certain chemical, organic, microbial, and other contaminants and about adequate testing and water analysis techniques, especially given the fact that so many new chemicals are being developed. This is a complex problem, requiring cooperation among governmental agencies, industry and agriculture concerns, and public interest groups to ensure water safety. The situation is made more complex by the fact that there is often limited understanding about the effects of these pollutants and at what levels they become harmful.

Once water enters the home, another source of possible contamination of drinking water comes from plumbing components. Lead, for example, is rarely found in the municipal water coming into a home. Yet water can be contaminated by the corrosion of plumbing materials found in some homes. Homes built before 1986 are more likely to have lead pipes, fixtures, and solder, though new homes are also at risk, as even legally "lead-free" plumbing may contain up to 8% lead in plumbing material. The most common problem is with brass or chrome-plated brass faucets and fixtures, which can leach significant amounts of lead into the water, especially from hot water. Home testing kits or professional testing facilities are available to test for contamination of water in the home.

In general, municipal tap water meets required safety standards, although, to ensure water quality, many residences also have some type of home water-purification system. Homes in rural areas that use their own well water usually have the water analyzed and tested for safety and have their own water-purification systems. Considering that our bodies are 60% water and that we naturally lose and consume approximately 2.5 qt (5 lb) of water each day, it is imperative that the water we drink be free from

Table 2–5   Contaminants and their Maximum Contaminant Levels (MCLs) (A sample of each contaminant category is shown. See the EPA Contaminant Levels for Drinking Water on-line at www.epa.com for the entire list.)

Contaminant Microorganisms	MCLG (mg/L)	MCL (mg/L)	Potential Health Effects from Ingestion of Water	Sources of Contaminant in Drinking Water
Cryptosporidium	0	TT	Gastrointestinal illness (e.g., diarrhea, vomiting, cramps)	Human and animal fecal waste
Giardia lamblia	0	TT	Gastrointestinal illness (e.g., diarrhea, vomiting, cramps)	Human and animal fecal waste
Contaminant Disinfection By-products	**MCLG (mg/L)**	**MCL (mg/L)**	**Potential Health Effects from Ingestion of Water**	**Sources of Contaminant in Drinking Water**
Chlorite	0.8	1.00	Anemia; nervous system effects in infants and young children	By-product of drinking water disinfection
Total trihalomethanes (TTHMs)	0	0.10	Liver, kidney, or central nervous system problems; increased risk of cancer	By-product of drinking water disinfection
Contaminant Inorganic Chemicals	**MCLG (mg/L)**	**MCL (mg/L)**	**Potential Health Effects from Ingestion of Water**	**Sources of Contaminant in Drinking Water**
Copper	1.3	Action level = 1.3	Short-term exposure: Gastrointestinal distress Long-term exposure: Liver or kidney damage	Corrosion of household plumbing systems; erosion of natural deposits
Lead	0	Action level = 0.015	Delays in physical or mental development in infants and children; potential slight deficits in attention span and learning abilities in children	Corrosion of household plumbing systems; erosion of natural deposits

Table 2–5 (*Continued*)

Contaminant Organic Chemicals	MCLG (mg/L)	MCL (mg/L)	Potential Health Effects from Ingestion of Water	Sources of Contaminant in Drinking Water
Carbon tetrachloride	0	0.005	Liver problems; increased risk of cancer	Discharge from chemical plants and other industrial activities
Polychlorinated biphenyls (PCBs)	0	0.0005	Skin changes; thymus gland problems; immune deficiencies; reproductive or nervous system difficulties; increased risk of cancer	Runoff from landfills; discharge of waste chemicals

Contaminant Radionuclides	MCLG (mg/L)	MCL (mg/L)	Potential Health Effects from Ingestion of Water	Sources of Contaminant in Drinking Water
Radium 226 and radium 228 (combined)	0	5 pCi/L	Increased risk of cancer	Erosion of natural deposits
Uranium	0	30 ug/L	Increased risk of cancer; kidney toxicity	Erosion of natural deposits

any harmful chemicals, disease-causing microbes, sediment, or harmful levels of radiation. Over a period of 20 days, a person will naturally lose, on average, more than 12 gallons (105 lb) of water and will replace that with more than 12 gallons of water.

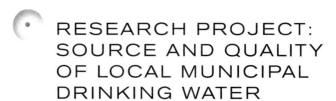

RESEARCH PROJECT: SOURCE AND QUALITY OF LOCAL MUNICIPAL DRINKING WATER

An interesting and valuable research project would be to learn as much as possible about the sources (e.g., aquifer, surface water) of your local municipal water supplies, treatment procedures, testing methods, and type of delivery system to homes and businesses (e.g., piping, water towers). You may find that the water comes from pure sources, with minimal potential for contamination from human activities. Or you may find that the water comes from sources with more potential for contamination. This knowledge can be very helpful, as it can provide information about what levels of home water purification would be necessary to make a client feel confident about the purity and safety of his or her water. You can also ask to receive notifications of any temporary contamination or other problems that may arise with the municipal water supply. Most people rarely take the time to do basic research on the source, quality, and purification of their local water supply. By doing this research yourself, you can share this information with your clients as appropriate. You can also provide interesting facts, such as the natural mineral content, combination of minerals, and pH level of the local drinking water. As discussed in Chapter 4, the information from this research on the source and quality of local drinking water can be shared with your clients as part a personal hydration consulting program.

SUMMARY

Understanding the hydrosphere and the hydrologic cycle is an important part of hydrotherapy education and further developing our understanding of the use of water as a therapeutic modality. The hydrosphere—the one dynamic water system on the planet—is the source for water, not only for use in hydrotherapy but also for all other human activities. Different expressions of the hydrosphere include oceans, lakes, rivers, mineral springs, groundwater, geysers, waterfalls, rain, snow, and ice. Learning about the dynamic behavior of water in the hydrosphere can provide a better understanding of the behavior of water during hydrotherapy treatments.

The hydrologic cycle describes the combined dynamic activity of the various systems of the hydrosphere. The total amount of water in the hydrosphere remains relatively the same and is in a constant state of circulation, purification, renewal, and distribution. The total human population, which is also part of the hydrosphere, at any given time, contains a total of about 66 billion gal of water. The hydrosphere is a unifying principle in nature, as all living systems are connected with the hydrosphere and depend on it for one of life's most essential resources—water.

Water systems of the hydrosphere form much of the beauty of our natural environment. Water in natural settings has been highly valued throughout time in every culture. The dynamic nature of the hydrosphere is constantly creating a beautiful changing display of clouds, rain, snowfall, and rainbows. People interacting with water in natural settings, whether for relaxation, rejuvenation, or healing, can experience profound health and wellness benefits. Much of our understanding of hydrotherapy comes from the health and wellness benefits that people have experienced throughout time from water in natural settings, such as the ocean, hot springs, and waterfalls.

Pollution from the activities of industry, agriculture, and individuals is causing damage to local and global water systems. Some of this pollution is exceeding the natural ability of these water systems to purify and renew themselves. Our water systems are also being harmed by the destruction of the environment and global warming. Because the hydrosphere has limits to its natural purifying and renewing activities, the only solution is to stop these harmful behaviors. Thus, there is a need for more effective education, legislation, and enforcement of laws to protect the hydrosphere. Therapists trained in hydrotherapy can also play an important role in protecting the hydrosphere by educating clients on the value of water for health and wellness and by supporting community, national, and global programs that work to protect the hydrosphere.

The hydrosphere is also the source of water used for daily hydration. All water used for hydration comes from some natural source, such as groundwater, lakes, or rivers. This water is usually treated to make it safe for drinking and other uses. Because every person needs to consume a considerable amount of water to stay hydrated (on average, 12 gal, over every 20 days), it is essential that the water be free from harmful levels of contaminants. Therapists can find information about the water coming from municipal water treatment facilities and determine the source of the water, mineral content analysis, and other information about the water. They can also ask to receive regular reports on water quality and any special notification of problems. This can be a valuable resource of knowledge to share with clients.

REFERENCES

(1)   Altman, N. (2000). *Healing Springs: The Ultimate Guide to Taking the Waters.* Rochester, VT: Healing Arts Press.

(2)   EPA Contaminant Levels for Drinking Water, available online at www.epa.gov.

REVIEW QUESTIONS

1. Describe the hydrosphere.

2. Describe the hydrologic cycle.

3. Why is the hydrosphere considered one interconnected water system?

4. Why are human beings a natural part of the hydrosphere?

5. Give an example of how knowledge of the use of water for hydrotherapy could have been gained from the experience of water in natural settings.

6. What are some of the everyday uses of water by people from sources in the hydrosphere?

7. What are some of the recreational uses of water?

8. List several ways human activity is damaging the hydrosphere. Discuss different ways to reduce or eliminate these problems.

9. Discuss how water, on a global scale, is purified by the hydrologic cycle and is naturally distributed to every region on Earth.

10. List several ways water is treated to make it safe for drinking, both by municipal treatment plants and by residential water purification systems.

Dynamic Fluid Anatomy and Physiology and Hydrotherapy

KEY TERMS

swedhana
cells

INTRODUCTION

Understanding the relationship between hydrotherapy and the human body is an essential element of hydrotherapy education. In hydrotherapy, we use water to produce therapeutic transformations for our clients, which means we also produce a change in how the body functions during and after the treatment.

This chapter, which reviews hydrotherapy from the perspective of anatomy and physiology, provides insights into the dynamic relationship between hydrotherapy and changes in the anatomy and physiology of the human body. By understanding this relationship, it is possible to see that hydrotherapy can be used to promote all health and wellness goals of our clients, including daily wellness, fitness, appearance and beauty, prevention, and healthful aging. The focus of hydrotherapy is often more on health problems, but through the proper use of hydrotherapy, treatments and programs can be applied to promote all of a client's health and wellness goals.

This textbook has been developed for therapists who have graduated from school or for students who are in school getting their professional therapist training and license. In their initial undergraduate training, students receive comprehensive training in anatomy and physiology, as this is an essential element in educating therapists about performing treatments on the human body. The purpose of

Table 3–1	Average Percentage of Fats (lipids), Proteins, and Carbohydrates in an Average Person	
Fats/lipids (mostly triglycerides) * Women have a higher percentage of fat than men. The ratio for fat-free mass for men and women is generally the same.		20%
Proteins * Men have a higher percentage of protein than women.		20%
Water		60%
Carbohydrates (stored glycogen)		2%

this chapter is to provide additional relevant, interesting, and practical information that will be of value for therapists in developing useful hydrotherapy knowledge and skills.

The average adult body is approximately 60% water, 20% fat (lipids), 18% proteins, and 2% carbohydrates (see Table 3–1).[1] Throughout this chapter, we are going to use as an example a human being who weighs 140 lb. Thus, our example client would have 84 lb (60%) of water, which equals 10 gal; 28 lb (20%) of fat (lipids), 25 lb (18%) of mostly proteins; and 3 lb (2%) of stored carbohydrates (glycogen). Obviously, different-sized people will contain different amounts of water (see Table 3–2). An interesting question is, where is

Table 3–2	Amount of Water in the Human Body*
Person's Weight	**Pounds of Water** **Gallons of Water**
125 lb	75 lb 9 gal
140 lb	84 lb 10 gal
155 lb	93 lb 11 gal
175 lb	102 lb 12.2 gal
200 lb	120 lb 14.4 gal

* Applies to people in a normal weight range.

Table 3–3   Location of Water in the Human Body

Location	Amount
Inside the approximately 100 trillion cells	66%
Interstitial fluid	26%
Blood plasma	7%
Other fluid systems	~1%

the 10 gal of water in the human body located, and what is it doing? Of those 10 gal, 66% is located inside the approximately 100 trillion cells of the human body, 26% is in the interstitial fluid that surrounds most of the cells of the human body, and 7% is found in the blood plasma.[2] There is also a small amount of water in other fluid systems of the body, such as the cerebral spinal fluid (100 mL), the aqueous humor of the eyes, and the synovial joints (see Table 3–3). All of the water in the body—the entire 10 gal—is in a state of constant dynamic circulation (see Figure 3–1), as will be seen in the discussion of the circulatory system later in this chapter.

ELEVEN SYSTEMS OF THE HUMAN BODY

Traditional education in anatomy and physiology deals mainly with gross anatomy and physiology, which divides the human body into 11 systems (see Table 3–4). These 11 major body systems are elements of one system—the human body, which is a complex, living system that requires the healthy integrated functioning of all the 11 systems. This chapter discusses each system from more of a dynamic, fluid, cellular system perspective. Finally, it includes a discussion of the various ways hydrotherapy can be applied in each of the 11 body systems.

Integumentary System: Skin

The skin is composed of the epidermis, or the outer layer of the skin, and the next layer, or the dermis. The subcutaneous layer, which is below the dermis, consists primarily of fat cells (adipocytes) that provide a layer of insulation between the skin and the body's core. The subcutaneous layer also adds a certain texture to the skin and is an important element of the skin's overall appearance.

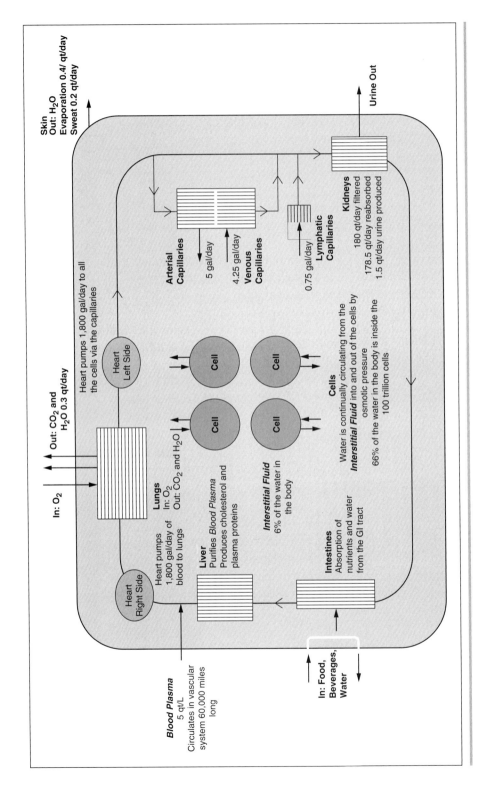

Figure 3–1 Total circulation of water in the human body.

Table 3–4 Gross Anatomy and Physiology: 11 Body Systems

Integumentary (skin)	Epidermis, dermis, hypodermis
Muscle	Skeletal, cardiac, smooth
Skeletal	Bone, ligaments, cartilage, joints, fascia
Cardiovascular	Heart and vascular system
Lymphatic and immune	Lymphatic vascular system, immune cells
Digestive	Total digestive system
Respiratory	Lungs (oxygen–carbon dioxide exchange)
Urinary	Kidneys, bladder
Endocrine	Thyroid, adrenal, etc.
Nervous	Central, peripheral, somatic, autonomic
Reproduction	Male and female

The skin has some important fluid dynamic elements (see Figure 3–2 and Plate 9). One such element is that the dermis and subcutaneous layer are highly vascular, which means large amounts of blood flows through them. Usually, only a small percentage (about 8%) of the body's blood is flowing through the skin; however, when an increase in the body's core temperature stimulates a cooling response, as much as 30% of the body's 5 qt of blood will be flowing through the skin. Increased blood flow to the skin allows heat to radiate from the blood, thereby reducing the body's temperature. In this process, the increased blood flow brings a greater flow of nutrients and oxygen to the skin cells.[3]

Another response of the body to increased core temperature occurs when the sympathetic nervous system stimulates the activity of the body's 4.5 million eccrine sweat glands to produce sweat, which produces an overall cooling effect. Sweat flows from the glands to the surface of the skin, where the water in the sweat evaporates. This evaporation absorbs heat from the body and releases the heat into the environment, thereby reducing the body's temperature. The human body can produce about 1 qt (1 L) of sweat per hour. In individuals who have acclimated to a warmer environment, the rate of sweat production can be as high as 2 qt (2 L) per hour.

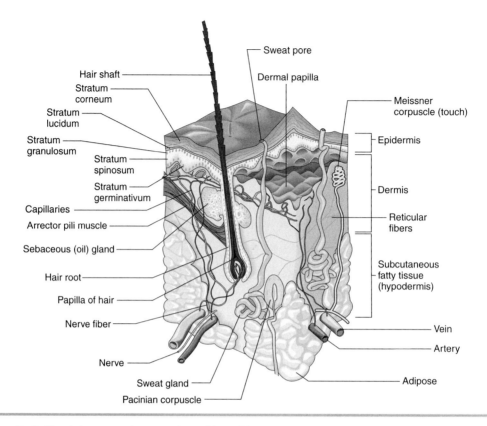

Hair shaft

Stratum corneum

Stratum lucidum

Stratum granulosum

Stratum spinosum

Stratum germinativum

Capillaries

Arrector pili muscle

Sebaceous (oil) gland

Hair root

Papilla of hair

Nerve fiber

Nerve

Sweat gland

Pacinian corpuscle

Sweat pore

Dermal papilla

Meissner corpuscle (touch)

Epidermis

Dermis

Reticular fibers

Subcutaneous fatty tissue (hypodermis)

Vein

Artery

Adipose

Figure 3–2 The integumentary system: The skin.

Hydrotherapy and the Integumentary System

Hydrotherapy treatments, including steam and hydrotubs, are used to increase the temperature of the skin and core body, which, in turn, increases blood flow to the skin. These treatments can be very useful in skin care, as the increase in blood flow results in an increase in the flow of nutrients and oxygen to the skin. These treatments also increase the metabolic activity of skin cells, which increases the rate of diffusion of substances and oxygen from the blood to the interstitial fluid and then to the cells. This means that products that are in contact with the skin and can diffuse into the skin will do so more quickly. Also, the effect of heat and moisture on the skin's surface loosens the contact of surface cells to the skin, allowing for a more even and deeper exfoliation process.

Sweating can be stimulated by the use of steam and warm/hot hydrotub treatments, which can produce a sweat flow rate of 1 to 2 qt (L) per hour. Inducing sweating, which has a long traditional use for detoxifying the body (especially the skin), is one of the oldest known hydrotherapy treatments. In the Ayurvedic tradition, sweating has been part of a detoxification program called **swedhana,** which has been used for thousands of years (see Chapter 8).

Combining heating of the skin with hydromassage can improve the skin's structural matrix at the dermis and subcutaneous levels, which can lead to improved appearance and texture of the skin. Although there are different types of connective tissue matrices in the dermis and subcutaneous levels, they are all basically made up of collagen fibers, elastin fibers, and a ground substance created by fibroblast cells. When these fibroblast cells and the connective matrix are heated and massaged using hydrotherapy, significant improvements in the structure and radiant look of the skin can be produced. Estheticians can use facial or full-body hydrotherapy treatments to promote the health and wellness of the skin.

Also, the skin, like most of the body systems, is affected by stress and tension in negative ways. Deeper levels of relaxation produced by most hydrotherapy treatments can reduce muscle tension and higher levels of stress hormones, which can have a beneficial effect on the healthy appearance of the skin.

Swedhana
A steam treatment in Ayurveda that induces sweating for detoxification.

Musculoskeletal System

In this section, the muscle and skeletal systems will be studied as one system. The skeletal system will be seen as including the bones, cartilage, ligaments, joints, tendons, and fascia. The muscles are the dynamic element of this total system, and their coordinated contraction is responsible for the precise movements of the body. What is of interest from a fluid dynamic perspective is that the body is 60% water and 20% fat/lipids (see Teaching Exercise 3–1), both of which are liquids. The fat is mainly composed of triglycerides stored in the body's fat cells (adipocytes) in a liquid state. The solid, structural system of the body, including the muscle proteins, is less than 20% of the body's total weight. This is important in that the body's structural systems must support the fluid weight of the body, which makes up approximately 80% of the body's weight. The combined weight of 80% of the body in the fluid state that needs to be supported by the solid structural system of the body, places significant compressive force on the body's structural system.

Hydrotherapy and the Musculoskeletal System

Because the body is about 80% liquid and because fat (lipids) are lighter than water, the human body is almost weightless in water. However, the structural system of the body is heavier than water. Thus, as a whole, the entire human body is, on average, 5% heavier than water. Although an average, normal-weight human will sink in water,

3-1 TEACHING EXERCISE

Amount of Liquids in the Human Body

For this exercise, refer to Figure 3–3.

1. Fill two 5 gal containers (or four 2½ gal containers) with water. This water represents the 10 gal of water in the body.

2. If possible, fill a 2½ gal container with vegetable oil. Vegetable oils are triglycerides similar to those in the human body. This represents the lipids in the body that are in a liquid state. The body normally has about 3.5 gal of lipids.

3. If possible, place these containers next to a skeleton model.

80% of the body's weight is in the liquid form. 60% (water) of this liquid is in a state of constant circulation. The skeleton and other structural elements must support the weight of the liquid component, which creates significant compression on the skeleton, joints, and cartilage disks.

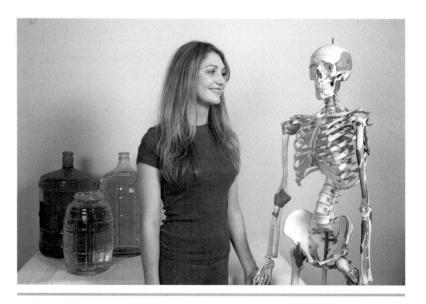

Figure 3–3 The body is 80% fluid: 60% water and 20% lipids.

he or she will feel weightless. The relationship between the principle of buoyancy and the human body is very important, as it can be used in different hydrotherapy treatments to produce different therapeutic changes. In some hydrotubs, especially those that are longer than the body, the client can lie fully extended, essentially removing the effects of gravity on the body. This means the structural system does not need to support the body's weight, making it possible for therapists to work with the body in ways that would not be possible on a normal massage table. For example, the body, when in water, can be rotated and stretched in various ways as a result of the total fluid environment. In addition, clients with certain types of restrictions, including pain, are often more comfortable and relaxed in water. Also, hydromassage done on specific areas of the client's body underwater can improve circulation and the functioning of different structural elements, such as the joints.

Steam therapy and warm/hot hydrotub treatments create heat exchange between the water and the body, increasing the temperature of the structural system. This increases the flexibility and the ability of the structural system to rotate and stretch, is especially effective for treatments involving the muscles and the total fascial matrix. It can also be used to improve passive range of motion done during or after the heating treatment. In addition, as people get older, there is more cumulative stress on the body's structural system and these types of treatments can be used to help improve structural systems as people age. Also, the deep relaxation produced by hydrotherapy can reduce excessive muscle tension in the body. Stress and anxiety have been correlated with greater muscle tension and a general sense of physical discomfort.

Cardiovascular and Lymphatic Vascular System

The cardiovascular and lymphatic systems are dynamic fluid systems that are key to the total circulation of fluids to and from the cells. The lymphatic vascular system helps drain the interstitial fluid surrounding the cells back into the cardiovascular system. In the human body, the combined cardiovascular-lymphatic system is greater than 60,000 mi in length (see Figure 3–4 and Plate 10).[4] The main exchange of nutrients, oxygen, and carbon dioxide takes place between the blood plasma and the interstitial fluid in the blood capillaries. There are more than 10 billion capillary beds in the body, and no cell in the body is more than five cells away from a capillary (exceptions are the cartilage disks and the skin's epidermis).[5]

The average person has 5 qt (5 L) of blood, which recirculates more than 1,440 times through the body each day. The heart pumps

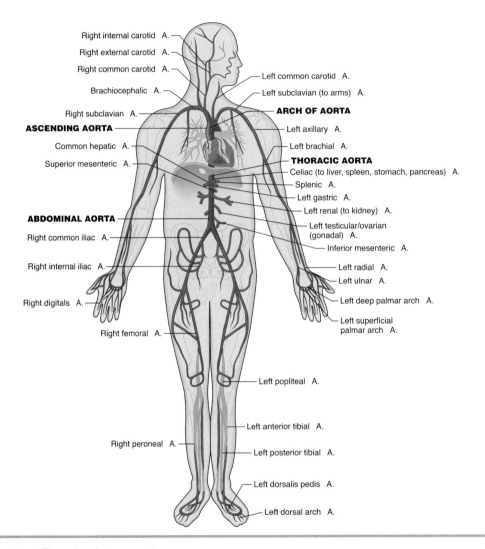

Right internal carotid A.
Right external carotid A.
Right common carotid A.
Brachiocephalic A.
Right subclavian A.
ASCENDING AORTA
Common hepatic A.
Superior mesenteric A.
ABDOMINAL AORTA
Right common iliac A.
Right internal iliac A.
Right digitals A.
Right femoral A.
Right peroneal A.

Left common carotid A.
Left subclavian (to arms) A.
ARCH OF AORTA
Left axillary A.
Left brachial A.
THORACIC AORTA
Celiac (to liver, spleen, stomach, pancreas) A.
Splenic A.
Left gastric A.
Left renal (to kidney) A.
Left testicular/ovarian (gonadal) A.
Inferior mesenteric A.
Left radial A.
Left ulnar A.
Left deep palmar arch A.
Left superficial palmar arch A.
Left popliteal A.
Left anterior tibial A.
Left posterior tibial A.
Left dorsalis pedis A.
Left dorsal arch A.

Figure 3–4 The circulatory system.

more than 1,800 gal of blood per day; actually, it pumps 3,600 gal, when you consider that the heart is really two pumps—the right and left sides (see Figure 3–5 and Plate 12).[6] More than 5 gal of blood plasma will flow from the blood into the interstitial fluid, allowing nutrients and oxygen to be delivered to the cells. Another 5 gal (0.75 gal of which will return as lymphatic fluid) will return to the blood via the blood capillaries and lymphatic system, carrying with it carbon dioxide, lactic acid, and other by-products of cellular metabolism. Of the approximately 5 qt (5 L) of blood in the vascular system, 60% is in the veins and venules (see Figure 3–6), 12% is in the vascular system in the lungs, 8% is in the heart, 15% is in the arteries and arterioles, and only 5% is in the total capillary system.[7]

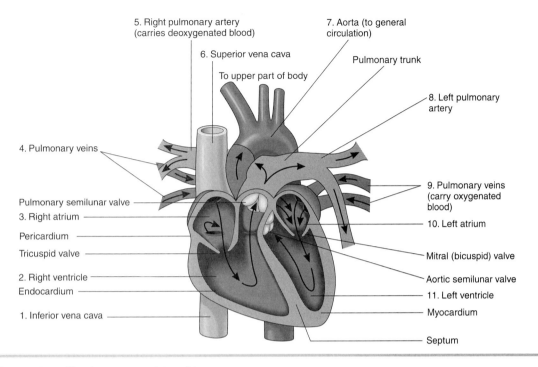

Figure 3–5 The heart consists of two pumps.

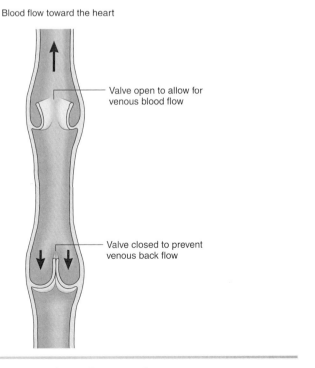

Figure 3–6 Veins and valves: One-way flow.

Hydrotherapy and the Cardiovascular and Lymphatic Vascular Systems

Heating hydrotherapy treatments, especially steam and warm/hot hydrotub treatments, increase circulation by increasing the heart rate and the force of the heart's contractions. This can significantly increase blood circulation to the skin and to cells of the body. As mentioned earlier, increasing the core body temperature also increases the metabolic activity of the cells, which, in turn, increases the need of oxygen in the cells. This need for more oxygen increases circulation to the cells. Increased body temperature also increases the rate of osmosis, which is an important part of the total circulatory process. Basically, heating hydrotherapy treatments have a stimulating effect on the total circulation of the body and have long been used as key element of many health and wellness programs.

Hydrotub treatments that include underwater hydromassage can be used to massage the body's vascular systems, providing a comfortable, but significant, level of pressure. This pressure not only stimulates circulation but also provides a massaging effect to the structure of the vascular system itself. Most parts of the vascular system, especially the capillaries, are very flexible and compressible. As this complex system ages, it is subjected to various stresses or injuries (e.g., bruises), in addition to normal wear and tear. Hydrotherapy allows the use of treatment modalities that work directly to help improve and maintain the health of the vascular system. Cardiovascular disease is a leading cause of death, especially among women. A healthy cardiovascular system is essential for healthy aging and prevention of disease.

Over time, factors such as compression from gravity, posture, and movement change the vascular system's natural alignment and symmetry so that it becomes less ordered. The hydromassage table and certain longer, deeper hydrotubs allow for unique stretching and rotating movements that work with the body as one integrated system that can lead to improvements in the alignment of the body's vascular systems. Hydromassage techniques can also have a positive effect on cellular alignment. Each of the 100 trillion cells of the human body has a natural alignment in relation to the rest of the cells of the body—a quite amazing fact—in the same way that each bone has a natural alignment in relation to other bones.

Immune System

The **immune system,** which is primarily a function of the white blood cells and the lymphatic vascular system, depends on the total circulatory system of the body to provide an effective immune response. The main white blood cells of the immune system include the monocytes, B-cells, T-cells, neutrophils, basephils, and eshophils, all of which circulate in the blood. When there is an infection, trauma, injury, or allergic reaction, these cells move from the blood to the affected area. The neutrophils are the first to respond to infections. Following this initial response, monocytes enter the area and mature into macrophages, which are responsible for much of the cleanup of the damaged areas. In case of an infection, killer T-cells migrate to the area of infection and respond to the specific microorganism causing the infection. B white blood cells (B-cells) produce antibodies that flow to the site of an infection to help destroy the specific germ that is causing the infection. The T-cells and B-cells will then "remember" the specific germs that caused the infection; if the same infection starts again, the T-cells and B-cells will kill the germ before infection develops.

Because an infection, trauma, or injury can occur anywhere in the body, a combined immune response from the white blood cells requires that these cells and antibodies travel to the site of infection or trauma via the body's vascular system. This very complex process depends on a normal, healthy functioning of the circulatory system. The lymphatic vascular system plays a special role in immunity, as the lymph nodes are sites where white blood cells purify the lymphatic fluid of microorganisms (germs), proteins, and other substances. The purified lymphatic fluid then flows back to the blood plasma.

Hydrotherapy and the Immune System

Heating hydrotherapy treatments, especially steam and hydrotub treatments, increase the temperature of the skin and the core of the body. An increase in the core body temperature increases the metabolic activity of the cells. For every 1°C increase in temperature of a cell, the cell's metabolic rate will increase by 12%.[8] Increasing the metabolic activity of the white blood cells has been shown to produce a more effective immune response, resulting in faster, more complete healing. Heating the core temperature also weakens the microorganisms (germs) creating the infection, which allows a more successful immune response.[9]

Hydromassage and heating treatment techniques can have a positive, stimulating effect on the total circulation of the body and also on the immune response. These techniques have a beneficial effect on the coordinated activity of millions of white blood cells participating in the immune response at the site of the trauma or infection. Healthy white blood cells and the total immune system are also one of the key defenses against cancer.

Regular hydrotherapy heating treatments have been used as an effective approach in the prevention of disease. Stimulating the immune system through heating treatments can help destroy some microorganisms (germs) and cancer cells before those cells can create an infection or other problems. It is important to note that most of the main holistic health and wellness traditions have historically used regular heating hydrotherapy treatments to aid in the prevention of disease and for healthy aging.

Digestive System

Everyday, in the process of digestion, the gland cells of the digestive system produce approximately 1.8 gal (7 L) of digestive fluids (juices).[10] These fluids, which include gastric acids, are mostly water. After the digestive process is complete, this water is reabsorbed into the blood plasma. The digestive process is coordinated mainly by the parasympathetic nervous system, which is more dominant when the body is in a resting or relaxed state. During digestion, because the body is not usually performing strenuous activity, there are fewer demands for water for circulation to muscle cells or for cooling the body. This means more water is available for the production of digestive fluids from the blood plasma and interstitial fluid.

Hydrotherapy and the Digestive System

The daily production of 1.8 gal of digestive fluids is one of the many uses of the body's 10 gal of water. A Balanced Hydration Program can help to ensure that there is adequate water available in the body, not only to produce the digestive fluids necessary for digestion but also to aid in all the body's other physiological activities that require water. Chapter 4 presents a Balanced Hydration Program that can be used to help clients maintain adequate levels of daily hydration.

The deep levels of relaxation produced by most hydrotherapy treatments also have a positive effect on the digestive system. Relaxation enlivens the parasympathetic nervous system that controls the digestive system and helps balance the effects of the sympathetic nervous system, which is generally overstimulated by the stresses of modern life. This form of relaxation therapy can produce immediate and long-term benefits for the functioning of the digestive system.

Respiratory System

In the respiratory system, the process of respiration begins with the diffusion of oxygen molecules in the lungs into red blood cells in the blood plasma. Most of these oxygen molecules attach to red blood cells, although a few diffuse in the blood plasma. Red blood cells then travel through the blood vessels to capillaries where the oxygen then diffuses into the interstitial fluid and then to the cells of the body. Most cells require a constant, continual supply of oxygen in order to survive and carry out normal cellular activities. If the flow of oxygen is stopped, cells can die within a few minutes. The healthy functioning of the vascular system and effective exchange of oxygen from the lungs to the blood are essential for healthy aerobic (oxygen) cellular respiration.

The exchange and transport of carbon dioxide from the body is basically the reverse process of oxygen being made available to the cells. The exchange of oxygen and carbon dioxide takes place in the more than 300 million alveoli of the lungs. The surface area of the combined alveoli is about 750 ft^2.[11] This means that the surface area of the lungs is 30 times greater than the surface area of the skin, which is approximately 22 ft^2. The wall of each alveolus is 0.5 micrometers (μm) wide; as a reference, the size of a red blood cell is 8 μm wide. The thinness of the walls allows oxygen to enter the bloodstream, as well as any other substance that we breathe in that can diffuse into the bloodstream. In this way, certain medicines, natural products, or even toxic substances, such as nicotine, are introduced into the blood via the lungs.

Hydrotherapy and the Respiratory System

Steam inhalation therapy can moisturize dry lungs during the cold winter. The steam also heats the lungs, thereby increasing the rate of diffusion and the exchange of oxygen and carbon dioxide with the blood. It also allows natural products mixed with the steam to dissolve into the bloodstream for delivery to the body's cells. Inhalation therapy can also help with the natural process by which the lungs purify themselves to get rid of microscopic particles that enter the lungs during respiration (see Teaching Exercise 3–2). It can also stimulate the large number of white blood cells in the lungs that help keep germs in the air from entering the bloodstream. Simple inhalation therapy treatments can be very beneficial for most clients and are easy and inexpensive to perform.

The relaxation produced by many hydrotherapy treatments can help promote relaxed breathing. Normal, correct breathing is a function of specific patterns of muscle contraction. Anxiety, stress, and tension increase unhealthy levels of muscle tension, which can interfere with or limit normal, relaxed breathing. Education and training on normal breathing can be done during certain hydro-therapy treatments when the client is deeply relaxed. Clients who

3–2 TEACHING EXERCISE

Air Pollution and the Respiratory System

The photo shows a part of a used home air filter that has been opened so that it is possible to see the effects of air pollution on the filter. The whiter areas are spots that did not come into contact with the air and are free of air pollutants. If possible, find a similar used filter and use it as a teaching demonstration with clients to illustrate the effects of air pollution on the lungs.

- **RESPIRATORY (LUNG) AND AIR POLLUTION**

    The lungs are exposed to the same levels of pollution that the air filter is exposed to. We are constantly breathing in a combination of natural pollutants, such as dust and pollen, and man-made pollutants, such as fine particles from the breakdown of material in residential homes.

- **STEAM INHALATION THERAPY—3 EFFECTS**

    1. Increase in moisture in the respiratory system as the steam condenses from vapor to liquid.

    2. Has a temporary heating effect on the respiratory system that increases the metabolic activity of the cells.

    3. Products can be added to the steam being inhaled that have therapeutic effects.

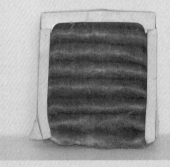

learn proper breathing patterns during a treatment can then work to restore that same normal breathing during regular activity. Another benefit of normal, relaxed breathing using the diaphragm is that it helps pump blood through the circulatory system and decreases the workload of the heart.

Urinary System

The urinary system is a highly fluid, dynamic system by which blood plasma is constantly purified and precise levels (homeostasis) of certain substances in the blood are maintained—for example, a sodium level of 142 mL/eq). Each day, the kidneys remove a total of 45 gal (180 L) of blood plasma from the blood at a rate of 125 mL/min. The kidneys then process this filtrate and return more than 99% back to the blood plasma. Less than 1% is removed in the form of urine, which is collected in the urinary bladder until it is expelled from the body by urination. On average, the kidneys produce 1.5 qt (1 L) of urine per day. For this process to function properly, the body must have normal levels of hydration. In addition, the blood pressure within the capillaries of the kidneys needs to remain about 55 mmHg.

Hydrotherapy and the Urinary System

The activity of the urinary system is a good example of a fluid dynamic system of the body and the normal functioning of the kidneys is essential for the total health of the body. The urinary system is very adaptive and when the body is dehydrated, the kidneys can compensate by producing urine using less water. Similarly, when there is excess water in the body, the kidneys remove it by producing larger volumes of diluted urine.

Chronic dehydration can stress the kidneys and increase the risk of developing kidney stones. In the other extreme, some individuals have died from drinking excessive amounts of water over a short period of time, which exceeded the kidneys ability to remove excess water. Drinking too much water can result in a dilution of sodium levels and cellular swelling (edema). For healthy aging of the kidneys and the prevention of certain health problems, maintaining normal daily hydration levels is very important. Using the Balanced Hydration Program taught in Chapter 4, a therapist can help a client maintain a balanced level of hydration throughout the day, while decreasing the intake of excessive calories and potentially harmful substances found in some drinking water and beverages. Using heating hydrotherapy treatments and hydromassage can stimulate the general circulation in the body which can also benefit the normal functioning of the kidneys.

Endocrine System

The endocrine system, along with the nervous system, is one of the main systems responsible for controlling and coordinating the activities of the 100 trillion cells of the human body (see Figure 3–7).

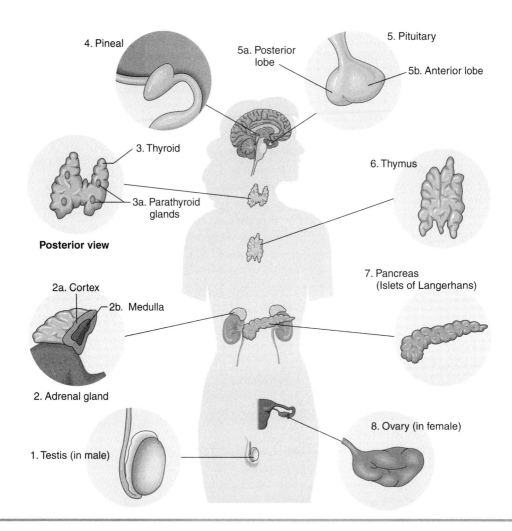

Figure 3–7 The endocrine system.

The various endocrine cells throughout the body produce many different major and minor hormones. Once an endocrine cell produces a hormone, such as a thyroid hormone, that hormone must then travel to cells at other locations in the body by way of the circulatory system. When the hormone reaches its target cell, it modifies the behavior of that cell. For example, the thyroid hormone increases the metabolic activity of a target cell.

The production and delivery of hormones is a complex process that works very efficiently when all the elements of the endocrine system and the vascular transport system are functioning normally. However, certain factors, including aging, vascular problems, demand for overproduction by endocrine cells, or an imbalance in production of the various hormones can disrupt and interfere with the integrated functioning of the endocrine system.

Hydrotherapy and the Endocrine System

Relaxation therapy, as produced by hydrotherapy treatment, can have profound, beneficial effects on the endocrine system. As mentioned, different hydrotherapy treatments are deeply relaxing and can produce a powerful calming effect. This calming effect, in turn, will decrease the production of hormones associated with high levels of physical, mental, and emotional activity—namely, cortisol and adrenaline. These hormones, which are also associated with stressful emotional states, decrease as levels of relaxation, calmness, comfort, and normal sleep increase. This relaxation can be beneficial not only for daily wellness but also for long-term, healthy aging. Overall, experiences of deep relaxation can help the endocrine system maintain a natural balance between high levels of stress and activity and calm and restful states. Relaxation therepy can also decrease high blood pressure and have other benefits for the circulatory system which plays a key role in movement of hormones in the body.

Research has shown that the relaxation produced by various techniques of massage also increases the production of the hormone oxytocin.[12] Increased levels of this hormone are correlated with an increased sense of comfort, connectedness, and well-being. During many hydrotherapy treatments, clients report experiencing a deep state of connectedness and well-being that seems enhanced by the effects of the water component of the treatment.

Nervous System

The nervous system, along with the endocrine system, is responsible for controlling and coordinating much of the activity of the 100 trillion cells of the body. A key function of the nervous system is also receiving sensory input and then sending those signals to the brain, where they are consciously perceived. The "experience" of a hydrotherapy treatment comes from the integrated sensory input of hearing, sight, taste, touch, and smell. Especially significant is the sense of touch from nerve endings in the skin, which allows the client to feel the sensations of different levels of pressure. Sensory input from the muscles, tendons, and joints as the client moves and stretches, combined with the sensory input of balance (inner ear), creates the special sensations of movement that occurs during hydrotherapy treatments. The skin is also very sensitive to hot and cold sensations. All of this combined sensory input allows for the rich and varied experiences of the many different types of hydrotherapy treatments.

In addition to creating the awareness of the outside world and movements of the body, these experiences are also processed by the autonomic nervous system (ANS), which automatically controls key physiological functions of the body, including heart rate, blood flow to specific organs, increase in production of certain hormones, and gland secretions. One division of the ANS, the sympathetic nervous system (SNS), controls increased blood flow and glucose for greater levels of physical and mental activity. The SNS can do this very quickly, especially in an emergency situation, by the immediate release of adrenaline and more slowly by the release of cortisol. The SNS is also simulated by feelings of pressure, stress, and anxiety. The parasympathetic nervous system (PNS) controls the more restful states of the body and facilitates rejuvenation of the body's energy resources by producing glycogen (the stored form of glucose in the body) and also controls much of the functions of digestion. When the PNS is more dominant, there is decreased heart and breath rate as well as decreased levels of adrenaline and cortisol (also known as stress hormones). In fact, when the SNS activity is greater, it inhibits the activity of the PNS and when the PNS activity is greater, it inhibits the activity of the SNS. Normally, during a 24-hour cycle, there is a natural balance of the activities of the SNS and PNS. However, in modern times, due to increased work and personal demands, as well as higher levels of stress and anxiety, the SNS is overstimulated and time spent resting and relaxing, which is controlled by the PNS, is less than normal. Higher levels of stress, anxiety, and exhaustion are highly correlated with an increase in physical, mental, and emotional health problems.

Hydrotherapy and the Nervous System

Hydrotherapy treatments and programs can be a highly effective as a form of relaxation therapy and part of a total stress management program. During hydrotherapy treatments, profound states of relaxation are produced that increase the activity of the PNS, decrease the activity of the SNS, and restore a balance functioning of the combined SNS and PNS activity.

During a hydrotherapy treatment, a client experiences various sensations of water including pressures and sensations of warmth (and cold). The client also experiences sensations of the body moving in various ways in water in hydrotubs (and on a hydromassage table) that enliven our past experiences of being in water and even our earliest memories of in the fluid environment of the womb (see Plate 16). Different hydrotherapy treatments provide different experiences; a shower treatment produces a unique set of sensations that is different from a steam or hydrotub treatment, but they are all related to our experiences of water. In addition to the experience of water, the therapist can also combine aromatherapy, music, touch (massaging), and light (color light therapy) to create unique patterns of sensory stimulation to enhance to effect of the treatment. Even the setting (décor) of the room can have an effect on the total outcome of the treatment. By providing a specific type of hydrotherapy treatment along with other modes of sensory stimulation, the therapist can produce profound, unique states of relaxation for the client. When these treatments are given on a regular basis, they can be an essential component of a total stress management program. These treatments also create powerful new emotional memories that become enlivened during similar treatments in the future, enhancing the total effect. In posttraumatic stress disorders, traumatic memories can be spontaneously remembered, producing similar physiological and emotional states. Conversely, in hydrotherapy treatments, positive emotional memories can also be enlivened by producing positive physiological and emotional states. There are many therapeutic benefits from hydrotherapy treatments for the nervous system, including balancing the SNS and PNS, and also in the creation of wonderful sensory and emotional experiences that are unique to hydrotherapy treatments.

Reproductive System

The reproductive system has many fluid dynamic aspects. One of the more interesting aspects is the growth and development of a baby from conception to birth. The development of the baby through the embryonic and fetal stages to birth takes place in a totally fluid environment. The developing baby essentially floats in the amniotic fluid for nine months, and only experiences gravity at the time of birth. Thus, our first experiences of buoyancy and floating come before we are born. Perhaps some of the special feelings of comfort and relaxation people feel during flotation treatments or when relaxing in warm water relates to our first experiences in the natural flotation environment of the womb, surrounded by sensations of warm water, wave motion, and a gravity-free environment. Although we may not consciously remember these experiences, they are some of our first memories.

Even a normal human sexual response has important fluid dynamic elements. The sexual response depends on the ability of the vascular system to direct a healthy blood flow to the genital areas to contribute to a normal state of sexual arousal. Although there are different causes of problems in this area, the inability to direct a normal blood flow under certain pressure and maintain that pressure for a specific period of time, inhibits and may totally prevent, a normal sexual response. This problem affects both men and women—the physiological process is basically the same, though there are basic anatomical differences. Well-known drugs are available that attempt to treat this problem by controlling the amount, pressure, and duration of blood flow to the genital areas. However, problems with sexual arousal related to blood flow are usually symptoms of much more serious problems with the cardiovascular systems that these medications do not address.

Hydrotherapy and the Reproductive System

Some types of hydrotherapy treatments can be helpful during pregnancy. These treatments often involve the principle of buoyancy and have the effect of reducing gravity on the mother's body. These treatments can be relaxing while also providing a temporary relief from the additional weight of pregnancy, which is mostly water weight. Hydrotubs that are longer and deeper are more suited for treatments with pregnant women. Heating treatments using steam, hot or cold water, or hydropressure are never appropriate (they are contraindicated) for pregnant women. Water-birthing, though not used often, provides unique conditions for giving birth in a warm, comfortable, gravity-free environment.

Also, as mentioned in the section on the nervous system, the profound relaxation of hydrotherapy treatments can help restore balance to the SNS and PNS activities of the autonomic nervous system, which can not only reduce stress hormone levels but also produce healthier functioning of the cardiovascular system. This in turn can be beneficial to the functioning of the entire reproductive system, including the human sexual response.

A DYNAMIC FLUID, CELLULAR, STRUCTURAL PARADIGM

This section presents a different paradigm of anatomy and physiology, a different way of seeing how the human body functions, that can help us understand why hydrotherapy works so well as a therapeutic modality. In hydrotherapy, we use water outside the body to transform the fluid dynamics of water inside the human body. In this paradigm, the human body is seen as a team of 100 trillion cells (*TeamCells*) that live in a totally dynamic, fluid environment. The human body is approximately 60% water and 20%

fat (which is also a fluid). The remaining 20% makes up the solid structural element of the body. Usually, we see the body as being more of a solid structure made up of muscles, bones, ligaments, fascia, and skin. However, when we look at the human body from another perspective, we see that the body is actually 80% fluid and is a very dynamic, fluid, cellular system with water as a key element. And the same basic principles of water that govern the behavior of water in the hydrosphere and the water we use in hydrotherapy treatments, are the same basic principles that govern the behavior of water inside the human body. Understanding this relationship provides unique insights into how hydrotherapy works, especially when we consider that water inside the human body is an essential element of almost every aspect of the physiology of the body.

This special way of seeing the functioning of the human body begins with a discussion of the cells of the body, which are mostly water and contain 66% (approximately 6.6 gal) of the water in the human body.

Cells of the Body

Every cell in the body requires continual circulation of water and nutrients, as well as the continual removal of the by-products of cellular metabolism. The activity of the cells is coordinated mainly through hormones and the nervous system.

The fundamental anatomy and physiology of all the different cells of the body is very similar, and all cells live in a similar fluid environment—the interstitial fluid. Cells, and the fluid environment in which they live, consist mainly of water. This environment is highly dynamic: The vascular system contains more than 10 billion capillary beds where fluid and nutrients move into and out of the interstitial fluid. To maintain the normal circulation of all the cells of the body, the heart must pump, on average, 3,600 gal of blood of each day.

When we look at the human body from this perspective, we see water—and all the natural ways in which it behaves—as one of the most fundamental elements of all of the activities of the cells of the body. When we see the amazing role water plays in virtually every aspect of the physiology of the human body, we gain a fundamental insight into the role of hydrotherapy as a modality for promoting health and wellness. In hydrotherapy, water is used in a controlled manner to produce physiological transformations, mainly in the cells and fluid systems inside the human body. By bringing water of different temperatures and different pressures into contact with a client's body, a therapist can produce changes in the metabolic activity of the cells and in the circulation to the cells. Through the use of hydrotherapy, it is possible to work with groups of cells, or even with all the cells at the same time. In the natural behavior of water, we find a unifying principle for the behavior of individual cells, as well as the coordinated, synergistic function of all of the 100 trillion cells of the body.

There are about 200 different types of **cells** (see Table 3–5 and Figure 3–8). The activity of the cells—both individually and collectively is responsible for all the primary physiological functions of the human body. For example, the activity of the different neurons allows us to perceive the world, to think, feel, and

Cells
The basic structural and functional unit of the body capable of performing all the activities vital to life.

Table 3–5   Types and Functions of Cells

Cells	Function (examples)
Skeletal, smooth, cardiac	Movement
Red blood cells	Oxygen delivery
White blood cells	Immune functions
Endocrine cells	Hormones; cellular communication
Gland cells	Production of digestive, sweat, and lubricating fluids
Neurons	Neural impulses and neurotransmitters
Epithelial cells	Skin, vascular, lining of GI tract
Hepatocytes (liver cells)	Production of bile, blood proteins, cholesterol
Adipocytes (fat cells)	Storage of triglycerides
Fibroblasts	Production of total fascial matrix, tendon, ligaments
Chondroblasts	Production of cartilage
Osteoblasts	Production of bone matrix
Osteoclasts	Dissolve bone matrix
Reproductive cells	Egg (ovum), sperm

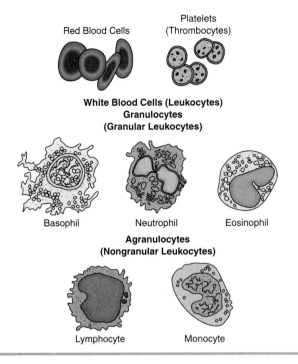

Red Blood Cells

Platelets
(Thrombocytes)

White Blood Cells (Leukocytes)
Granulocytes
(Granular Leukocytes)

Basophil   Neutrophil   Eosinophil

Agranulocytes
(Nongranular Leukocytes)

Lymphocyte   Monocyte

Figure 3–8 Examples of cells.

understand. The activity of muscle cells (fibers) allows us to perform all simple and complex movements. The circulation of the 25 trillion red blood cells (25% of all cells) brings oxygen to all the other cells in the body. Basically, whatever we do in terms of moving, experiencing, thinking, and feeling—plus all that the body does that we are not always aware of—is being done by the cells of the body. Thus, the health and wellness of the cells is fundamental to the health and wellness of the total person. Anything that interferes with or limits the normal function of the cells will have a negative impact on how well we think, feel, and perform. (See Teaching Exercise 3–3.)

The Anatomy and Physiology of the Cells

Most of the different types of cells of the body have a similar anatomy and physiology, although with differences that provide the unique physiological functioning for that specific type of cell. (See Figure 3–9 and Plate 11.) For example, even though a sweat gland cell and a neuron cell are similar in many ways, one cell produces a fluid secretion and the other produces neural impulses.

3–3 TEACHING EXERCISE

Cells in a Fluid Environment: The Interstitial Fluid

1. Use different shapes of balloons to represent the different shapes and sizes of cells in the body.

2. Fill each balloon with water that is close to 98°F–99°F.

3. Place a water balloon in a container of water that will easily hold that balloon. The water in the container, which should also be close to 98°F–99°F, represents the interstitial fluid that surrounds every cell in the body.

4. While holding the cell (balloon) underwater, visualize that every cell in the body lives in the fluid environment of the interstitial fluid. Visualize that there must be constant circulation of interstitial fluid to each cell, bringing substances to and removing substances from the cells.

What is keeping the water inside the cells and the interstitial fluid at a constant temperature of 98.6°F? It is the metabolic activity of each of the 100 trillion cells that generates heat.

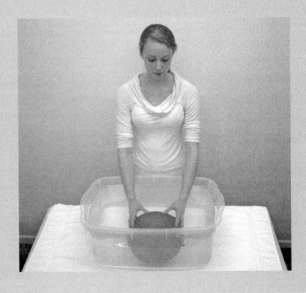

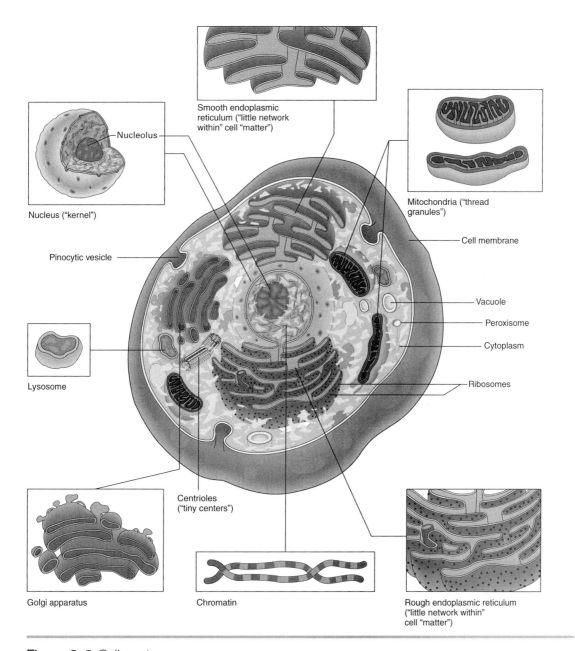

Figure 3–9 Cell anatomy.

The following are the key elements of cell anatomy and physiology that are common to almost every cell in the body.

- Plasma membrane: This is the barrier between a cell and the interstitial fluid (the environment that surrounds every cell in the body). The plasma membrane selectively allows the passage of substances into the cell from the interstitial fluid and out of the cell into the interstitial fluid.

- Cytosol: This is the fluid portion of the cell that contains many dissolved substances, such as oxygen and electrolytes. Most cells are about 70% water. The main exception is adipocytes (fat cells), which store triglycerides (fat) and which are 28% water.

- Mitochondria: These are responsible for converting glucose and fatty acids to produce energy in the form of ATP molecules. This energy is then used for most of the cell activities, such as building proteins and creating muscle contractions.

- Ribosomes, endoplasmic reticulum, and Golgi body: These elements function together as a "factory" to produce most of the proteins, lipids, hormones, neurotransmitters, and other substances that will be used by the cell or exported from the cell to be transported to and used by other cells. Much of their activity is under the control of RNA and DNA.

- Lysomes, peroxisomes, and proteasomes: These organelles are responsible for removing substances that are either no longer needed or possibly harmful to the cell. They digest the substances and convert them to simpler substances that can either be used by the cell or be removed from the cell.

- Nucleus: The nucleus contains the primary information, in the form of DNA, that is responsible for controlling most of the cell's activity, including cellular division. Cellular division is one of the most dynamic activities of cells taking place in the body. For example, more than 2 million new red blood cells are produced every second.

CELL SIZE: One challenge with applying the cellular paradigm is that we do not "see" cells. We can easily see skin, eyes, and structures of a dissected body, such as muscles and bones, but we do not see cells in the same way. However, modern technology allows us to see photos—and even videos—of all the cells of the body, as well as the elements within the cells, such as the mitochondria and nucleus. Cells are not actually large or small; rather, they are very complex, living structures, and their size is merely relative to something else.

Most cells are about 10 μm in diameter. As a reference, the diameter of bacteria is about 1 μm, and a centimeter is 10,000 μm.

TEAMCELLS: Cells function individually and collectively. Any activity of the body—for example, muscle contraction—is the result of the combined activity of many different types of cells, including muscle cells and neuron cells. Collectively, all the cells of the body are responsible for the total, holistic functioning of the body to maintain all the essential homeostatic functions, including body temperature, blood pressure, pH levels, electrolyte balance, blood volume, osmolarity, oxygen, and carbon dioxide levels, and much more. It is as if there are small teams of cells that form larger teams of cells that collectively form one team that is the human body, similar to the concept of tissue, organ, system, and total organism. Thus, a person's health and wellness is directly related to the health and wellness of the individual cells and how those cells behave synergistically as a team to produce an integrated functioning of the whole body.

Because cells, and the fluid environment in which they live, are primarily water, hydrotherapy can produce profound beneficial changes in the behavior of these fluid systems, thereby creating significant health and wellness transformations for the client. Even a hot or cold compress, which may seem to have an effect on a small area of the body, is actually transforming the functioning of billions of cells in the skin, subcutaneous layer, and even the deeper muscle layer. Hydrotherapy treatments like a hot (104°F/40°C) hydrotub can transform the activity of basically every one of the 100 trillion cells in the body by increasing the skin and core temperature.

Dynamic Fluid Matrix

The human body is made up of several, interconnected dynamic fluid systems. As mentioned earlier, the body is approximately 60% water, and all the fluid elements of the body (e.g., blood and interstitial fluid) are mainly water. All of these fluid elements are in a state of constant, dynamic circulation. This also helps us to understand the relationship between the behavior of water used in different forms of hydrotherapy, the changes produced in the body, and the benefits that result. This special way of looking at the anatomy and physiology of the human body can provide many insights not only into the understanding of hydrotherapy but also into the functioning of the human body.

The key components of the fluid matrix are the blood plasma, interstitial fluid, lymphatic fluid, and cerebral spinal fluid. Together, these components contain 34% of all the water in the body. The other 66% of water in the body is located inside the 100 trillion cells. The following are key dynamic principles of the fluid matrix:

- The heart pumps, on average, 3,600 gal of blood each day. The vascular system reaches more than 10 billion capillary beds, where blood plasma exchanges fluids with interstitial fluid and then passes it on to cells. No cell in the body is more than 5 cells from a capillary. In addition, the 25 trillion red blood cells, as well as a much smaller number of white blood cells, are circulating continually within the blood plasma.

- Every day, on average, 5 gal of blood plasma flows from the capillaries into the interstitial fluid to provide cells with nutrients, oxygen, hormones, and other substances. Each day, 4.25 gal of interstitial fluid returns back to the blood plasma via the capillaries and 0.75 gal of interstitial fluid returns via the lymphatic system. This allows the removal of by-products of cellular metabolism, such as carbon dioxide, lactic acid, hydrogen ions, and ammonia, from the interstitial fluid and the purification of the interstitial fluid by the lymphatic system.

- Each day, the kidneys filter more than 45 gal of blood plasma from the blood, process it, and produce about 1.5 qt of urine. All of the fluid that was processed by the kidneys, minus the 1.5 gal used to produce urine, is returned to the blood plasma. This process takes place at a rate of about 125 mL/min.

- Each day, about 480 mL of cerebral spinal fluid (CSF) is produced by special cells that convert interstitial fluid into CSF. The normal production and circulation of CSF is essential to healthy functioning of the brain and spinal cord.

- There are some other, very small amounts of circulation to areas such as the synovial joints and the aqueous humor of eyes.

- There is continual circulation between the fluid inside the cells and the interstitial fluid that surrounds them. (See Figure 3–10.)

Structural Matrix of the Body

The structural matrix of the body, which contains mostly protein (in the form of collagen, elastin, and muscle contractile fibers) and crystallized bone matrix, represents about 20% of

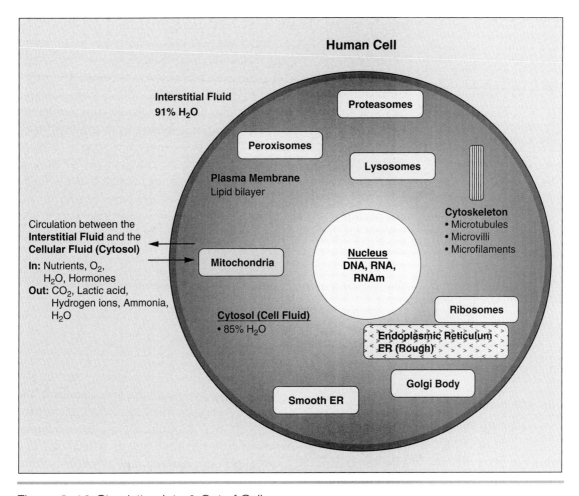

Figure 3–10 Circulation Into & Out of Cells.

the body's weight. These are the nonfluid, solid structural elements of the body. The following are the key structural elements of the body:

- Bones
- Cartilage
- Ligaments
- Tendons
- Fascial matrix
- Muscle proteins (mainly myosin, actin, and titan)

It is interesting to note that all of these structural elements function together as an interconnected (integrated) system. This system moves, rotates, compresses, and stretches as one. Also note that this integrated system must support and balance the total weight of the body, 80% of which is made up of fluid elements—water and fat (lipids). This places significant compressive forces on the structural system, especially the joints and cartilage disks. One principle of water that is used in hydrotherapy is buoyancy, which allows a human body in water to be temporarily free from gravity which allows a therapist to work on the body in a unique environment. Also, a heating hydrotherapy treatment that increases the core temperature of the body makes tendons, ligaments, and the fascia more flexible and stretchable,[13] which can also have the added benefit of improving the alignment of blood vessels, nerve fibers, and muscle fibers.[14] This, combined with more relaxed, easy-to-stretch muscles, allows the therapist to work with the combined structural and muscle system in various ways to produce therapeutic changes that would not be possible on a normal treatment table.

 ## SUMMARY

The chapter began with a discussion of the anatomy and physiology of the human body from the perspective of gross anatomy, the 11 systems of the body, and hydrotherapy. The information provided is supplemental to the formal training on anatomy and physiology that therapists receive during their initial education. The chapter ends with a discussion of anatomy and physiology from the perspective of the dynamic, fluid cellular nature of the body. During hydrotherapy, a therapist brings water into contact with the body to produce beneficial changes in the body. Because the human body is approximately 60% water, many of the changes created by the use of water outside the body produce changes in the behavior of water inside the body. Because the same basic principles of water outside the body apply to the behavior of water inside the body (e.g., buoyancy, heat capacity), much can be understood regarding the use of water as a therapeutic modality.

This chapter also offered suggestions on how different hydrotherapy treatments can be used to produce beneficial therapeutic effects on the 11 different systems of the body. Any beneficial change produced by a hydrotherapy treatment will produce a corresponding change in the anatomy and physiology of the body. Thus, developing an understanding of the anatomy and physiology as it relates to hydrotherapy treatments is part of comprehensive hydrotherapy education.

■ REFERENCES

(1) Tortora, G., & Grabowski, S. (2003). *Principles of Anatomy and Physiology* (10th ed.). New York: John Wiley & Sons, p. 992.

(2) Tortora & Grabowski, *Principles of Anatomy*, p. 992.

(3) Guyton, A., & Hall, J. (2004). *Textbook of Medical Physiology* (10th ed.). Elsevier, p. 823.

(4) Tortora & Grabowski. *Principles of Anatomy*, p. 660.

(5) Guyton & Hall. *Textbook of Medical Physiology*, p. 163.

(6) Tortora & Grabowski. *Principles of Anatomy*, p. 660.

(7) Tortora & Grabowski. *Principles of Anatomy*, p. 702.

(8) Guyton & Hall. *Textbook of Medical Physiology*, p. 820.

(9) Tortora & Grabowski *Principles of Anatomy,* p. 942.

(10) Tortora & Grabowski *Principles of Anatomy,* p. 890.

(11) Tortora & Grabowski *Principles of Anatomy,* p. 818.

(12) Turner, R. (1999, Summer). Preliminary research on plasma oxytocin in normal cycling women: Investigating emotion and interpersonal distress. *Psychiatry* 62(2): 97–113.

(13) Alter, M. (2004). *Science of Flexibility* (3rd ed.). Champaign, IL: Human Kinetics, p. 50.

(14) Alter, *Science of Flexibility,* p. 49.

■ SUGGESTED READINGS

Alter, M. (2004). *Science of Flexibility* (3rd ed.). Champaign, IL: Human Kinetics.

Guyton, A., & Hall, J. (2004). *Textbook of Medical Physiology* (10th ed.). Elsevier.

Tortora, G., & Grabowski, S. (2003). *Principles of Anatomy and Physiology* (10th ed.). New York: John Wiley & Sons.

■ REVIEW QUESTIONS

1. List some of the different systems of the human body and give an example of a fluid dynamic element of each of these systems.

2. Describe how hydrotherapy can be used as a therapeutic treatment in each of the above examples.

3. Explain where the approximately 10 gallons of water is located in the human body.

4. Explain how this water is in a continual state of circulation.

5. How does the endocrine system depend on the healthy circulation of the body?

6. How does the deep relaxation produced by hydrotherapy treatments affect the endocrine system?

7. How does the sensory input from a hydrotherapy treatment influence the functioning of the nervous system?

8. Why can the human body also be considered a dynamic fluid cellular system?

9. What percentage of the body is fluid?

10. What percentage is solid (structural)?

11. Explain the relationship between the water used during a hydrotherapy treatment and the changes it produces in the dynamic fluid and cellular systems inside the body?

The Balanced Hydration Program: A Key to Health and Wellness

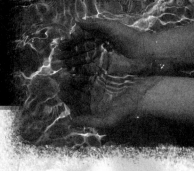

KEY TERMS

Balanced Hydration   osmolarity   osmoreceptor
  Program   thirst center   baroreceptor

INTRODUCTION

A normal, and ideally optimal, daily level of hydration is fundamental for the health and wellness of every human being. This chapter presents the **Balanced Hydration Program,** which allows therapists to develop a personalized hydration program for their clients. The information in this chapter explains the principles of hydration, which will help therapists evaluate each client's current daily patterns of hydration and make practical recommendations for adjustments and improvements. Balanced hydration is a key component of hydrotherapy. It combines an understanding of the behavior of water in the human body and how the body naturally and automatically loses predictable amounts of water each day, with suggestions on how to replace the water that is lost by consuming drinking water, beverages, and food to maintain normal hydration and prevent dehydration.

The chapter includes a discussion of the fundamental points of hydration. This discussion, which is based on modern knowledge of anatomy and physiology, scientific research on hydration, and some current formulas for maintaining normal levels of hydration, is relevant to gaining a comprehensive understanding of the principles of hydration. The practical application of this knowledge is in the Balanced Hydration Program, a systematic program for developing a personalized hydration program. This program can benefit

Balanced Hydration Program
A systematic, personalized hydration treatment.

every client, can be used immediately, and requires no investment in equipment or products, other than a few simple items for teaching demonstrations.

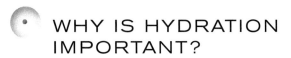

WHY IS HYDRATION IMPORTANT?

Hydration is fundamental to health and wellness because the human body is a dynamic, fluid, cellular system. In Chapter 3, we learned that the human body is approximately 60% water and that this water is the main component of the body's 100 trillion dynamic cells, the blood, and the interstitial fluid that surrounds the body's cells. We also discussed how all the water in the body, which is approximately 10 gal, is constantly circulating as part of the blood, the interstitial fluid, and the fluid inside the cells. The body needs to maintain precise volumes of water not only in the blood plasma, interstitial fluid, and within each cell, but also in the cerebral spinal fluid, aqueous humor (eyes), and other fluids. Maintaining these precise volumes depends on ensuring that the body has adequate levels of hydration. However, maintaining adequate levels of hydration is complicated by the fact that each day, we naturally and automatically lose approximately 2.5 qt/L (2.5 L) of water, which represents 6.25% of the total amount of water in the body.

Maintaining normal, and ideally optimal, levels of hydration provides many benefits and is essential for achieving all of a client's health and wellness goals. Proper hydration also prevents dehydration, which has been associated with decreased physical and mental performance, as well as with more serious health problems, such as kidney stones, gallbladder problems, and even cancer.[1] Finally, a Balanced Hydration Program allows clients to take more control and personal responsibility for their health and wellness.

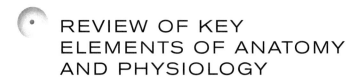

REVIEW OF KEY ELEMENTS OF ANATOMY AND PHYSIOLOGY

The following is a brief summary of the dynamic fluid nature of the human body. This summary gives an insight into why maintaining normal hydration levels in the human body is so essential to health and wellness.

Dynamic Fluid Elements
of the Human Body

- The human body is approximately 60% water (see Figure 4–1 and Plate 13).

- 66% of this water is in the 100 trillion cells of the body, 27% is in the interstitial fluid that surrounds the cells, and 7% is in the blood plasma (Figure 4–1). The volume of water in the cells, interstitial fluid, and blood plasma must be maintained at very precise levels.

- The heart pumps 1,800 gal of blood per day. (Actually, if you consider the heart to be two pumps—left and right sides—it pumps 3,600 gal a day.)

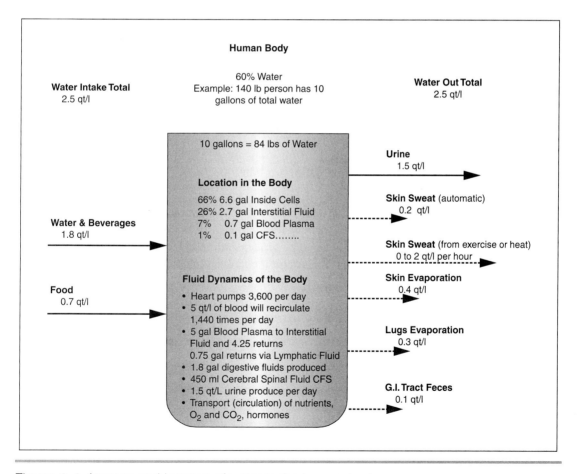

Figure 4–1 Amount and location of water in the human body.

- The total amount of blood in the body is 5 qt (5 L), which recirculates 1,440 times per day through the vascular system, which is more than 60,000 mi long.

- Each day, 5 gal flows through the capillaries from the blood plasma to the interstitial fluid, bringing nutrients, oxygen, and hormones to the cells. There are more than 10 billion capillary beds in the human body, and most cells are no more than 5 cells' distance from a capillary.

- Each day, 4.25 gal returns to the blood plasma through the capillaries from the interstitial fluid, carrying by-products of cellular metabolism that must be removed from the body.

- Each day, 0.75 gal, or 3 qt (3 L), returns via the lymphatic system, removing proteins in the interstitial fluid and allowing for purification of the lymphatic fluid in the lymph nodes.

- The kidneys process more than 45 gal of blood plasma a day and produce about 1.5 qt/L of urine, which is then eliminated from the body.

- The digestive system produces about 1.8 gal of digestive fluids (juices) a day, mostly made up of water, which are reabsorbed after being used.

- The body naturally and automatically loses approximately 2.5 qt (2.5 L) of water per day, which represents 6.25% of the total amount of water in the body. This is what must be replaced at regular intervals throughout each day to maintain a balanced level of hydration.

From this list, it is easy to see why it is so essential to keep the body's hydration at normal levels. Even minimal levels of dehydration can have an adverse effect on the body's activities, especially when you consider that all of these activities are happening at the same time and that each requires a certain amount of water. This helps us understand why dehydration has been shown to produce decreased physical and mental performance, health problems, and even death.[2] Figure 4–2 (Plate 14) shows a person standing next to 10 gal of water (the average amount of water in the body) and 2.5 gal of vegetable oil lipids (triglycerides), which are very similar to the lipids (fat) in the human body. This is approximately the same as the amount of lipids (fat) in the human body.

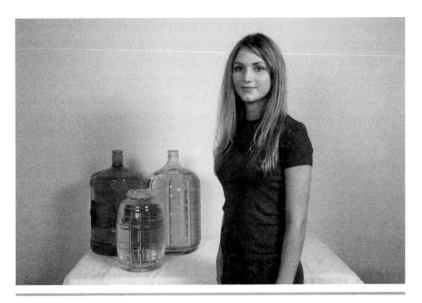

Figure 4-2 The human body contains 60% water and 20% lipids (fat).

 PRINCIPLES OF HYDRATION

This section describes the main elements of hydrotherapy that are key to understanding hydration, dehydration, and programs for maintaining balanced hydration. These elements include natural water loss and daily water intake from drinking water, beverages, and food.

 NATURAL WATER LOSS
FROM THE HUMAN BODY

Fundamental to understanding a program for normal (optimal) hydration is knowing the amount of water that the body loses and that must be replaced. The human body does *not* store extra water, so each day we must replace the *total* amount of water that the body loses in order to maintain balanced hydration. Today, through scientific research and studies, we have a good understanding of not only how much water the body loses each day but also how that water is lost. With this information, we have the basis for knowing how much water needs to be replaced each day. Any excess water intake, above the amount required to maintain the body's normal fluid levels, will be eliminated in the form of urine. However, although our bodies can remove considerable amounts of excess water in the form of urine, overconsumption (intake) of water can lead to potential health problems, which will be discussed in more detail later in this chapter.

Amount of Daily Water Loss

Using precise measuring techniques, scientific studies have determined that each day, an average-size person weighing about 140 lb naturally loses about 2.5 qt (2.5 L) of water.[3] This represents an average loss of about 3.5 oz (110 mL) each hour, although the loss is somewhat less during sleep (see Table 4–1). Obviously, the amount of daily water loss is relative to body size—that is, a smaller person will, on average, lose less water than will a larger person (see Figure 4–3). Any water loss through sweating due to exercise or heat will add anywhere from a small amount to several quarts (liters) to a person's total daily water loss. Sweating is one of the body's main cooling mechanisms—as sweat evaporates from the skin, heat is lost and the body is cooled. A significant amount of heat is removed from the body for every ounce (milliliter) of sweat. As with normal daily water loss, the loss of water through sweating must be completely replaced to maintain balanced hydration. The timing of normal water replacement should be at regular intervals throughout the day to prevent dehydration; water loss from sweating should be replaced as quickly as possible, as sweating produces rapid water loss over a short period of time (see Figure 4–4).

Table 4–1   Average Daily Water Loss and Gain

Water Loss (automatic)	Water Gain
Total: 2.5 qt/L per day	Total: 2.5 qt/L per day or more
1.5 qt/L urine	1.6 qt/L from fluids: water, beverages
0.4 qt/L evaporation (skin)	0.7 qt/L from solid food
0.2 qt/L perspiration (skin)	0.2 qt/L metabolic water (water produced by the body)
0.3 qt/L evaporation (lungs)	
0.1 qt/L fecal moisture (GI tract)	
Additional water loss is mainly by sweating for evaporative cooling of the body.	If more water is gained than needed, the excess water will be removed by the kidneys in the form of urine.

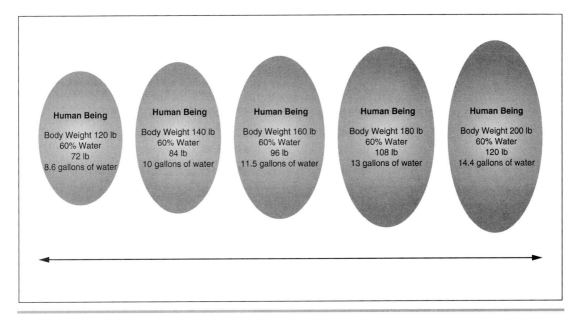

Figure 4–3 Body size and amount of water.

Another way of understanding water loss is that the body loses a specific, measurable amount of water molecules each day in both the liquid and the vapor (gas) form. The number of water molecules that are lost must be replaced from total daily water intake, which includes drinking water, beverages, and food. In Chapter 1, we learned that 1 mol of water equals 18.02 g/mL of water and that each mole contains 6.23×10^{23} water molecules. The average daily water loss of 2.5 qt (2.5 L) equals about 139 mol of water or $139 \times 6.23 \times 10^{23}$ water molecules. The intake of water molecules from drinking water, beverages, and food contributes water molecules to hydration by replacing the water molecules lost each day. Water, in any form or amount, represents a measurable number of water molecules.

How the Body Loses Water

In addition to knowing how much water the body loses, it is also important to know how the body loses that water. Each day, the human body naturally and automatically loses water in five ways. Our bodies lose approximately 1.5 qt (1.5 L) in the form of urine, 0.4 qt (0.4 L) in the form of evaporation from the skin, 0.2 qt (0.2 L) in the form of sweat from the skin, 0.3 qt (0.3 L) in the form of evaporation from the lungs, and 0.1 qt (0.1 L) in the form of fecal moisture from the gastrointestinal (GI) tract (Table 4–1).

NOTE: QT AND L ARE ALMOST THE SAME, SO QT = L.

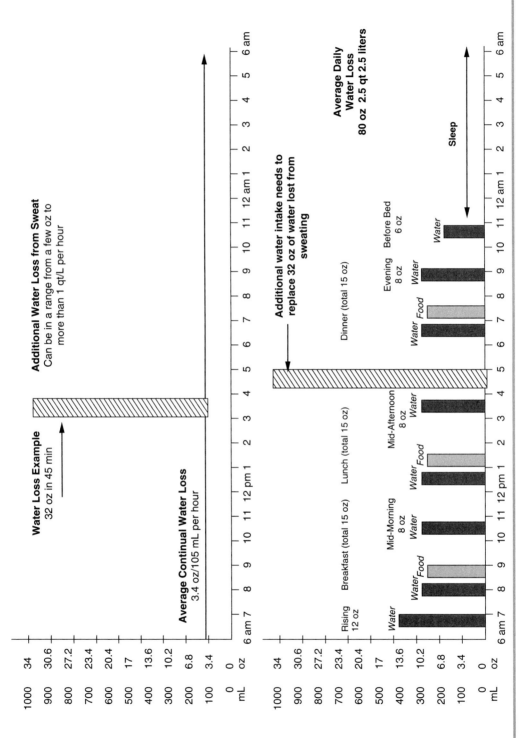

Figure 4–4 Daily water loss and gain.

We lose some water in the form of sweat, even if we don't exercise or are not in a hot environment. During strenuous physical activity or in hot weather, the rate of sweating can increase from a small amount up to 1 qt (1 L) per hour or greater. This means the rate of water loss can go from an average of about 3.5 oz (110 mL) per hour to more than 1.1 qt (1100 mL) per hour or greater, representing more than a 10-fold increase in water loss due to sweating (Figure 4–4). This is a very important point: Our need to rehydrate dramatically increases with sweating. Sweat also contains various levels of electrolytes, including sodium (salt) and potassium. If a person is producing a high rate of sweat, it may be necessary for him or her to replace the lost sodium and potassium in addition to the lost water (see Table 4-2 for adequate daily intake for sodium and potassium). Sports drinks have been developed to replace both water loss and sodium and potassium losses. After about a week, a person will typically become more acclimated to increased physical activity or exposure to a hot climate and will be able to produce more sweat per hour with less sodium loss. This increases the efficiency of cooling and decreases the loss of sodium.

During certain spa and wellness treatments that increase the body's core temperature, sweating is produced at levels of 1 qt (1 L) per hour or greater. These treatments include full-body steam treatments, saunas, and immersion in hot water hydrotubs. It is important that clients rehydrate following these treatments so that they can receive maximum benefits from the treatment without any of the negative side effects of dehydration. It can also be of value for clients to drink some water before the treatment, knowing that water is going to be rapidly lost due to sweating (Figure 4–4).

Table 4–2	Adequate Daily Intake and Upper Limit for Sodium and Potassium	
	Adequate Intake (AI)	**Upper Limit (UL)**
Sodium		
Sedentary adults	1.5 g/day (3.8 g salt)	2.3 g/day (5.8 g salt)
Active adults	Greater than 1.5 g/day (can exceed 10 g/day)	none
Potassium		
Sedentary adults	4.7 g/day	none
Active adults	4.7 g/day	none

TOTAL WATER INTAKE FROM DRINKING WATER, BEVERAGES, AND FOOD

As mentioned earlier, people do not have control over how much water their bodies naturally lose, as this is automatically regulated. However, we do have control over the amount, timing, source, and quality of our water intake each day. Over time, every person has developed learned patterns of behavior regarding water intake. Through additional education on hydration, these patterns can be changed and improved.

Most of our behavior regarding intake of water through fluids and food is learned from the way we were raised and from changes we have made since then. For most people, these learned patterns of consumption are not based on conscious attempts to stay hydrated or to follow a specific hydration program. Therefore, water loss is not always well balanced by water gain. However, through education on balanced hydration, including an evaluation of daily water intake behavior, it is possible to make recommendations that can result in improvements in a person's daily hydration. This will be of value for your clients' general health and wellness and will also help in attaining specific treatment goals, such as improved daily wellness, appearance, healthy aging, disease prevention, and fitness. Obviously, improved hydration has many positive benefits!

Scientific research, through measurements and surveys, has determined that just as there are predictable patterns of water loss, there are also predictable patterns of water gain (intake) by human beings. Scientific surveys show that in the United States and Canada, the average total intake of water from all sources is, on average, 3.7 qt (3.7 L) per day for men and about 2.7 qt (2.7 L) per day for women. About 80% of the total water intake comes from water in drinking water and beverages, and about 20% comes from water in food. Thus, each day, men consume, on average, about 3 qt (3 L) of water from drinking water and beverages and about 0.75 qt (0.75 L) of water from food. Women consume about 2.2 qt (2.2 L) of water each day from drinking water and beverages and about 0.5 qt (0.5 L) of water from food. As we will see later in this chapter, a report from the National Academy of Sciences that was based on these surveys, set the adequate daily water intake level (AI) at 3.7 L for men and 2.7 L for women.[4]

Each day, our bodies also produce about 0.2 qt (0.2 L) of water that is known as metabolic water. Metabolic water is water that the human body produces mainly through the metabolic activity of the cells as they convert glucose, lipids, and proteins into energy. The creation of ATP (energy) molecules, mainly through oxidation of glucose molecules by the cells' mitochondria, produces energy, carbon dioxide (CO_2), water (H_2O), and heat. The 0.2 qt (0.2 L) of metabolic water molecules contributes to the body's overall hydration.

WATER LOSS AND GAIN: EVERY 20 DAYS

Over a period of 20 days, a person's average total water intake is more than 12 gal (or about 100 lb) of water. Over those same 20 days, a person will lose more than 12 gal of water. This intake and loss of water is greater than the entire amount of water in the human body, which averages 84 lb (10 gal). Because of the large amount of water we take into our bodies each day, month, and year, it is essential to not only balance water loss and water gain for normal hydration but also to choose the highest-quality sources of water intake in the form of drinking water, beverages, and food. It is also important to have a healthy balance between the amount of water intake from plain drinking water versus that from beverages. Many people prefer beverages over drinking water for staying hydrated. However, many of these beverages, especially soft drinks, contain high amounts of calories and are also sources of potentially harmful (toxic) substances.

DEHYDRATION

Levels and Risks

As was discussed in Chapter 3 and summarized above, the human body is a complex, dynamic, fluid cellular system that needs to constantly maintain adequate levels of hydration. Scientific research has shown that dehydration levels of even 1% can produce decreased physical and mental performance. It is possible that dehydration at levels of less than 1% can place stress on the body's various fluid cellular systems.

Scientific research shows that dehydration is correlated with the following conditions:[5]

- Decreased cognitive functioning at dehydration levels of 2% or greater.
- Decreased ability to perform aerobic tasks.

- Compromised cardiovascular, thermoregulatory, central nervous system, and metabolic functions—One or more of these alterations will decrease endurance-exercise performance when dehydration levels exceed 2%.
- Heat strain—A dehydration level of only 1% of body weight has been reported to elevate core body temperatures during exercise. Heat exhaustion has been shown to occur sooner when a person is dehydrated than when he or she is euhydrated (normally hydrated).
- Increased heart rate when standing or lying down in temperate conditions. This is in proportion to the level of dehydration.
- Death—This can occur at dehydration levels of 10% or greater, especially when there are other stressors, such as excessive heat, involved.
- Increased risk of urinary tract infections.
- Increased risk of developing kidney stones.
- Increased risk of developing colon and bladder cancer.

Measure of Dehydration

The following are three measurements of hydration and dehydration.

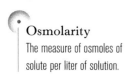

Osmolarity
The measure of osmoles of solute per liter of solution.

- The best physiological measurement of hydration and dehydration is blood plasma **osmolarity.** Normal blood plasma osmolarity is in a range of 280–290 mOsomol/kg. Blood plasma osmolarity below this range is an indicator of dehydration.[6]
- A visible indicator of dehydration is urine color. Normally urine is a pale yellow color. Urine that is darker than normal is an indication of dehydration. For example, the first urine eliminated in the morning is usually darker than normal, as there has been no water intake for about 8 hours. According to *The Dietary Reference Intakes* study from the Institute of Medicine (IOM), "Although not nearly as precise as biochemical measurements, urine color can give crude indications of hydration status."[7]
- Because our bodies produce urine at a constant level of approximately 100 mL per hour, people usually urinate at regular intervals throughout the day and night. If there has been overconsumption of water and beverages, urine output will increase. If water and beverage consumption decreases,

urine output will decrease, as will the time intervals between urination. Longer intervals between urination and a urine production rate below 30 mL/hr, indicate that a person is probably dehydrated.[8]

Areas of the Body Affected by Dehydration

Scientific research has shown that as the body becomes dehydrated, the levels of dehydration are greater in some organs of the body than in others. Muscles will show a level of dehydration of 40%, the skin of 30%, and both the viscera and the bones of 14%. It is important to note that there is minimal dehydration of the brain and liver. This shows that all the systems of the body do not become equally dehydrated as dehydration develops. Thus, because dehydration has a greater effect on muscles, it will impair physical performance. Estheticians have long known that good hydration is essential for the healthy appearance and aging of the skin. Dehydration of the viscera and the bones can effect digestion and many other essential bodily functions. The body limits dehydration of the brain, liver, and blood to protect the functioning of these vital organs and systems.

WATER INTOXICATION AND HYPERHYDRATION: HOW MUCH IS TOO MUCH?

Overconsumption of water above the body's hydration needs will result in excess water being removed from the body by the kidneys in the form of dilute urine. As we have seen, our bodies do not store extra water. Thus, if we consume more water than is needed, the body will quickly eliminate it. Our bodies have an amazing capacity to eliminate up to about 20 qt (20 L) per day of excess water intake through urine.

However, excess water consumption over a short period of time can cause the dilution of sodium levels in the blood plasma and interstitial fluid, which can lead to a condition known as water intoxication. Normal sodium levels in the blood plasma are maintained at levels very close to 142 mEq/L. When sodium levels fall below 125 mEq/L, hyponatremia (low sodium) can occur, which can lead to dizziness, nausea, mental confusion, or even death. Water intoxication is very rare because of the body's ability to excrete large amounts of urine each day. However, two deaths from water intoxication were reported in California. The first was in a fraternity hazing incident in which a member was forced to drink excessive amounts of water. In another case, a radio show game required contestants to drink large amounts of water; the winner was the last person to use the bathroom (urinate). One of the contestants, a mother of three children, died during the competition. In addition to these cases, several marathon runners have also died from excess water intake during an event.

The National Academy of Sciences published a report in 2004 (see below) establishing the recommended dietary allowances for water. According to that report, "Because healthy individuals have a considerable ability to excrete excess water and thereby maintain water balance, a Tolerable Upper Intake Level (UL) was not set for water. However, acute water toxicity has been reported due to rapid consumption of large quantities of fluids that greatly exceed the kidney's maximal excretion rate of approximately 0.7 to 1.0/hour."

The effects of hyperhydration (overhydration), except at very high levels that result in water intoxication, are not well understood. Some health professionals recommend against drinking high volumes of water that exceed the body's hydration needs. However, other health professionals recommend drinking large amounts of water—above the hydration needs of the body while still remaining below the levels that produce the noticeable effects of water intoxication—as part of a detoxification program. Because the kidneys will eliminate any excess water in the form of urine, the value of consuming excessive amounts of water is questionable—at least as far hydration is concerned. In addition, overhydration can be potentially harmful, especially for people with certain health conditions, such as high blood pressure.

Overhydration is an aspect of hydration that has not been thoroughly researched. However, as more relevant information becomes available, it should be possible to gain a better understanding of what levels and under what conditions excess water intake can be harmful.

 ## BALANCED HYDRATION AND THE TIMING OF WATER INTAKE

Another fundamental principle of hydration is the rate of water loss over a 24-hour period. Knowing this rate will help therapists determine the rate at which water must be replaced to maintain normal (optimal) hydration levels. The body loses water at a rate of about 110 mL/hr. As has been stated, there can also be a significant increase in water loss—greater than 1,000 mL/hr—from sweating due to exercise or heat. By knowing the natural rate of water loss from the body, it is possible to develop more precise formulas for water replacement.

Timing of Water Consumption: Learned Behavior and Thirst

The key principle regarding the timing of water intake is to balance water loss with equal or greater water intake at regular intervals throughout the day. If too much time passes between water loss and water intake, dehydration will develop because the body is continually losing water through evaporation and the formation of urine.

A regular pattern of water intake for most individuals includes taking in water at breakfast, lunch, and dinner. During these meal-times, we take in water from drinking water, beverages, and food. Between meals, we usually take in additional water from drinking water, beverages, and snacks.

One of the most important times to hydrate is soon after waking up. While we sleep, our bodies lose water through the formation of urine and through evaporation from the skin and lungs. By the time we wake up, natural water loss could have led to a level of dehydration as high as 1%. When you interview clients about their hydration patterns, it is especially important to note when they begin to consume water after waking and approximately how much they consume at that time. Consuming some water before going bed can also help maintain balanced hydration, especially if there is a long break in water consumption between dinner and going to bed. However, it is important to avoid overconsumption of water before going to bed, as doing so will increase the formation (volume) of urine during sleep.

For most people, learned behavior patterns govern their daily patterns (timing) of water intake. People follow the same basic patterns for timing of meals, snacks, and drinking water and beverages. For many people, the sensation of thirst is not a major factor in hydration, as people often have enough water intake on regular intervals to rehydrate. However, when the sensation of thirst is stimulated, it produces a powerful conscious motivation to drink water or beverages. However, although the sensation of thirst will definitely motivate a healthy individual to drink water as he or she becomes dehydrated, relying on this sensation may not be sufficient to maintain a normal, balanced level of hydration. The goal of the Balanced Hydration Program is to make sure that there is sufficient water intake at regular intervals to maintain normal hydration (Figure 4–4).

Thirst

The sensation of thirst, which is our conscious desire for water, is a powerful natural force that motivates and urges us to consume water. The **thirst center,** located in the hypothalamus of the brain, governs our urge to drink. Dehydration produces increased osmolarity (sodium concentration) in the blood, a decreased volume of blood and blood pressure, and, at higher levels of dehydration, dryness of the mouth and the mucous membranes. These changes generate input to the thirst center, which, in turn, creates the sensation of thirst. The following physiological changes lead to an increase in the sensation of thirst (see Table 4–3).

Thirst center
The portion of the brain, found in the hypothalamus, that governs the urge to drink.

Osmoreceptor
Neuron in the hypothalamus that is sensitive to changes in the blood's osmolarity.

Baroreceptor
Neurons that are sensitive to changes in blood pressure.

- **Osmoreceptors** in the hypothalamus are sensitive to changes in the blood's osmolarity. The normal level of sodium in the blood is 142 mEq/L. When there is decreased water volume in the blood plasma (dehydration of the blood plasma) and a blood plasma sodium level of about 2 mEq/L above normal, the thirst mechanism is activated, producing the sensation of thirst. This sensitive, natural "metering" effect of dehydration responds to small increases in dehydration.

- **Baroreceptors,** which are found in some arteries, are neurons that are sensitive to changes in blood pressure. A drop in blood pressure stimulates the baroreceptors to send signals to the thirst center, which, in turn, stimulates the sensation of thirst. An increase in water intake increases the volume of water in the blood and blood pressure.

- A decrease in blood volume and blood pressure also causes an increase of the hormone angiotensin II in the blood, which stimulates the sensation of thirst.

- Neuron receptors detect dryness in the mouth and mucous membranes of the esophagus and will elicit the sensation of thirst.

Table 4–3   Sensation of Thirst

- Increased osmolarity (sodium level) in the blood plasma
  Normal level: 142 mEq/L
  An increase of 2 mEq/L stimulates the thirst sensation
- Decreased blood volume and blood pressure
- Increase of the hormone angiotensin II (produced by decreased blood volume and blood pressure)
- Dryness of mouth and the mucous membranes of the mouth and the esophagus

SOURCES OF TOTAL WATER INTAKE: "YOU ARE WHAT YOU DRINK"

The first section of this chapter covered the principles of hydration from a scientific understanding of how much and at what rate the body loses water. The following section discusses the sources of water that we all use on a daily basis to replace the water that we naturally lose each day. Some of these points are included in the Balanced Hydration Program for developing a normal (optimal) hydration program for your clients.

As mentioned above, we typically consume a large amount of water each day through drinking water, beverages, and food to keep hydrated. Because we can choose from a variety of sources of drinking water, beverages, and food, we each have a degree of personal control over our hydration behavior. The following is a list and brief explanation of the primary sources of water intake (see Figure 4–5).

Natural Water **(nothing added)**		Tap Water. Purified Tap Water.
Bottled Natural Water **(nothing added)**		Spring Water Mineral Water Purified Tap Water
	Bottled Beverages	Soft Drinks (Caffeinated and Noncaffeinated)—sugar or artificial sweeteners Sport Drinks Energy Drinks—high caffeine Enhanced Water—vitamin water, electrolytes, minerals, herbs Teas and Herbal Drinks Beer and Wine Juices from natural sources—can contain many additives
	Tea and Coffee	Prepared at time of use. Milk, flavors, and sweeteners can be added. High caffeine.
	Juices	Fruit and vegetable prepared at time of use.
	Food (Natural)	Fruits, Vegetables, Chicken, Fish, Meat, Grains, Nuts (90% to 4%) Water
	Food (Processed)	Bread, Chips, Cookies, Candy, etc. (Generally lower water content than natural foods)

Figure 4–5 Water sources for hydration.

Sources of Drinking Water Intake

The following is *not* a recommendation for water intake. Rather it simply describes some of the most common sources from which people get their daily water intake. When consulting with clients, you will review their current daily hydration program and note the various sources they are using for total water intake. Based on that information, you will be able to make appropriate recommendations. The primary sources for hydration are:

Tap Water

Tap water is municipal water that flows out of faucets in homes and businesses. It is used for drinking and cooking.

Purified Tap Water

Most households that use tap water for drinking and cooking purify the tap water before using it. To better understand what must be done to effectively purify the water, it is advisable to learn as much as possible about the water that is coming into the home (see Chapter 2). Your local municipal water company can provide detailed information on drinking water, including whether the source of the water is from aquifers, groundwater, lakes, or rivers. The water company also has detailed information on the water's mineral content and publishes regular reports on water analyses for unhealthy levels of naturally occurring minerals, viruses, bacteria, parasites, toxic chemicals, and gases. The water company can also provide information about the levels of chlorine (used as a disinfectant) and fluorine added to the water, as well as about the quality of the pipes that bring water from the treatment plant to homes and businesses. In addition, the company can provide a list of resources for testing water to determine whether there is any possible contamination from pipes and fixtures within a home.

As a therapist, it is a good idea to research this information to help your clients determine the best way for them to purify their water. You should also talk with your clients about their special concerns. For example, some clients may only be interested in removing chlorine and fluorine from the water. Others, however, may have additional concerns that would require more thorough purification. Keep in mind that municipal water quality will vary from area to area. It is possible that some temporary problems with municipal drinking water may arise, such as scheduled flushing of city water lines with water containing higher chlorine levels. This information may be of interest to your clients.

You may find it helpful to keep an e-mail list of your clients (you may already have this for updates on your services) so you can send them updates on the quality of the municipal water supply based on the treatment plant's published reports. You can also alert your clients to any warnings the plant may issue concerning any immediate problems. Your e-mails could also include other useful information, such as a reminder to change the filter on any water purification systems and inspirational reminders about staying hydrated—*There is no vacation from your hydration!*

This research and reporting provides an additional way to maintain an active connection with your clients while also providing a valuable service.

Bottled Water

This refers to water bottled from natural sources without the addition of any chemical additives. The main forms of bottled water are listed below.

SPRING WATER: Spring water is water that has been bottled at the source of a spring. It often bears the name of the spring. A spring is considered a place where water comes to the Earth's surface under natural pressure and is not pumped from the ground. Water from springs used for bottling usually comes from deep underground water sources. These springs often have some historical story or tradition connected with them, and they are often promoted for their purity, mineral content, or other qualities. You may find it interesting and educational to learn how different bottled waters are promoted. Some informative research would be to purchase a few bottles of spring and mineral water from Europe, the United States, and other locations and not only drink the water but also read the information presented on each company's Web site.

MINERAL WATER: Although all bottled spring water has dissolved minerals in it, mineral water is water that has a mineral content above the level of 250 parts per million (ppm) of total dissolved solids. Mineral water comes from a high-mineral-content spring or from a well drilled into an aquifer that has a high mineral content. When the mineral content in water from natural sources is very high (greater than 500 ppm), it is usually not suitable for drinking. When reading the mineral analysis for bottled water (this information is usually on the company's Web site or on the bottle), look for the total dissolved solids. There are several well-known mineral water brands—mainly from Europe—that are available on the market today.

Both spring water and mineral water may be naturally carbonated from carbon dioxide in the ground. This is different from soft drinks, which are artificially carbonated.

BOTTLED AND FILTERED TAP WATER: Some very popular bottled waters are tap water drawn from municipal treatment plants. The water is further purified in various ways, depending on the bottling company. The water is promoted as pure drinking water that has undergone rigorous purification processing to ensure that it is free from any harmful substances. The bottle's label usually names the location of the municipal treatment plant that is the source of the water.

Sources of Water Intake from Beverages

Milk and Juice

Milk and natural juices are mostly water. Whole milk is 89% water, and orange juice is 88% water. There are several options to consider when choosing a brand, such as whether they are organic, how they are processed and bottled, and whether there are any additives. Although these beverages are sources of nutrients, they can be high in calories and glucose (natural sugar in juice and milk).

Coffee and Tea

Detailed survey data show that coffee is the most consumed beverage after filtered tap water and bottled water. Most of your clients will drink coffee or tea. Coffee and tea, other than herbal tea, both contain caffeine. Because excessive intake of caffeine is harmful, most therapists and alternative health practitioners suggest that caffeine intake be limited or eliminated completely. The general understanding is that caffeine acts as a strong diuretic and causes the water intake from coffee (e.g., 8 oz) to contribute minimal to no water toward rehydration. Some say it may even produce a negative effect in terms of contributing water toward hydration. Scientific research, however, indicates that caffeine is a mild diuretic. The report by the National Academy of Sciences, states that scientific research confirms that beverages with caffeine should count toward daily hydration.[9] This is a relatively new recommendation and can be considered in developing or adjusting hydration formulas. If any of your clients are interested in reviewing scientific research on the diuretic effects of caffeine, please refer them to the section on caffeine in the National Academy of Sciences' report, which is available on-line for free (see Suggested Readings at the end of this chapter).

Not only the effects of caffeine must be considered when determining a person's water intake, but also the water source used to produce the coffee or tea as well as the quality of the additives used for flavoring. Because people who drink coffee consume, on average, more than 65 gal of coffee a year, considerations about the quality of the water and other added ingredients is important.

Soft Drinks

After coffee, caffeinated and noncaffeinated soft drinks are the most consumed beverages. As with coffee and tea, an important consideration, in addition to determining the amount consumed, is in regard to the quality of the water and other ingredients used in the soft drinks. Soft drinks can contain high levels of glucose or artificial sweeteners, as well as preservatives. Other factors to consider include the quality of manufacturing and shipping and whether the drink comes in plastic bottles, aluminum cans, or glass bottles. In most soft drink brands, the combination and quality of ingredients can be unhealthy, especially in the amounts that many people consume. Recent scientific research, published in the July 2007 edition of *Circulation*, correlates drinking an average of two soft drinks a day with a significant increased risk for cardiovascular disease.[10] Research also shows that when people are free to choose what to drink, they usually choose a beverage that has a sweet taste.[11] Soft drink manufactures have taken advantage of this natural behavior trait. It is interesting to see how many brands of soft drinks and other sweetened beverages are offered at supermarkets—often at very low prices.

Enhanced Water

Many beverages, including sports drinks, that are now on the market consist of water with vitamins, minerals, electrolytes, herbs, and other substances added to enhance certain health benefits. These beverages are usually low calorie and have some form of sweetener, such as sugar or natural juice, to increase their palatability. Although these beverages are promoted for their health benefits, it is important to check that their claims are realistic. It is also important to consider the added ingredients, the source of the water, the manufacturing process, and the beverage container. When working with your clients, you should determine whether there is something more natural that offers the same beneficial ingredients or whether naturally pure water would be a better choice. For example, sports drinks are developed to be used by people with very high rates of sweating for long periods of time. However, these drinks are marketed to everyone, even people who are not experiencing excess sweating. To consume sports drinks other than when there is excessive sweating means a person is taking in extra sugar, sodium (salt), and possibly potassium that the body does not need.

Table 4–4   Percentage of Water in Foods

Apple	84%	Pea	82%
Banana	74%	Pear	84%
Broccoli	91%	Potato	75%
Carrots	88%	Raisin	14%
Chicken	67%	Rice (cooked)	68%
Fish	73%	Rice (uncooked)	12%
Grape	81%	Spinach	92%
Lettuce	96%	Steak	60%
Mushroom	83%	Walnut	4%
Orange	84%	Watermelon	92%

Food

Food is a major daily source of hydration and nutrition. Most food contains a high percentage of water, accounting for about 20% of our daily total water intake (see Table 4–4). Most people follow a regular schedule (timing) of breakfast, lunch, and dinner, with some snacks in between. This regular schedule makes it possible to calculate the general timing of water intake from food. It is interesting to note that water in food is water in the liquid form—as moisture in food. Thus, food, in a sense, is a solid beverage. In a few foods, such as ice cream, the water contained is in the solid (frozen) state; but in general, anything in the frozen state that is placed in the mouth melts before it is swallowed.

Drinking Water Versus Beverages for Hydration

On average, a person will consume more than 250 gal of combined fluids a year. For every person, this intake is a combination of drinking water and water contained in beverages. The general recommendation is to make drinking water (plain, pure, natural water with no additives) the primary source for hydration. Plain water does not contain any calories and is easily absorbed by the body's GI tract. Plain water also does not contain artificial flavors, sweeteners, preservatives, or other synthetic additives. However, some beverages—especially from natural sources like milk and fruit and vegetable juices—contain important and essential nutrients that are not found in drinking water. For example, recent scientific research shows that people who consume fruit and/or vegetable juice on a regular basis show a decreased risk of Alzheimer's disease.

Even though almost everyone agrees that drinking pure, plain water for daily hydration is important, there are many different perspectives about the ratio of intake from drinking water versus that from drinking beverages. Most of your clients—and most people in general—do not base their ratio of daily water and beverage consumption on any formulas or recommendations; rather it is based on what they have learned growing up and what they enjoying drinking. By the time a person is an adult, these patterns of water and beverage consumption are firmly set. The Balanced Hydration Program, in the next section, allows you to use information from the client to evaluate his or her total daily water intake, including the ratio of drinking water to beverages. With this program, you will be able to make helpful recommendations regarding the ratio of drinking plain water and beverages.

 # CURRENT HYDRATION PROGRAMS AND FORMULAS

This section includes a brief review of two of the most popular formulas currently used for hydration. Also included is a review of a 2004 report by the National Academy of Sciences that determined the adequate daily water intake for people of different ages to maintain normal hydration levels and to avoid dehydration. This government study contains references to most of the current scientific research on hydration and dehydration, as well information from large surveys about the hydration behavior of the general population of North America.

Formula 1: Drinking Eight 8-Ounce Glasses of Water a Day

The 8 × 8 (sometimes the 10 × 8) is a popular hydration formula that recommends drinking eight (or sometimes 10) 8-ounce glasses of water a day. This is equal to 2 qt (2 L), or 64 oz, of water intake. If the general need is to replace 2.5 qt (80 oz) of water each day, and if about 20% (16 oz) is replaced from food, then that leaves about 64 oz of water that needs to be replaced by drinking water and beverages. So, 64 oz of water intake is a good approximation of the hydration needs of an average-size person. However, the water needs of each person varies in relationship to his or her size, with smaller people needing less water intake and larger people requiring more.

Even though this is a simple formula, it has been interpreted in many different ways. Some say that the 8 × 8 refers only to drinking water and does not include other beverages. Others say that some types of beverages can be included but not others. Almost everyone using this formula feels that drinks containing caffeine or alcohol act as diuretics, do not contribute to hydration, and therefore should not be counted. In addition, most people using this formula do not include water from food as counting toward hydration. The problem is that drinking 64 oz of water in addition to other beverages and food that people consume could lead to excessive water intake. As mentioned earlier, it is not fully understood how much excess water intake is harmful. What is known is that any excess water intake above the body's hydration needs will be eliminated as urine to maintain homeostasis of the body's fluid levels.

The simple version of the 8 × 8 hydration formula does not take body size into account. As noted earlier, water requirements vary according to the size of a person. A person who weighs 200 lb will require more water intake for hydration than will a person who weighs 120 lb. In addition, water loss from sweating would, of course, increase the water needs by the amount of water lost as sweat (see Figure 4–3). Research into the origin of the 8 × 8 formula indicates that the formula cannot be attributed to a specific person and was not based on scientific research, but was more of popular idea that became accepted as a valid formula for daily hydration.[12]

Formula 2: Half the Body Weight Equals the Recommended Ounces of Daily Water Intake

Another popular hydration formula for the total amount of daily water intake is to take an individual's body weight and divide that by 2. This number gives the amount of ounces of water that person should consume each day. For example, if you weigh 150 lb, then you would need to consume 75 oz of water a day. As with the 8 × 8 formula, some say that water from all beverages should count, whereas others say only drinking water should count. If only drinking water is allowed to count toward hydration, then there may be excess water intake at different levels, as discussed in the 8 × 8 formula. Most people using this formula state that beverages that contain caffeine, such as coffee and some soft drinks, should not count, because caffeine has been thought to act as a diuretic. This formula does take into account body size as a major factor in determining water intake requirements. However, hydration needs are not necessarily precisely linear; a person who weighs 240 lb will not necessarily need twice as much water as a person who weighs 120 lb. Although hydration formulas can offer general guidelines, daily water needs vary even for people of the same size due to individual differences.

If a client is overweight and possibly obese, adjustments must be made for different hydration formulas. Increase in weight due to increase in body fat does not proportionally increase the body's hydration needs. Although there will be some increased water needs for this person, this is usually less than the difference between differences in normal body weights. This area needs much more research. Regardless, for overweight people, it is important to be cautious about any recommendations that could lead to excessive water intake, as obesity is often associated with stress on the cardiovascular system and higher blood pressure. Overconsumption of water temporarily increases the blood volume above normal, which could increase the person's blood pressure. If a client has any serious medical conditions, especially with the cardiovascular system, any recommended changes in his or her total daily water intake should be approved by a physician. For example, if a person's normal weight is 140 lb but he or she currently weighs 195 lb, that person will be 40% heavier than normal. But this same person will not have an increased 40% hydration need.

The Institute of Medicine's Formula for Adequate Daily Water Intake

NOTE TO READER: THIS IS THE MOST COMPREHENSIVE REVIEW AND EVALUATION OF SCIENTIFIC RESEARCH ON HYDRATION AND WAS USED TO SET AN OFFICIAL ADEQUATE INTAKE (AI) LEVEL FOR WATER. THE REPORT CONTAINS THE OFFICIAL GOVERNMENT GUIDELINES FOR HYDRATION. IT IS BASED ON ALL AVAILABLE SCIENTIFIC RESEARCH AND HYDRATION THEORIES FROM LEADING SCIENTISTS. THIS REPORT CAN VIEWED IN FULL ON-LINE AT THE NATIONAL ACADEMIES PRESS (WWW.NAP.EDU) FOR FREE. ANYONE WHO WISHES TO PURSUE A MORE INDEPTH STUDY OF THE PRINCIPLES OF HYDRATION SHOULD READ THIS REPORT. ALSO, BECAUSE OF THE IMPORTANCE OF THIS REPORT, MORE DETAILED INFORMATION HAS BEEN PROVIDED IN THIS SECTION.

The 2004 report on hydration by the Institute of Medicine, (a department of the National Academy of Sciences), set an official adequate intake (AI) level for water. This report is titled *The Dietary Reference Intakes: Water, Potassium, Sodium, Chloride, and Sulfate,* The report found that, on average, the total daily intake of water for men is 3.7 qt (3.7 L), and for women, it is 2.7 qt (2.7 L). These amounts are considered to be more than adequate to balance the body's normal daily water loss, which averages 2.5 qt (2.5 L). Based on the findings of this report, the IOM set the AI level for total water at 3.7 qt (3.7 L) for men and 2.7 qt (2.7 L) for women daily. However, this amount does not include water intake needed to balance additional water loss through sweating.

The report examined all available relevant scientific research and made recommendations based on the collaborative finding. The National Academy of Sciences issued the following summary of the report:

> The vast majority of healthy people adequately meet their daily hydration needs by letting thirst be their guide, says the newest report on nutrient recommendations from the Institute of Medicine of the National Academies. The report set general recommendations for water intake based on detailed national data, which showed that women who appear to be adequately hydrated consume an average of approximately 2.7 liters (91 ounces) of total water—from all beverages and foods—each day, and men average approximately 3.7 liters (125 ounces) daily. These values represent adequate intake levels, the panel said; those who are very physically active or who live in hot climates may need to consume more water. About 80 percent of people's total water comes from drinking water and beverages—including caffeinated beverages—and the other 20 percent is derived from food.
>
> We don't offer any rule of thumb based on how many glasses of water people should drink each day because our hydration needs can be met through a variety of sources in addition to drinking water. While drinking water is a frequent choice for hydration, people also get water from juice, milk, coffee, tea, soda, fruits, vegetables, and other foods and beverages as well. Moreover, we concluded that on a daily basis, people get adequate amounts of water from normal drinking behavior—consumption of beverages at meals and in other social situations—and by letting their thirst guide them.

This report refers to *total* water, which includes the water contained in beverages and the moisture in foods, to avoid confusion with drinking water only.

Total water intake at the reference level of 3.7 liters for adult men and 2.7 liters for adult women per day covers the expected needs of healthy, sedentary people in temperate climates. Temporary underconsumption of water can occur due to heat exposure, high levels of physical activity, or decreased food and fluid intake. However, on a daily basis, fluid intake driven by thirst and the habitual consumption of beverages at meals is sufficient for the average person to maintain adequate hydration.

Prolonged physical activity and heat exposure will increase water losses and therefore may raise daily fluid needs. Very active individuals who are continually exposed to hot weather often have daily total water needs of six liters or more, according to several studies.

While concerns have been raised that caffeine has a diuretic effect, available evidence indicates that this effect may be transient, and there is no convincing evidence that caffeine leads to cumulative total body water deficits. Therefore, the panel concluded that when it comes to meeting daily hydration needs, caffeinated beverages can contribute as much as noncaffeinated options.

Some athletes who engage in strenuous activity and some individuals with certain psychiatric disorders occasionally drink water in excessive amounts that can be life threatening. However, such occurrences are highly unusual. Therefore, the panel did not set a UL (upper limit) for water.

Key Points of the Institute of Medicine Report

Two key concepts in the report are the adequate intake (AI) level and the tolerable upper limit (UL). Regarding the AI level set for water, the report states:

Individual water requirements can vary greatly, even on a day-to-day basis, because of differences in physical activity and climates. To a lesser extent, dietary factors also influence water requirements, as the osmotic load created by metabolizing dietary protein and organic compounds, as well as by varying intakes of electrolytes, must be accompanied by adequate *total* water consumption. Hence, there is no single daily total water requirement for a given person, and needs vary markedly depending primarily on physical activity and climate, but also based on diet. It would be misinterpreting for setting the AI to state that there is a "requirement" for water at the level of the AI. The AI does not represent a require-ment; it is an amount that should meet the needs of almost everyone in a specific life stage group under the conditions described.[13]

Regarding the UL for water, which is the highest average daily intake that likely poses risk of adverse effects for most individuals, the report states: "Because healthy individuals have considerable ability to excrete excess water and thereby maintain water balance, a Tolerable Upper Intake (UL) was not set for water. However, acute water toxicity has been reported due to rapid consumption of large quantities of fluids that greatly exceed the kidney's maximal excre-tion rate of approximately 0.7 to 1.0 L/hour."

The report does not present a specific hydration formula. Instead, it states that Americans and Canadians, on average, are consuming enough water each day to balance average daily water loss and thereby maintain normal hydration. In addition, it states that water loss from sweating can be considerable and that addi-tional water intake is necessary to rehydrate after sweating. The report makes a general statement about excessive water intake on the human body by explaining that the body can eliminate consid-erable amounts of excessive water; therefore, the report does not set an upper limit.

Regarding dehydration, the report states that if for any reason a person does not replace the total daily water loss with an equal amount or greater of total water intake, dehydration will result, with negative health consequences. The list of scientific studies in the report references the specific problems associated with dehydra-tion. There is also a brief section on water intoxication, a serious health condition that can result from overconsumption of water in a short period of time.

The report concludes that, in general, people consume enough total water intake to stay hydrated. However, it also states that for those who consume less than this amount, dehydration can occur. Based on the report, the AI level for water is set at 3.7 qt (3.7 L) per day for men and 2.7 qt (2.7 L) per day for women. The report makes it very clear that the AI for water is not a requirement; it simply states that people, on average, consume these amounts of total water each day, which is usually enough to balance average daily water loss of 2.5 qt (2.5 L) per day.

Some of the report's findings and recommendations, such as caffeinated beverages counting toward hydration, vary from the recommendations offered by popular hydration formulas. Regarding caffeine, many hydration formulas state that caffeine is seen as a diuretic that results in a net water loss. Another finding of the report that is opposite to other common formulas is the statement that "following your sensation of thirst is what will keep you hydrated." Many other hydration formulas state that by the time you feel thirsty, you are already dehydrated.

The two hydration formulas and the IOM report present some guidelines and education for daily hydration. They also provide valuable information and insights about hydration and about the popular current theories on hydration. Over time, as more information is gathered—both scientific and from other sources—about the important aspects of hydration, hydration programs and formulas will continue to evolve.

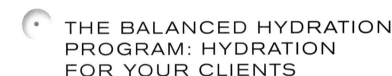

THE BALANCED HYDRATION PROGRAM: HYDRATION FOR YOUR CLIENTS

Developing a Balanced Hydration Program with an individual client involves four steps: interview, evaluation, recommendations, and follow-up. You may want to refer to Figure 4–6 as you consult with your clients.

> **NOTE:** THE ON-LINE COMPANION FOR THIS TEXTBOOK WILL PROVIDE THE INTERVEIW AND RECOMMENDATION FORMS TO DOWNLOAD AND PRINT. THERE WILL ALSO BE A SECTION FOR THE BALANCED HYDRATION PROGRAM THAT GIVES MANY EXAMPLES OF WORKING WITH CLIENTS, A REVIEW OF KEY POINTS OF THE PROGRAM, AND A CALCULATION PROGRAM TO AUTOMATICALLY CALCULATE TOTAL DAILY WATER INTAKE, ETC.

Step 1: Interview

During a hydration counseling session with your client, ask your client questions about his or her daily patterns of total water intake from drinking water, beverages, and food. Use the client interview form to record data and feedback and make notes. This form (see Figure 4–7) is not intended for the client to fill out; rather it is for you to note relevant information during the client interview.

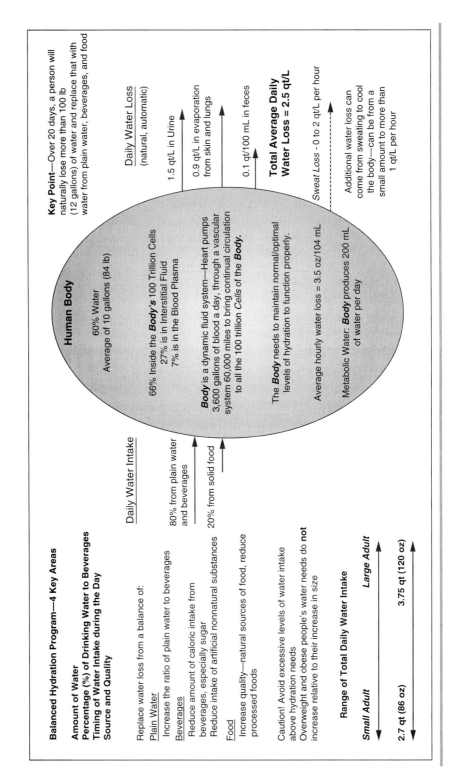

Figure 4–6 Principles of water loss and gain.

Balanced Hydration Program Interview Form

Client Name: _____   Date: _____   Note: All amounts on form are in ounces (oz.)

Client's own feedback and evaluation of the daily hydration behavior and improvements they feel they could make

_____

1. After Waking (Before Breakfast)

Amount of Plain Water: _____

Amount of Beverages: _____

Types of Beverages:

_____

2. At Breakfast

Amount of Plain Water: _____

Amount of Beverages: _____

Types of Beverages:

_____

3. Mid-Morning

Amount of Plain Water: _____

Amount of Beverages: _____

Types of Beverages:

_____

4. Lunch

Amount of Plain Water: _____

Amount of Beverages: _____

Types of Beverages:

_____

5. Mid-Afternoon

Amount of Plain Water: _____

Amount of Beverages: _____

Types of Beverages:

_____

6. Dinner

Amount of Plain Water: _____

Amount of Beverages: _____

Types of Beverages:

_____

7. Mid-Evening

Amount of Plain Water: _____

Amount of Beverages: _____

Types of Beverages:

_____

8. Before Bed

Amount of Plain Water: _____

Amount of Beverages: _____

Types of Beverages:

_____

Figure 4–7 Client interview form. (*Continues*)

Total Daily Water Intake

Total Plain Water: _____

Total Beverages: _____

Total Daily Fluid Intake: _____ **(63–90)** (Normal Range)

(Total Beverages + Drinking Water)

Total Water intake from Food _____ **(17–24)**

Total Daily Metabolic Water __**6**__

Total Daily Water Intake _____ **(86–120)** (Normal Range)

Daily Solid Food Intake

Comments: Note that the 20% of our daily total water intake comes

from (solid) food. This represents approximately 18 oz of water each day

Daily **Timing** of Water Intake Note: _____

_____

_____

Calculate the Percent (Ratio) of Drinking Water to Total Daily Fluid Intake

Divide the Total Plain Water by the Total
Daily Fluid Intake + Drinking Water: _____ %

Range of Total Daily Water Intake

Small Adult   *Large Adult*

2.7 qt (86 oz)   3.75 qt (120 oz)

Figure 4–7 Client interview form.

1. The first step is to ask the client about the amount and source of plain water and beverage intake during each of the eight time periods each day. Also, note if the client's daily (solid) food intake is a normal balanced diet, or possibly more of a dry food diet (more processed foods). Normally, 20% of our water intake comes from a normal balanced diet, but the percentage could be lower with a dryer diet.

2. Next, have the client provide as much feedback as possible, both positive and negative, about his or her daily hydration behavior. This feedback is very helpful, because most people are aware of the positive and negative things they are doing each day to stay hydrated and what changes they feel they need to make. The client's understanding of his or her own daily hydration program, along with the amounts of total water intake during the day, represents the baseline, or starting point, upon which recommendations for changes are made. In follow-up with the client, you can compare progress against this original baseline data.

Step 2: Evaluation

From the information you obtain from the client interview, you will be able to evaluate the client's general patterns of total daily water intake as the basis for making recommendations.

First, make the following calculations using the Balanced Hydration Inteview Form

1. Add the amount of intake of **Plain Water** from each of the eight daily time periods and write the number in the **Total Plain Water** column. Do the same for the daily intake of **Beverages** (note this in the column).

2. Add the **Total Plain Water** plus the **Total Beverages** to find the **Total Daily Fluid Intake** (note this in the column).

3. Determine the percent (%) of **Plain Water** of the **Total Daily Fluid Intake.** Do this by dividing the **Total Daily Plain Water** by the **Total Daily Fluid Intake.** (Note this in the % column.)

4. Determine if approximate amount of **Total Water Intake from Food** (solid food) is in a range from 17 oz to 24 oz for a normal diet depending on the size of a person. Just estimate the amount between 17 oz to 24 oz based on the general size of the person (from small, medium, to large).

NOTE: IF THE DIET IS MADE UP OF MORE DRYER, PROCESSED FOOD, THIS NUMBER WOULD BE LOWER.

5. The **Total Daily Metabolic Water (**water we gain from daily metabolic activity) is already entered for you at 6 oz (approximately 200 ml.) This is a relatively small amount and 6 oz is considered to be the average for everyone.

6. Add the **Total Daily Fluid Intake** plus **Total Water Intake from Food** plus **Total Daily Metabolic Water** to get the **Total Daily Water Intake**. Note this in the column.

Total Daily Water Intake

Based on the recommendations of the IOM as discussed above, the Adequate Intake for adults is in a range between 2.7 qt for women (smaller adults) to 3.7 qt for men (larger adults). In analyzing your client's Total Daily Water Intake, you want to see:

- What your client's Total Daily Water Intake is and where it fits in this range between 2.7 qt and 3.7 qt. Mark this on the line in the Range of Total Daily Water Intake box (judge where it fits on the line). It is possible that it could be less than 2.7 qt or greater than 3.7 qt. Note this number on the Amount Line in the Range of Total Daily Water Intake box.

- Next, estimate your client's (normal) size in a general range from small, medium to large. Normal size means, not their weight, but what their size would generally be at relatively normal weight. For example, woman are generally a smaller size than men. Note the client's size on the Size Line in Rangel of Total Daily Water Intake box (judge where it fits on the line).

NOTE: THE AMOUNT WATER NEEDED FOR SOMEONE WHO IS OVERWEIGHT OR OBESE, DOES NOT INCREASE RELATIVE TO THEIR INCREASE IN WEIGHT.

- Evaluate if the client's Total Daily Water Intake in a normal range relative to their size. The following are some examples: A medium size person has a Total Daily Water Intake of 3.5 qt. This would be in a normal range. A small size person has a Total Daily Water Intake of 3 qt. This would be in a normal range.

- A small size person has a Total Daily Water Intake of 1.7 qt. This would be in a low range. A large size person has a Total Daily Water Intake of 2.7 qt. This would be in a low range. There are more examples and further discussion on the Online Companion for this textbook.

NOTE: THESE NUMBERS ARE GENERAL ESTIMATES TO DETERMINE IF A CLIENT'S TOTAL DAILY WATER INTAKE FALL IN A NORMAL RANGE OR OUTSIDE THAT RANGE. SOME CAUTION MUST BE USED IN THESE ESTIMATES AS CLIENTS MAY PROVIDE INCORRECT DATA AND SIZE ESTIMATES COULD BE DIFFICULT IN SOME CASES.

Percentage of Drinking Plain Water to Beverages

Analyze if the percentage of water intake from **Plain Water** compared to **Beverages** is a healthy range. In general, at least 50% of our fluid water intake should be from **Plain Water.** Even though water from beverages contributes toward daily hydration, it can also include high levels of calories and possible intake of food additives, preservatives, etc. Some beverages, such as natural fruit and vegetable juices, milk, and herbal teas, can be positive nutritional sources. The main goal is to improve the ratio of **Plain Water** intake to **Beverages.**

Timing

From input on the amount of intake of **Plain Water** and **Beverages** during the eight periods of the day, it should be possible to determine whether water is consumed at regular intervals throughout the day to balance the water that is constantly being lost. Most clients' water intake is at regular intervals throughout the day. However, some clients have long intervals between water intake that may lead to various levels of dehydration. Note in the section on **Timing** if there are any possible concerns with the timing of water intake.

NOTE: WATER LOSS DUE TO SWEATING FROM PHYSICAL ACTIVITY, EXPOSURE TO A HOT CLIMATE, OR STEAM TREATMENT CAN VARY FROM A SMALL AMOUNT TO MORE THAN 1 QT (1 L) PER HOUR. THIS WATER NEEDS TO BE REPLACED AND BALANCED BY AN EQUAL AMOUNT AS SOON AS POSSIBLE. EXCESSIVE LOSS OF SWEAT OVER LONGER PERIODS OF TIME MAY REQUIRE ADDITIONAL INTAKE OF SODIUM AND POTASSIUM TO BALANCE ELECTROLYTE LOSS.

Source and Quality

Make notes of the types of beverages used by the client for daily hydration. Some clients will consume more high-quality beverages, but many will consume beverages of a lower quality. There are many cases of people who stay hydrated consuming large amounts of soft drinks and very little if any water. Remember that enhanced drinks are considered beverages as they contain additives other than water.

Remember food is the source of, on average, 20% of our daily hydration. There is a wide range of food sources from a more balanced diet of vegetables, fruits, grains, etc., to a diet of mostly processed food. Make notes about food intake, including source and quality, that may be of value in making recommendations.

Step 3: Recommendations

Use the Balanced Hydration Program Recommendation Form to note recommendations to the client (see Figure 4–8). After evaluating the information from the Interview Form, recommendations for the client can be made regarding improvements in his or her daily hydration behavior. It is important to recommend changes that can be more easily made rather than more drastic changes in the client's daily hydration behavior. Small changes over an extended period of time can be more effective than major changes over a short period of time. Our patterns of Total Daily Water Intake from plain water, beverages, and food are learned patterns over a lifetime, and are not always easy to change, especially major changes. The Balanced Hydration Program is designed to be an ongoing program over an extended period of time with periodic sessions to evaluate the progress of the client. Small steps of improvement over an extended period of time can add up to major positive changes, especially for clients that appear to have more negative daily hydration behavior. It is also important to remember that there are four different areas that client's can make improvements in their daily hydration. The amount of daily water intake is only one area.

When possible, use Teaching Exercise 4–1 when explaining to clients the principles of hydration and making recommendations.

The following are the four different areas of recommendations for daily water intake for maintaining balanced daily hydration (see Figure 4–9):

- **Amount:** Based on your evaluation of the client's daily total water intake relative to his or her size, make recommendations for increasing (or decreasing) the amount, if necessary. In general, the recommendation to increase water intake would be to consume more drinking water either at meals or during intervals between meals. The amount of additional drinking water depends on the amount estimated to be lacking. When you meet your client during follow-up meetings, you can use his or her feedback to evaluate whether the recommendation appears to be producing the desired effect. Further adjustments can then be made as needed.

Balanced Hydration Program Recommendation Form

Client Name:_____ Date:_____

Daily Total Hydration Goal:_____ Goal of Ratio (%) of Plain Water to Beverage:_____

Current Total Daily Water Intake_____ Current Percentage (%) of Plain Water to Beverages_____

Additional Suggestions:_____

After Waking (Before Breakfast)
Plain Water (Amount, Source): _____

Beverages (Amount, Source): _____

_____

Breakfast
Plain Water (Amount, Source): _____

Beverages (Amount, Source): _____

_____

Mid-Morning
Plain Water (Amount, Source): _____

Beverages (Amount, Source): _____

_____

Lunch
Plain Water (Amount, Source): _____

Beverages (Amount, Source): _____

_____

Mid-Morning
Plain Water (Amount, Source): _____

Beverages (Amount, Source): _____

_____

Dinner
Plain Water (Amount, Source): _____

Beverages (Amount, Source): _____

_____

Mid-Evening
Plain Water (Amount, Source): _____

Beverages (Amount, Source): _____

_____

Before Bed
Plain Water (Amount, Source): _____

Beverages (Amount, Source): _____

_____

Figure 4–8 Balanced Hydration Recommendation Form.

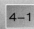

4-1 TEACHING EXERCISE

Demonstrate How Much Water Is Lost Each Day and Must Be Replaced

AMOUNT OF WATER NATURALLY LOST EACH DAY
Show client the 2.5 qt (2.5 L) of water in a container and explain that this is how much water his or her body will automatically lose each day, even if he or she does not sweat due to physical activity or a hot environment. (Explain that water lost to physical activity or a hot environment is an additional amount.) Explain that each day, your client must replace at least the amount of water lost. Your client will see that 2.5 qt (2.5 L) of water is a large amount.

AMOUNT OF WATER NATURALLY LOST EACH HOUR
Show client the small measuring cup with 3.5 oz (110 mL) of water. Explain that the body is continually losing water at a rate of about 3.5 oz (110 mL) per hour.

AMOUNT OF WATER LOST FROM SWEATING
Explain that a cooling mechanism the body uses is sweating. When the body temperature increases (mainly due to physical activity or a hot climate/environment), the body produces sweat for cooling. The greater the body temperature, the greater the rate of sweating. Tell your client that it is possible to have a sweat rate of 1 qt (1 L) per hour. Fill a container with 1 qt (1 L) of water to demonstrate the amount of sweat that could be lost. Explain to your client that this amount of water must be replaced to maintain proper hydration. This water should ideally be replaced as soon as possible within the time of sweating.

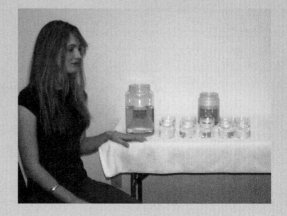

4-1 TEACHING EXERCISE (*Continued*)

A loss of 1 qt (1 L) of sweat would produce an average dehydration level of 1.4% until water intake balances the water loss.

Small Glass (3.5 oz/110 mL): Amount of water naturally lost each hour

Tall Glass (32 oz/1 L): Amount of water that can be lost during about 1 hour of exercise

1 Gallon Container: Add (2.5 qt/2.5 L): Average total amount of water lost naturally each day. Water lost from sweating due to physical activity or being in a hot environment would be extra. An example would be to combine the 2.5 qt (2.5 L) naturally lost each day with the 1 qt (1 L) additional loss by sweating, for a total daily loss of 3.5 qt (3.5 L) of water.

- **Timing:** If your evaluation shows that there are long intervals between the client's water intake, recommend drinking water at regular intervals to balance continual water loss. Under normal conditions, a person loses about 110 mL (4 oz) of water each hour. Because time spent sleeping is the longest interval between water intakes, there should be adequate water intake after waking (including breakfast) to balance water lost during sleep. Water loss due to sweating represents rapid water loss and can be greater than 1 qt (1 L) per hour. A person can lose several quarts (liters) of water per day due to exercise or exposure to a hot climate. It is essential that this water loss be replaced as closely as possible to the time of water loss (Figure 4–4).

- **Percentage (%) of Drinking Water to Beverages:** For some clients, it will be obvious that they are drinking mostly beverages during the day and very little water. Some clients will have a more balanced ratio. Start with gradual changes, for example, by having the client substitute one beverage with the same amount of water. Over several months, a client could significantly improve this ratio of plain water to beverages, which could have very positive health and wellness benefits. A higher ratio of drinking water to beverages means that a person is consuming fewer calories and the numerous additives in many beverages.

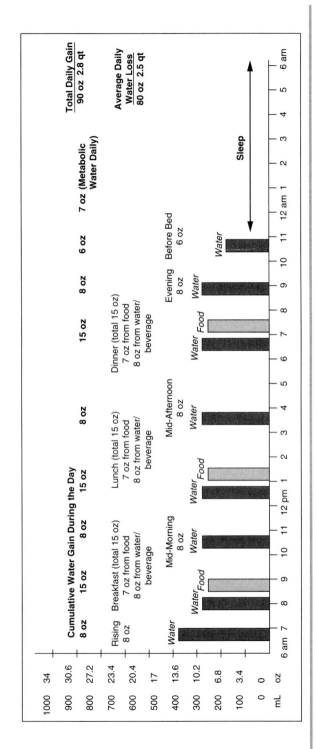

Figure 4–9 Balanced hydration.

Remember that most patterns of daily consumption of beverages is learned behavior that is repeated automatically (unconsciously) each day and take time to change. A ratio of 50% plain water to 50% beverages would be a good initial goal for people drinking mostly beverages and the ratio of plain water could be increased over time.

- **Source and Quality:** There are a wide range of sources for drinking water, beverages, and food. From all these possible options, your client has developed a regular, learned pattern of total daily water intake. Main focus of your recommendations should be to see that your client uses quality sources of drinking water, beverages, and food. Drinking water should be as pure as possible, which normally requires some level of purification. Beverages, that high in additives such as artificial sweeteners, food colors, and preservatives, should be gradually reduced. This can also apply to beverages with high amounts of substances such as sugar, salt, and caffeine. Try making gradual changes. For example, replace one processed food item with a natural item, for example, a piece of fruit. Replace a soft drink with a natural juice drink or plain water (see Figure 4–10). Small changes over an extended period, for example 6 months, can add up to major improvements. The Balanced Hydration Program is designed for regular sessions to provide a client with feedback and encouragement to make positive lifestyle changes. As mentioned, the fact that people naturally prefer to drink something that "tastes good" is one of the greatest challenges to normal balanced hydration.

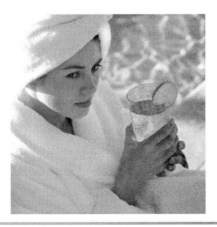

Figure 4–10 Drinking water *(image copyright iofoto, 2008. Used under license from Shutterstock.com).*

Research has shown that drinks that have a sweet taste are generally preferred. Thus, virtually all beverages sold today are sweetened in some way. Motivating people to change their patterns of beverage and consumption can be very difficult, even if they know it is better for them.

Step 4: Follow-Up

Follow-up is an important part of a personalized Balanced Hydration Program. Try to make a schedule of periodic sessions over an extended period of time, for example, once a month for six months. Make notes of your recommendations and then follow up on their success in making positive changes in your client's daily hydration behavior. Based on feedback from clients, you can make adjustments to their hydration program. Just by putting attention on hydration behavior can inspire a client to make significant, positive changes. Even clients who are already following a good hydration program can benefit by learning more about the principles of daily balanced hydration. Through the Balanced Hydration Program, the therapist becomes, in a very real sense, the client's "hydration coach." The motivation and support you provide can help the client make positive changes in his or her personal hydration behavior.

It is important to note that many therapists already have developed their own approach to hydration, both for themselves and for what they recommend to their clients. Whatever this approach may be, the Balanced Hydration Program can be adjusted to work with that program. The Balanced Hydration Program gives a structured, educational format along with teaching demonstrations and opportunities for client feedback and follow-up—all with the goal of making improvements in the client's daily hydration. Some improvements may be small and some may be more dramatic, but any improvements makes the program worthwhile. Finally, in the process of consulting with clients, one learns by teaching, which may result in improvements in one's own personal hydration program.

 ## SUMMARY

Balanced daily hydration is not only essential for daily wellness but also for the attainment of all health and wellness goals, such as healthful aging, prevention of diseases, appearance, beauty and fitness. By maintaining a Balanced Hydration Program, people can enjoy the many benefits it offers, while avoiding health problems associated with different levels of dehydration. The Balanced Hydration Program allows you to evaluate the current hydration patterns of your clients, to discuss with them the principles of balanced hydration using teaching demonstrations to illustrate key points, and to motivate and inspire them to improve their daily hydration routine.

The goal of a hydration program is to develop healthy hydration behaviors. The optimal functioning of all the systems of the body depends on normal fluid levels, which must be maintained through proper hydration. What makes daily hydration challenging is that the human body is constantly and automatically losing water approximately 2.5 qt/l per day. And the body can lose dramatically more water during sweating due to physical activity or a hot environment. Dehydration, at a level of even 1%, has been scientifically shown to produce a decrease in physical and mental performance and more serious health problems.

We have minimal control over the amount of water lost each day, as it is a natural process, but we do have control over the amount of total daily water intake from drinking water, beverages, and food. We also have control over the timing of total water intake and the sources and quality of our drinking water, beverages, and food. Water intake should occur at regular intervals throughout the day. Clients should also be informed about good choices for the source and quality of drinking water, beverages, and food, and about maintaining a healthy ratio between consumption of drinking water versus other beverages.

This chapter discussed two popular formulas currently used for determining the amount of total water intake—the 8 × 8 formula and the drinking an amount of water equal to half your body weight in ounces. In general, these formulas provide enough total fluid water intake, but depending on how the formula is used, it can also lead to excessive levels of water intake. However, there are many variations on these formulas, and any hydration program should be specifically adjusted for each client's weight and other special needs.

According to the 2004 report by the National Academy of Sciences Institute of Medicine, scientific surveys on food and water consumption in the United States and Canada show that men, on average, have a total water intake of 3.7 qt (3.7 L) per day, and women take in 2.7 qt (2.7 L) per day. These surveys also show that 80% of this intake comes from drinking water and beverages; the other 20% comes from food. The report concludes that this amount more than exceeds the normal daily water loss (not including sweating) and that, in general, people are staying adequately hydrated. The report lists several scientific studies that show the serious health consequences of a person becoming dehydrated for either a short time or chronically. The report set the adequate intake (AI) level for total daily water intake at 3.7 qt (3.7 L) for men and 2.7 qt (2.7 L) for women, though this is not a required level.

The Balanced Hydration Program consists of an interview, evaluation recommendations, and follow-up sessions with clients to make improvements to his or her daily hydration program. The goal of the program is to provide useful information about a client's daily patterns of hydration behavior and to make suggestions for improvement.

Each day, clients have control over four main areas of hydration:

- Amount of daily total water intake
- Percentage (%) of drinking water to beverages
- Timing of daily total water intake
- Source and quality of daily total water intake

By working with your clients in each of these four areas, you can help guide your clients to make better daily hydration choices. Improving a client's daily hydration behavior can produce many significant benefits in a client's overall health and wellness benefits.

The information in this chapter is not intended to replace a hydration formula or program that a therapist may already be using. Instead, it is intended to provide additional useful information and tools that will be helpful in providing clients with a better understanding of the basics of hydration and motivating them to make positive changes.

REFERENCES

(1) Institute of Medicine, Board of Health and Nutrition. (2004). *The Dietary Reference Intakes: Water, Potassium, Sodium, Chloride, and Sulfate.* Author, p. 124.
(2) IOM, *Dietary Reference Intakes,* p. 120.
(3) IOM, *Dietary Reference Intakes,* p. 88.
(4) IOM, *Dietary Reference Intakes,* p. 73.
(5) IOM, *Dietary Reference Intakes,* pp. 105–118.

(6) IOM, *Dietary Reference Intakes,* p. 92.

(7) IOM, *Dietary Reference Intakes,* p. 99.

(8) IOM, *Dietary Reference Intakes,* p. 99.

(9) IOM, *Dietary Reference Intakes,* p. 133.

(10) Dhingra, R., Sullivan, L., Jacques, P., Wang, T., Fox, C., Meigs, J., D'Agostino, R., et al. Soft drink consumption and risk of developing cardiometabolic risk factors and the metabolic syndrome in middle-aged adults in the community. *Circulation July 2007* (116): 480–488.

(11) IOM, *Dietary Reference Intakes,* p. 102.

(12) Valtin, H., Drink at least eight glasses of water a day. Really? Is there scientific evidence for 8 × 8?, *Am J Physoil Regulatory Integrative Comp Physiol 2002* (283): 993.

(13) IOM, *Dietary Reference Intakes,* p. 144.

SUGGESTED READINGS

Guyton, A. C., & Hall, J. E. (2005). *Textbook of Medical Physiology* (11th ed.).

Tortora, G. J., & Grabowski, S. R. (2003). *Principles of Anatomy and Physiology* (10th ed.). New York: John Wiley & Sons.

The Dietary Reference Intakes: Water, Potassium, Sodium, Chloride, and Sulfate, Institute of Medicine, Board of Health and Nutrition, Feb 2004.

REVIEW QUESTIONS

1. What is the approximate percent of water in the human body?

2. Where are the three main areas where this water is located in the body?

3. List the main physiological functions of water in the human body.

4. Can the body store water?

5. Describe a few health problems associated with dehydration.

6. How much water does the body naturally lose each day?

7. Name three ways the body naturally loses water.

8. What are the three general categories of daily sources of water intake?

9. List some problems associated with drinking beverages.

10. What percentage of our daily water do we get from food?

11. What does the IOM recommend as the AI (adequate intake) for water? What is the IOM recommendation for UL (upper limit) of water intake?

 For additional information on Hydrotherapy, visit our on-line companion at http://www.milady.cengage.com

Understanding the Key Elements of Hydrotherapy Treatments

KEY TERMS

Moor mud	Vichy shower	aquatic therapy pool
hydrosol	Swiss shower	Ayurveda
mineral salts	handheld shower	colon therapy
thallasotherapy	WATSU	
wet room	Kneipp therapy	

INTRODUCTION

This chapter describes the key elements common to the hydrotherapy treatments presented in this textbook. This information will provide therapists with a comprehensive understanding of the role each element plays in a hydrotherapy treatment and will present a hydrotherapy "treatment formula" that describes how all the elements function together. This chapter also includes an overview of the different treatments that will be described in more detail in Chapter 7.

Hydrotherapy treatments offered in a private practice, wellness center, or spa may consist of a single treatment, may be part of a combination package of treatments, or may be included in a series of treatments over an extended period of time. Hydrotherapy treatments may also be part of a total health and wellness program that includes treatments done at home. Other hydrotherapy programs that require special education at approved educational institutions (e.g., WATSU®) will also be discussed.

A wide range of hydrotherapy treatments and programs will be presented (see Figure 5–1), from simple to more complex, that will provide a greater understanding of the possible range of treatments

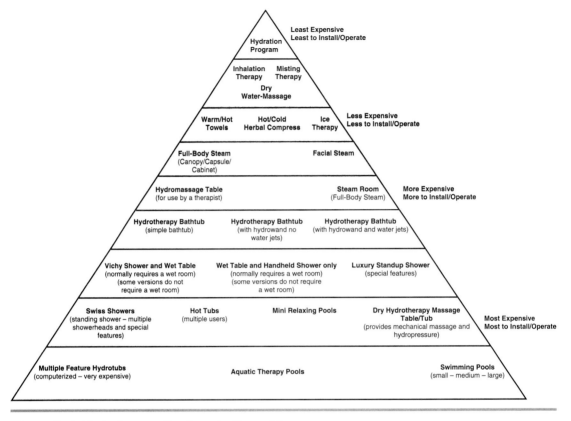

Figure 5–1 Hydrotherapy Treatments Pyramid.

and programs that can be offered. Some treatments and programs require simple inexpensive equipment and can be offered immediately, for example, inhalation therapy, and some require more complex equipment and training. But each treatment, whether simple or complex, uses the natural behavior of water to produce profound health and wellness transformations. The Balanced Hydration Program requires no equipment and can be offered to any client (see Chapter 4). Treatments using misting or inhalation therapy, as well as some forms of hydromassage, are inexpensive and easy to implement. Steam therapy using steam canopies that fit on a massage table allow personalized steam treatments without the expense of a steam room. Simple bathtubs can be used for some hydrotherapy treatments as well as more expensive hydrotubs with multiple features. Given all of the different options for hydrotherapy treatments and programs, it is possible to add hydrotherapy as an element to any health and wellness program. These are some of the same treatments that have been a fundamental part of all the great health and wellness traditions throughout history, including traditions from Greece, Rome, Japan, India, Germany, France, and other European countries.

KEY ELEMENTS OF HYDROTHERAPY TREATMENTS

This chapter provides a detailed description of the common elements of hydrotherapy treatments. These key elements can be expressed in an easy-to-remember "treatment formula" (see Table 5–1 and Figure 5–2). Each element is an essential part of a hydrotherapy treatment, and by maintaining a high quality of each element, the total beneficial effect of the treatment will be enhanced. For example, using the best hydrotherapy equipment and quality natural products will produce greater benefits. Having a greater understanding of the health and wellness goals of the client and having the treatment performed by a therapist who is properly trained will produce better results. The proper design and décor of the treatment room will contribute to the successful outcome of the hydrotherapy treatment. Each element contributes something important to the treatment, and when each element is fully expressed, the beneficial outcome of each treatment can be truly remarkable. As the ancient Greek saying states, "The whole is greater than the sum of its parts." Knowledge of each of these elements will also help to gain a better understanding of each of the hydrotherapy treatments presented in Chapter 7.

Table 5–1	Hydrotherapy Treatment Formula
Hydrotherapy Treatment = (Client + Therapist) + (Product + Equipment + Water) + Steps + Facility	

- Client
- Therapist
- Water
- Equipment
- Products
- Facility
- Steps: Pretreatment, Beginning, During, End, Post

Hydrotherapy Treatment Formula

Hydrotherapy Treatment = (Client + Therapist) + (Product + Equipment + Water) + Steps + Facility

Time

Transformation – Goal (Intention)

Hydrotherapy Treatment

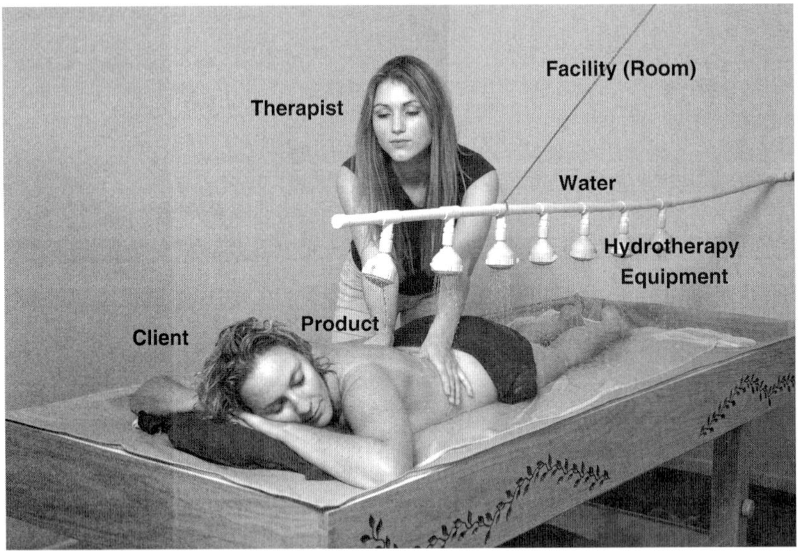

Figure 5–2 Hydrotherapy Treatment Formula.

Client

To help clients achieve and maintain their individual health and wellness goals, a range of treatment programs, including hydrotherapy, have been developed over time. Many of these treatments are performed in health and wellness settings by trained therapists. By understanding the health and wellness goals of each client, as well as how client's needs vary with age and gender, it is possible to make recommendations to him or her for programs best suited to their needs.

- **Gender:** Hydrotherapy treatments appeal to both men and women. The design of hydrotherapy treatments and treatment packages can be tailored toward either gender, depending on the spa menu. For example, full-body esthetic treatments for skin care using steam and hydrotubs tend to be more popular with women, whereas combinations of steam therapy with sports massage are often more popular with men. However, most hydrotherapy treatments are designed for both genders and creative approaches to promote these treatments to all clients can make them popular with both genders (see Chapter 11).

- **Age:** Hydrotherapy treatments can appeal to clients of any age. Many hydrotherapy treatments, including steam, hydrotub, and hydromassage table treatments, are very gentle, comfortable, and effective. These treatments can have a special appeal to older or even elderly clients, who often do not get "typical" massage treatments because of their age but who could greatly benefit from gentler forms of treatments. More treatments that include hydrotherapy need to be developed for this age group. In addition, spas and wellness programs could offer programs for retirement communities, as many people who are retiring are knowledgeable about the value of alternative health programs. Similarly, spas could offer packages for parents and their children, which would create more hydrotherapy treatment options for children of any age.

- **Client's Health and Wellness Goals:** All health and wellness programs have been developed to help clients achieve their health and wellness goals. Each person is unique and will have his or her own combination of health and wellness goals and by a proper evaluation of these goals, recommendations can be made for specific hydrotherapy treatments and programs (see Chapter 7). One of the most important points about hydrotherapy is that it can be an effective therapeutic modality to help clients achieve *all* of their health and wellness goals (see Table 5–2). The following is a description of clients' key health and wellness goals.

DAILY WELLNESS: People want to feel good; they want to have optimal physical, mental, and emotional energy; balance; motivation; and creative skills to deal with daily demands and challenges. Different spa and wellness programs are designed to help clients maintain this daily continuum of wellness. Hydrotherapy treatments can be very helpful in pursuing this goal, as they can

Table 5–2   Health and Wellness Goals

Wellness Goals	Health Goals
Daily wellness	Symptoms
Appearance and beauty	Rehabilitation
Fitness	Major medical conditions
Healthy aging	
Prevention	
Enhancement	

provide profound relaxation therapy, healthy stimulation of cellular metabolism and circulation, optimal daily hydration, healthy structure alignment, and coordinated muscle pattern functioning. Most clients have profound experiences of relaxation and wellness during a hydrotherapy treatment which helps to balance an overstimulated nervous systems.

APPEARANCE AND BEAUTY: Personal appearance is a priority for most clients. Many spa and wellness programs are designed to help clients attain this goal. Different hydrotherapy treatments can promote the health and appearance of the skin of the entire body, not just the face. It can also promote healthy aging of the skin, assist in weight-management programs, and provide relaxation therapy. Clients will not only look better, they will also feel better.

FITNESS: Fitness leads to greater energy, endurance, performance, and coordination, which can all be of benefit in sports programs and everyday life. Certain hydrotherapy programs can enhance the development and maintenance of greater levels of fitness. For example, steam therapy promotes detoxification and stimulates cellular metabolism, hydromassage relaxes muscles and promotes healthy circulation to muscles, and relaxation therapy balances the effects of strenuous exercise and sports activities. Fitness also applies to mental, emotional, and spiritual fitness. Thus, a total concept of fitness deals with maintaining optimal levels of performance in all these areas.

HEALTHY (ANTI) AGING: Healthy aging is based primarily on the healthy aging of the body's cells. As discussed in Chapter 3, the cells of our body are mainly responsible for most of the activity of our bodies, including movement, perception, thinking, feeling, and appearance. Promoting healthy aging of our body's cells is a fundamental aspect of healthy aging. Various hydrotherapy treatments can promote healthy blood circulation to the 100 trillion cells of the human body, stimulate cellular metabolism, maintain optimal hydration of the cells and the other fluid systems of the body, and promote proper cellular alignment. As mentioned earlier, cells have precise alignment relative to other cells and to the blood capillaries that maintain circulation, which can be improved through different forms of hydromassage. Hydrotherapy treatments can also be used to detoxify the body, a treatment that is increasingly important due to the exposure to food, air, and water pollution. Equally important is the profound relaxation provided by hydrotherapy treatments, which can help keep the nervous system and the hormonal (endocrine) system balanced as we age.

PREVENTION: Most health problems can be prevented before they ever occur, a fact that has been verified by extensive scientific research. Hydrotherapy treatments can provide effective tools for maintaining health and wellness and for managing the daily impact of exposure to stress, toxins in water and food, and pollution in the environment. It can also help prevent problems created by certain occupations, such as sitting in front of computers for long periods or performing repetitive movements, both of which can have negative cumulative effects. In addition, different levels of dehydration have been scientifically correlated with a variety of health problems. The Balanced Hydration Program (see Chapter 4) can help clients maintain normal levels of hydration and prevent dehydration. Hydrotherapy offers many options, especially when combined with other wellness programs, for promoting the prevention of major health problems. Eliminating major health problems before they ever occur is one of the greatest benefits of a well-designed holistic health and wellness program.

ENHANCEMENT: Hydrotherapy treatments can be of value in programs that seek to unfold and enliven latent human potential. There is a general understanding that human beings have far more physical, mental, emotional, and spiritual potential than what is being expressed. Today, many people are actively pursuing their full potential in various areas, whether it be artistic, physical, mental, emotional, or spiritual. Hydrotherapy treatments not only promote general health and wellness but also help us to unfold and express more of our full potential. During many hydrotherapy treatments, including special hydrotub treatments such as flotation and personally designed steam treatments, people have reported unique experiences, including greater creativity, greater connection with nature, expanded spiritual awareness, and feelings on deeper emotional levels. The deep relaxation of many hydrotherapy treatments, combined with the use of special products, light, and music, can enliven new levels of awareness.

SYMPTOMS: People often experience high levels of stress and tension, back pain, and other forms of discomfort associated with the muscular skeletal system and other health problems. Many massage therapy and bodywork techniques help people control and minimize these negative symptoms. The relaxation produced by hydrotherapy can also help reduce feelings of stress and tension. This physical relaxation can also help with the treatment of muscle, joint, and body alignment problems. The heating effects of hydrotherapy can help make the body more flexible and easier to stretch, which can, in turn, help with certain massage and body treatments. Problems associated with these types of symptoms are one of the main reasons clients seek programs and treatments to help alleviate or eliminate these discomforts and hydrotherapy can significantly enhance treatment options for effectively dealing with these problems.

REHABILITATION: Once an individual has recovered from an initial accident, injury, surgery, or other problems, symptoms may continue that require additional rehabilitation. Hydrotherapy can assist in the rehabilitation process when included in programs given by massage therapists, occupational and physical therapists, or other types of bodyworkers. The ability of hydrotherapy to safely heat and cool the body in a carefully controlled manner and to produce significant levels of relaxation, both on the mental and physical levels, can create conditions that enhance the speed and completeness of rehabilitation. For example, some simple hydrotubs allow the client's body to be fully extended (horizontally) in the water, creating a gravity-free environment and allowing the therapist full access to the client. Steam therapy, done using a steam canopy, allows steam treatments to be done on any massage table. Hydrotherapy, when used properly, offers an alternative and effective approach for rehabilitation of problems, many of which are chronic from injuries that have never completely healed.

MAJOR MEDICAL CONDITIONS: Historically, hydrotherapy programs have had a long tradition of use, in combination with other medical approaches, in treating major medical conditions (see Chapter 8). Today, in several European countries and in Japan, hydrotherapy programs are often a component of medical programs under the supervision of trained, professional medical staff. For example, treatments at Thermes de Vichy Callou, in Vichy, France, require a doctor's prescription, are done in conjunction with other medical modalities, and are paid for by national health insurance. Treating major medical conditions with hydrotherapy requires special training and must be done under strict medical supervision. Therefore, hydrotherapy treatments that treat specific major medical conditions will not be covered in this textbook. However, the basic training in the theory and technique to perform a broad range of the hydrotherapy covered in this textbook provides a basic education in hydrotherapy that could be used by a therapist to perform various treatments under the supervision of a professional medical staff. For more information, see the section on the treatment of major medical conditions using hydrotherapy in Chapter 10.

Therapist

A therapist is a key element in the hydrotherapy treatment formula. The therapist controls all elements of the hydrotherapy treatment and is responsible for ensuring that the treatment is done properly and effectively. The outcome of the treatment depends on the therapist's knowledge and skills. The client is essentially a passive element during treatment and can relax, knowing that the treatment is being performed by a trained professional. Because hydrotherapy treatments can produce dramatic changes in the functioning of a client's physiology (e.g., raising the core temperature of the body), these techniques should be done by therapists with proper training in both the complex nature of the human body and hydrotherapy.

Most professional therapists can incorporate hydrotherapy as a treatment modality, including massage therapists, estheticians, fitness instructors, cosmetologists, yoga instructors, bodyworkers, and occupational and physical therapists.

Water

Water is the essence of a hydrotherapy treatment. Hydrotherapy education allows a therapist to develop a special relationship with water and the ability to use water in multiple ways to produce specific therapeutic transformations. Usually, water is brought into external contact with the client's body, as in a hydrotub treatment, underwater massage, or shower treatment. Sometimes, however, the water is used internally in inhalation or hydration treatments. Often, natural products, such as essential oils, can be combined with the water, especially in hydrotub and inhalation treatments. By using the fundamental principles of the behavior of water (e.g., buoyancy, heat exchange, movement, solvent, and suspension), a skilled therapist using water can produce significant, positive, therapeutic health and wellness transformations for clients.

Hydrotherapy Equipment

Hydrotherapy equipment, an essential element of most hydrotherapy treatments, allows a therapist to bring water into contact with the client's body in carefully controlled ways. For example, steam therapy treatment requires a steam canopy, steam cabinet, or steam room. A hydrotub treatment requires some type of simple bathtub, hydrotub, or hot tub. The specific instructions for different hydrotherapy treatments, provided in Chapter 7, include recommendations for the hydrotherapy equipment that should be used for each treatment. This textbook does not mention specific equipment manufacturers, as companies are constantly changing and new equipment is being developed. However, the Hydrotherapy Equipment Resource Guide in the Appendix suggests sources for researching different types of hydrotherapy equipment in trade magazines, at trade shows, and on the Internet. The following is some important information to consider when choosing hydrotherapy equipment (see also Table 5–3).

Client Comfort

Relaxation is one of the greatest benefits of hydrotherapy, and many of the therapeutic effects of the treatments are due to the profound relaxation produced. Thus, if clients are uncomfortable on a specific type of hydrotherapy equipment, much of the benefit of that treatment can be lost. Even if the primary goal of

Table 5–3   Hydrotherapy Equipment Considerations

- Client comfort
- Design: Therapist-friendly, effective control of water temperature, pressure
- Durability: Problem free, adequate warranty, easy to repair
- Hygienic and safe
- Education: Installation, how to use, treatments, menu planning

a treatment is something other than relaxation, such as detoxification, the treatment can still produce deep relaxation, which can add to the treatment's total beneficial effect. Thus, it is important that hydrotherapy equipment be designed to be in harmony with the structure of the human body and be as comfortable as possible.

When considering different brands of hydrotherapy equipment, it is important to try each brand of equipment, to determine which system is the most comfortable. Some hydrotherapy equipment is often designed more for its "spa look," especially in the spa field, than for the client's comfort. Yet, clients will always benefit more from equipment that is more comfortable rather than equipment that looks good.

Design

Hydrotherapy equipment should have therapist-friendly design features. This means the equipment should allow the therapist to work effectively on the client. Thus, well-designed hydrotherapy equipment should allow therapists maximum accessibility to their clients during the treatment. The hydrotherapy equipment should also include features that allow for precise control over the temperature, pressure, or other key behaviors of water during a treatment.

More hydrotherapy equipment is now being developed that is robotic in nature. These equipment systems require minimal or no interaction between the client and the therapist during the treatment. Although such hydrotherapy equipment may have value in certain spa and wellness programs, it cannot replace the complex interaction that takes place between client and therapist. Treatments that involve working on the human body require that the therapist have the skills necessary to work with the complex nature of the human body as well as how hydrotherapy treatments produce unique changes in the physiology. Most hydrotherapy treatments, to be safe and to produce the maximum benefits, require the skills of a professionally trained therapist.

Durability

Just as a good massage table will last for many years of use, hydrotherapy equipment should have a long lifetime with minimal maintenance and repairs. Equipment should come with a good warranty. Once the warranty is over, it should still be possible to quickly and inexpensively fix any problems with the equipment. This is especially important for equipment with major electrical or computerized components.

When choosing equipment—especially expensive equipment—ask for references from people who already own or are using the equipment. In addition, carefully evaluate any claims the manufacturer makes about how profitable the equipment will be. Sometimes equipment manufacturers provide very unrealistic projections about how many treatments a spa or wellness center will do per day and how profitable the equipment will be.

Hygienic and Safe

It should be possible to easily clean and disinfect all surfaces of hydrotherapy equipment, especially any hydrotherapy system that recirculates water during treatment, such as hydrotubs, pedicure baths, and hot tubs. The manufacturer must verify that these systems can be adequately disinfected between treatments and must include cleaning and disinfecting instructions. Recirculating pumps and pipes, if not disinfected properly, offer an ideal environment for the growth of harmful microorganisms, especially bacteria (see Chapter 6). Additional research should be done to determine whether the equipment is safe, especially in terms of getting onto (into) and out of (off of) the equipment, especially equipment that is wet and slippery.

Treatment Suggestions and Menu Planning

Manufacturers of hydrotherapy equipment normally provide support for installation and training in the proper use of the equipment. This is usually done by printed materials, DVD presentations, and on-line support. The manufacture should also provide similar instructions on how to perform various treatments using the equipment as well as suggestions and support for developing marketing materials and treatment menus. This can include photos of the equipment as well as creative descriptions of the treatments that can be used to help develop these promotional materials.

Products

Products, an important element of most hydrotherapy treatments, have been used in all hydrotherapy traditions. These products include herbs, special oils, and mineral salts. Natural products, when combined with water or applied to the client's body, produce a special synergy between the products, the water, and the client, creating special, beneficial effects. As an example, the Japanese have long used special products in their therapeutic bath treatments.

Ayurveda also has rich tradition in the use of many different types of herbs and oils in various hydrotherapy treatments.

A wider range of natural products are now available than ever before. Many companies offer special products that can be used during hydrotub, steam, and shower treatments. Most of these companies offer education on how to use their products during treatments to get the maximum benefit from the product. Most of these products are for skin care, though there are some specifically for relaxation of muscle tension and muscle and joint problems.

Trade shows and magazines for the spa, aesthetic, and massage professions provide a good resource for researching treatments and products that can be used with different hydrotherapy equipment. You can also search the Internet for special products. The Hydrotherapy Product Resource Guide in Appendix C provides additional information on products for use in hydrotherapy treatments. Note that the Appendix does not list specific product manufacturers, as new companies continue to develop and existing companies often change their products.

This section covers the general product categories commonly used during hydrotherapy treatments (see Table 5–4). As mentioned earlier, most companies provide detailed education on the use of their products. For example, a company that sells a seaweed product for a bath treatment, will specify how much product to use, how long the bath should be, the benefits of the bath, and suggested temperature of the water.

Herbal Preparations

Many herbal products are available for use during hydrotherapy treatments. These products may use a single herb or, more often, may be several herbs in combination to produce specific health and

Table 5–4   Natural Products and Hydrotherapy Treatment
• Herbal preparations
• Moor mud
• Essential oils: Aromatherapy
• Hydrosols: Aromatherapy
• Natural oils: Massage and skin care
• Seaweed and algae products
• Mineral salts
• Clay (Mud)

wellness benefits. These products usually dissolve in water or can be mixed into the water during the treatment. Many therapists with experience in using natural herbal products often design their own herbal preparations. For example, mixing a gallon of St. John's wort tea with water for a hydrotub treatment produces a very subtle, but relaxing, effect for the client.

Moor Mud

A special type of natural product used in hydrotherapy treatments at many spa and wellness centers is a form of nutrient-rich peat created by the gradual transformation of herbs, plants, and flowers that have been submerged under pressure underground. In the correct climatic and biological conditions, this plant matter, which is free from the decaying effects of oxygen, undergoes a ripening process over thousands of years into a rich, black organic substance, known as **Moor mud.** During this process, the organic and inorganic substances within the plants are assimilated into the mud, resulting in an herbal complex with wonderful therapeutic properties. Some of the best-known sources of Moor mud are in Austria and are sometimes certified as medical-grade.

Moor mud
Rare form of nutrient-rich peat that has been created by the gradual transformation of herbs, plants, and flowers, which have been submerged underwater or underground.

Essential Oils

These natural oils are often used as part of hydrotherapy treatments for aromatherapy or some other purpose, depending on the goal of the treatment. Different essential oils are often used with steam therapy or hydrotub treatments. Most steam therapy equipment includes a feature that allows for essential oils to be mixed with the water that creates the steam. Another use of essential oils is to blend it with carrier oil that is massaged onto the client's skin before the client receives a steam or hydrotub treatment. The heat from the steam or water then increases the rate of absorption (diffusion) of the oil by the skin.

As mentioned, one of the greatest benefits of many hydrotherapy treatments is the deep and unique state of relaxation they can produce. This state of relaxation can be further enhanced by the use of aromatherapy. Most therapists have some formal training in the use of aromatherapy and essential oils that will allow them to chose specific essential oils for use in different treatments. (See Suggested Reading at the end of this chapter.) Designing hydrotherapy treatments that include aromatherapy can be a very creative process.

Hydrosol
Water-soluble essence of plants (as compared with essential oils, which are the oil essence of the plant).

Hydrosols

Hydrosol is the water portion that remains during the production of essential oils and contain the "water essence" of the plant. They contain many of the therapeutic properties as the oil portion and they can dissolve in water. They can be added to bath treatments, and some steam treatments, and can be used as an ingredient in misting sprays. They can be used for aromatherapy and produce various natural fragrances during the hydrotherapy treatment. There are many types of natural hydrosols available, many of them organic. Just a few examples are lavender, orange flower, lime, lemon, basil, cucumber, peppermint, and rose. The use of hydrosols, like essential oils, offers many special ways to be creative when developing hydrotherapy treatments.

Massage and Skin Care Oils

Many natural massage and skin care oils can be used with hydrotherapy. Oils are not water-soluble and, thus, when massaged onto the skin, will not easily wash off during a steam, shower, or hydrotub treatment. Some of this oil will remain on the skin, which can have moisturizing and other skin care benefits. Some oils can be absorbed by the skin, and the increased heat of a steam treatment or hot water hydrotub treatment can increase the rate of absorption of these oils. Many types of skin care treatments benefit from the increased rate of absorption of these oils.

Seaweed and Algae Products

Some species of seaweed, a nutrient-rich plant that grows naturally in the ocean, have been found to have therapeutic uses, especially for skin care. Another natural product from both sea water and fresh water is algae, which can also be used for skin care during hydrotherapy treatments. Some of these products can be placed on the skin during a steam treatment, while others are best placed in the water during a hydrotub treatment. The water and heat of hydrotherapy enhances the interaction between the seaweed or algae products and the skin.

Mineral Salts

Natural **mineral salts** have been used for centuries and are well-known for having beneficial effects on the skin, muscles, and joints and for promoting a sense of well-being. These natural mineral salts are often used during hydrotherapy treatments—usually hydrotub treatments. Examples of mineral salts include natural ocean salt from such locations as Bali, the North Sea, and the Atlantic Ocean off the coast of Brazil; Dead Sea salts from Israel; and mineral salts from other dry seas and lake beds. Epsom salt, a pure mineral compound (magnesium sulfate), has been traditionally used in bath treatments to enhance relaxation, soothe tired muscles, and for certain skin care

Mineral salts
Natural minerals salt that easily dissolve in water, for example calcium, magnesium, sodium and chloride.

benefits. Some hydrotherapy treatments add about 35 g of sea salt to every liter of water in a hydrotub to produce approximately the same concentration of sea salt as is found in the ocean. **Thallasotherapy** treatments, which use ocean water, are popular at some spa and wellness centers located near the ocean.

Clay

Natural clay, also sometimes referred to as mud, has long been used for therapeutic purposes. Traditional European hydrotherapy spas use clays in many of their skin care and medical treatments. Treatments using natural mud (clay) from the local area, are popular at some natural hot springs, for example, Calistoga in Northern California. Some clay products are applied to the skin before a hydrotherapy treatment begins and some can be placed in the water during a hydrotub treatment. The use of clay in hydrotherapy will continue to increase, especially as more sources of clay become available from various sources around the world, each with its own tradition of therapeutic benefits.

Hydrotherapy Facility

The spa or wellness facility is a component of a hydrotherapy treatment. Hydrotherapy treatments must be done in a treatment room—often a dedicated hydrotherapy room—that is part of a larger treatment facility. Some hydrotherapy treatment rooms are **wet rooms,** which allow water to flow from a wet table onto the floor and drain to a central floor drain. Other hydrotherapy treatments, however, do not require a wet room; these include steam treatments in a steam canopy, cabinet, or capsule. Some wet table and Vichy shower treatments can even be done on special equipment designed for use in a normal treatment room. Whether the hydrotherapy treatment room is a wet room or not, there are many special considerations for these rooms including proper ventilation, safety precautions for walking on wet floors, and the ability to properly clean and dry surfaces that become wet.

Many spas and wellness centers include various water elements in their decor. Water fountains may be found in the reception areas and in individual rooms. The center may be playing relaxation and nature CDs that include the sounds of water such as ocean waves, rain, streams, and waterfalls. Photographs of natural water settings may be displayed on the walls, and some spas even have painted murals with water themes. A water theme can add another element to the use of water for health and wellness (see Chapter 11).

Some facilities also include the principles of feng shui in their design, especially the use of flowing water. According to feng shui, the healthy flow of water in a building is necessary to promote a healthy chi, or life force, for the health and wellness of all the people in the building.

Some luxury spas and resorts have made significant investments in developing aesthetically pleasing designs that often include water themes. Many of these high-end facilities will have special themes, such as Hawaiian, Roman, Japanese, or Balinese. The elaborate and beautiful decor of these resorts is considered to be an essential component of the total spa experience.

Steps of the Treatment

Every hydrotherapy treatment presented in Chapter 7 consists of specific, step-by-step procedures. Nearly every treatment is taught using the same sequence of steps: pretreatment, beginning the treatment, treatment, end of the treatment, and post-treatment. The following is a brief description of each element of the sequence.

Pretreatment

Pretreatment usually includes preparing the equipment for use in the treatment. For example, filling a hydrotub with water at a certain temperature and adding any natural product or turning on a steam generator so that the steam will be ready at the beginning of the treatment.

Beginning the Treatment

This step usually begins as the client enters the room. The therapist usually assists the client into or onto the hydrotherapy equipment, such as a hydrotub or wet table. The client may have already changed into a bathrobe, towel, or bathing suit (if this makes him or her more comfortable). Or the client may change in the room before the therapist enters. Draping procedures are basically the same as those used for massage therapy and full-body skin care treatments; however, these procedures may require more creativity in keeping the client covered and warm during hydrotherapy treatments. The most important considerations in terms of draping are to ensure client comfort and to follow all local and state regulations.

Treatment

Each hydrotherapy treatment described in Chapter 7 includes step-by-step procedures that will produce the desired therapeutic transformation for the client. Some treatments are simpler, while others are more complex. During the treatment, the therapist will bring water into contact with the client in a controlled manner for a specific amount of time along with other procedures, for example, massage. The skill of the therapist plays a significant role in the beneficial outcome of the treatment. The client should be able to completely relax knowing that a knowledgeable therapist is in control of every step of the treatment.

End of the Treatment

The end of the treatment may be a transition from the treatment to another treatment or a period of resting before leaving. This transition should always be as comfortable as possible. It is recommended to assist the client from (off) the hydrotherapy equipment to the next treatment room or resting room.

Post-Treatment

This step usually involves cleaning and disinfecting the hydrotherapy equipment and surfaces, including the floor and anything else to prepare the room for the next treatment.

 ## PROGRAM OPTIONS

Many hydrotherapy treatments can be done as a single treatment and it is also possible to combine a hydrotherapy treatment with other types of treatments. Most spa and wellness centers offer treatment packages, which is a combination of two or more treatments, including hydrotherapy, massage, full-body skin care, and hair and scalp treatments. Combining several treatments can produce a special synergy, creating a totally unique treatment with special benefits, similar to combining natural products to create a synergistic blend with totally unique properties and benefits.

Combinations of Hydrotherapy with Other Treatments

The following are suggestions for combining different types of hydrotherapy treatments with other treatments:

Steam Therapy Combinations

- **Steam and massage:** Steam treatments are usually done before the massage treatment, as they relax the client, stimulate circulation, and warm the fascial and musculo-skeletal systems. Steam therapy can be combined with most massage therapy modalities.

- **Detoxification:** Steam therapy treatments can be combined with other detoxification approaches, such as massage, herbal cleanses, and inhalation therapy. When detoxification is the primary goal, massage is sometimes done before the steam treatment, as is done with the Ayurveda steam and massage treatment for detoxification.

- **Esthetics and skin care:** Steam therapy can be combined with exfoliation treatments, as it heats the epidermal layers of the skin, facilitating the process of exfoliation. It can also be combined with certain body-wrap treatments, as it enhances absorption of the product. Steam therapy can also be an effective preparation of the skin before applying a full-body skin product, as there will be greater circulation to the skin and absorption of the product.

- **Cosmetology and hair and scalp:** Steam therapy treatments, especially those that steam the head and scalp, can be a great preparation for a hair and scalp treatment. Steam therapy increases circulation to the scalp and heats the hair, which increases the absorption of products into the hair and scalp. Today, many hair salons are a combination of a salon and day spa that offers or could offer steam therapy.

- **Weight-management programs:** Steam therapy treatments have been proven to be beneficial for weight-management programs, as they increase the total metabolic activity of the body. This increase burns more calories and has a stimulating effect on the body's total metabolism, which can produce both immediate and more lasting benefits for weight management.

- **Stress-management programs:** Many steam hydrotherapy programs produce profound levels of deep relaxation. This form of relaxation therapy can be added as a key component of total stress-management programs.

- **Yoga, Pilates, and bodywork:** Steam therapy not only relaxes the body but also heats the body's fascial matrix. Heated, relaxed muscles can allow the body to stretch more deeply and easily during yoga, Pilates, or bodywork treatments.

Hydrotub Therapy Combinations

Hydrotubs range from simple bathtubs to more complex versions with multiple features. There are virtually unlimited possibilities of hydrotub treatments, especially considering all the products, music, and color light elements that can also be included. The following are several examples of possible hydrotub therapy combinations.

- **Massage:** Hydrotub treatments are very relaxing, which means they are good preparation for a massage. If the water in the hydrotub is heated above body temperature, it will warm the connective matrix of the bones, muscles, tendons, ligaments, and fascia, which will then stretch more easily and be more flexible.

- **Hydromassage:** A hydrowand for underwater massage in a hydrotub provides a therapist with a very effective massage procedure for many different forms of massage, including lymphatic, vascular, and shiatsu. These treatments are also an excellent preparation for traditional massage treatments.

- **Esthetics and skin care:** A warm hydrotub has a heating effect on the skin and significantly increases blood circulation to the skin. This can be very effective preparation for the application of skin care products after a bath. Some products can be added to the water to interact with the client's skin during the treatment. Other non-soluble products that will not easily wash off can be applied directly to the client's skin before he or she relaxes into the heated hydrotub water. A heated hydrotub bath can also be a used as a preparation for an exfoliation treatment.

- **Cosmetology and hair and scalp:** Hydrotub treatments can also be part of a special package that includes a hair and scalp treatment followed by hair styling. Special products can be applied to the client's hair and scalp as they relax in a hydrotub. These products are then rinsed out with a handheld shower. This can be a great preparation for a styling session.

Flotation Therapy Combinations

Flotation therapy using a flotation tank or a hydrotub designed to allow flotation can combine well with other treatments including:

- **Massage:** Flotation therapy produces a profound sense of relaxation and can be used as preparation for most massage therapy treatments.

- **Spa and wellness packages:** Flotation treatments can be included as an element of relaxation therapy in half-day or full-day spa packages.

Shower Therapy Combinations

- **Massage:** Shower therapy, including horizontal (Vichy), vertical (Swiss), and handheld shower treatments, is a great postmassage treatment. Shower therapy not only bathes and rinses any product from the client but also adds another level of hydromassage to the regular massage treatment.

- **Esthetics and skin care:** A horizontal (**Vichy shower**), vertical (**Swiss shower**), or **handheld shower** treatment is very effective at the end of a full-body esthetics treatments, when product should be removed from the client's body. These treatments also produce a hydromassaging effect on the body. A normal shower by the client in a traditional shower stall at the end of a treatment does not produce the same total beneficial effect, though it will rinse the product from the body.

- **Cosmetology and hair and scalp:** Shower treatments can also be part of a special package that includes a hair and scalp treatment and hair styling. Special products can be massaged into the client's hair and scalp as he or she lies on a wet table. This product is then rinsed using a handheld shower before the styling. One of the most client-pleasing hydrotherapy treatments is getting a hair and scalp massage, in combination with a handheld shower, which happens as a natural part of a hair and scalp treatment given by a cosmetologist.

Hydromassage Table Combinations

- **Massage:** Most traditional forms of massage can be done on a hydromassage table, which allows therapists to combine the features and benefits of hydrotherapy with traditional forms of massage.

- **Esthetics and skin care:** It is possible to combine some a esthetic treatments with the hydromassage table. For example, some facials can be done on the table, which also increases the client's level of relaxation. It is possible to use the heat of a hydromassage table to enhance the benefits of a full-body skin care treatment, such as exfoliation and body wraps. This is a unique way to combine a hydrotherapy element with a full-body skin care treatment.

Vichy shower

A horizontal shower with multiple showerheads (approximately seven) that showers over a client lying on a wet table, often as the client is also being massaged. The origin of the treatment is from Vichy, France.

Swiss shower

A vertical shower system with multiple showerheads (approximately ten) that showers a client on all sides, including the head, as the client stands.

Handheld shower

The use of a handheld shower by a therapist to massage a client on a wet table with water or to rinse product off the client.

Extended Treatment Program: Series of Treatments

To achieve and maintain most health and wellness benefits from hydrotherapy treatments, one treatment session is generally not enough. To set treatment goals for your client and to be able to realistically attain those goals, it is essential to determine how many treatment sessions will be necessary. Most clients realize that it will take several treatment sessions to obtain the desired benefits and are willing to commit to the program.

Holistic Health and Wellness Programs

Many spa and wellness centers are beginning to offer more holistic health and wellness programs. These are total programs offered to help clients achieve and maintain all their health and wellness goals. These programs include nutrition, exercise, breathing, hydration, and regular health and wellness "tune-ups," including massage, detoxification, and skin care, as well as retreat sessions. Historically, great holistic health and wellness traditions, including Ayurveda from India, have all included hydrotherapy as a key element of their total program. This continues today in modern Ayurveda and Japanese programs, in the Kneipp program popular in Germany, and in other successful programs used in France and other European countries. This long tradition of the successful use of hydrotherapy in total holistic health and wellness programs and the current developments in hydrotherapy, including a better understanding of the behavior of water in relationship to the human body, demonstrates that hydrotherapy will continue to be a key part of modern holistic health and wellness programs.

Home Program

After a treatment session at a spa or wellness center, clients are usually given a continuing treatment program to perform at home. For example, if the client has had a skin care treatment, the therapist will instruct the client on how to continue with a home program. Clients are given instructions for different treatments, including the use of various products, such as essential oils, herbs, and music CDs (for relaxation), for their home programs. These home treatments, can be helpful in maintaining and enhancing the benefits of treatment sessions at the spa or wellness center.

Home treatments are also important for the financial success of a spa or wellness business, as sales of products and other items are a significant contribution to the total income. Also, successful home programs keep clients connected to the spa or wellness center that recommend the program.

Some simple home hydrotherapy treatments include those which use a bathtub or shower in combination with certain natural products. Inhalation treatments could be recommended, with the client using safe, inexpensive inhalation therapy equipment. The Balanced Hydration Program, presented in Chapter 4, is another daily hydrotherapy program that includes periodic follow-up, evaluation, and recommendations by a therapist.

DIFFERENT TYPES OF HYDROTHERAPY TREATMENTS

As discussed in this chapter, there are many types of hydrotherapy treatments, from simple and effective treatments that require no equipment to treatments that require very expensive and complex equipment and everything in-between. With the wide range of hydrotherapy treatments available, it is possible for therapists to begin to offer hydrotherapy as part of their total treatment program or expand their existing hydrotherapy program. The following is a list of the basic categories of hydrotherapy treatments (see Figure 5–3).

- Immersion (bathtub)
- Steam
- Shower
- Hydromassage table
- Misting
- Compresses
- Daily hydration program
- Special hydrotherapy programs

Hydrotherapy treatments for each of these categories (with the exception of special hydrotherapy programs) will be presented in Chapter 7.

Hydrotherapy Treatments—Examples

Immersion (Bathtub)

Hydrotub, Simple Bathtub, Hydrotub
- Relaxation
- Detoxification
- Skin care
- Exfoliation Preparation
- Flotation
- Underwater Hydromassage
  - Lymphatic
  - Cellular
  - Shiatsu
- Massage and Bodywork
- Cellular and Vascular Alignment
- Hydro-Yoga
- Sound: Music, Primordial Sounds
- Foot Bath
  - Reflexology
  - Pedicure

Compresses
- Hot, Warm
- Cool, Cold
- Herbal compresses
- Ice: cryotherapy for treatment of sprains, contusions

Steam

Canopy/Cabinet/Steam Room
- Relaxation
  - Breathing
- Detoxification
- Skin care and Products
- Skin care – exfoliation
- Massage preparation

Inhalation: Mouth and Nose
- Moisture for exposure to dry, cold air
- Purification (detoxification) or respiratory lining
- Product delivery to lungs

Balance Daily Hydration
- Hydration Program Amount, Timing, Sources of water for hydration

Hydromassage Tables
- Relaxation
  - Breathing
- Traditional forms of massage
- Special Hydromassage Table forms of massage
- Skin care – full-body, facials

Special Hydrotherapy Education
- WATSU®
- Ayurveda
- Kneipp®
- Colonics
- Aquatic Therapy Pools
- Physical and Occupational Therapy

Shower

Horizontal Shower (Vichy Shower)
- Relaxation
- Contrast Hot and Cold
- Skin care
- Skin care – exfoliation
- Hydromassage
- Combined with Manual Massage
- Lymphatic Massage

Vertical Shower (Swiss Shower)
- Relaxation
- Contrast Hot and Cold
- Hydromassage
- Lymphatic Massage

Handheld Shower
- Relaxation
- Contrast Hot and Cold
- Hydromassage
- Lymphatic Massage
- Hair and Scalp Massage

Misting
- Cooling
- Product application
- Aromatherapy
- Wetting Skin

Figure 5–3 Hydrotherapy treatments.

SPECIAL HYDROTHERAPY PROGRAMS

Some special treatment programs that use hydrotherapy as an essential component require special, certified training through approved educational institutions. For example, for a therapist to offer WATSU® treatments, he or she must be trained and certified by an educational institute certified to teach WATSU®. The following is a brief discussion of some of these popular programs.

WATSU

Harold Dull began developing **WATSU** in 1980, floating his Zen shiatsu students in the warm pool at Harbin Hot Springs (California) while applying stretches and special movements (see Figure 5–4). In this program, the therapist and client are in a WATSU® pool with the water at a neutral temperature (the client should not get heated or cooled during the session). The therapist holds the client in various positions while creating movement through the water at the same time. The therapist maintains contact with the client throughout the treatment, and some stretching and rotating movements are involved. The treatment creates a profound sense of well-being, relaxation, and

WATSU
Form of hydrotherapy in which the therapist works with the client in a special pool, taking the client through a series of passive flowing motions.

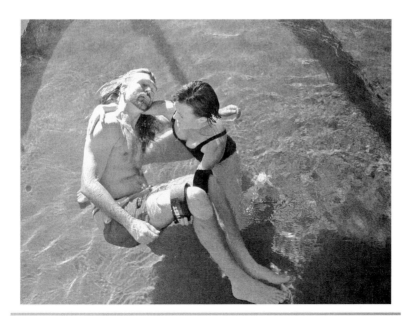

Figure 5–4 WATSU treatment *(courtesy of Grace Jull).*

emotional balance, as well as a greater sense of connection with nature. Buoyancy is one of the key water principles involved in WATSU, and the sensations created by being held, supported, and moved through the water produce very unique, positive experiences.

The transformation that takes place in a one-hour WATSU session is quite remarkable. Also remarkable is the growing popularity of WATSU in different countries and spas around the world. This very special form of hydrotherapy is continuing to evolve, and different, extended forms of WATSU are being taught by educational institutes approved to teach these programs. These programs can sometimes qualify for CEU credits. For information on educational resources for WATSU, please contact the Worldwide Aquatic Bodywork Association at www.waba.edu.

Aquatic Integration

Aquatic integration theory was developed by Cameron West, a certified massage therapist and adapted physical education teacher. Aquatic integration is a new approach to hydrotherapy that combines Eastern meridian and point work with myofascial release, proprioceptive neuromuscular facilitation, and breathwork. It is effective in restoring sensory perception, motor control, increasing range of motion, reducing muscular spasms, and for pain management. For more information on education for Aquatic integration, please visit www.aquaticintegration.com.

Kneipp Holistic Health Program

This program was developed by Father Sebastian Kneipp (1821–1897), who was born in Bad Worishofen in southeastern Germany. At the age of 15, he became sick with tuberculosis. Through intuitive insights and a natural connection with nature's healing process, he was able to cure himself by using simple hydrotherapy techniques, herbs, and exercises. Kneipp believed that nature provides everything needed to maintain optimal health, wellness, and fitness. He went on to develop a holistic healing program, **Kniepp therapy,** that could be used by anyone and was affordable to everyone. In his approach, the client is actively involved and takes personal responsibility for managing his or her own health and wellness. The program is based on the following natural principles:

Kneipp therapy
The holistic program of health and wellness that includes hydrotherapy, founded by Father Sebastian Kneipp in around 1875. The program is the foundation for modern hydrotherapy programs in Germany.

- Nutrition: A healthy, natural, and balanced diet
- Exercise: An active daily program that combines moving the body, sports activities, and strength training, all preferably done outdoors in natural settings

- Natural herbal medicinal remedies: The use of many natural herbs for different medicinal and wellness applications

- Hydrotherapy: Kneipp developed many hydrotherapy treatments, most using simple hydrotherapy equipment, including bath treatments (see Figure 5–5), single-hose showers, pouring water on the body, walking in hot and cold foot pools, and immersing the arms in cold and hot water. Special herbal preparations, including herbal compresses, are used in some of these treatments.

- Appreciation and connection with nature: Kneipp had a great appreciation of nature and the value of maintaining a conscious connection with nature. Therefore, a theme of the Kneipp program is to develop greater appreciation and connection with nature by spending time in beautiful natural settings. Visitors to Bad Worishofen can see this theme expressed in the many large and beautiful parks and herbal botanical gardens with special trails for nature walks (see Chapter 8).

At present, there is limited education on Kneipp programs available in English; most education is offered in Germany. However, there is usually one course in English every year. For more information, contact the Sebastian-Kneipp Schule in Bad Worishofen, Germany, at www.kneippschule.de.

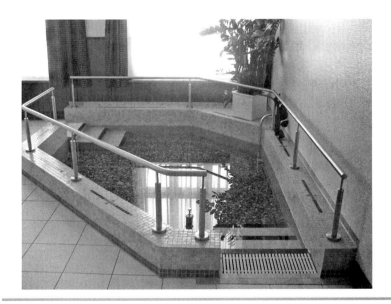

Figure 5–5 Kneipp hydrotherapy foot bath *(compliments of Edelweiss Hotel–Kneipp Therapy, <www.hotel-edelweiss.de>).*

Aquatic Therapy Pools

There have been recent developments in the designs of small hydro-therapy pools that include special features. These **aquatic therapy pools** are designed for physical therapy, sports conditioning, fitness, and the eldercare market. Aquatic therapy pools focus on maximizing water's therapeutic properties to accelerate rehabilitation and provide a nearly stress-free medium for exercise. Special training is provided by the manufacturers of this equipment. For information on resources for aquatic therapy pools, please search using the keyword "aquatic therapy pools" on the Internet.

Ayurveda

Ayurveda is a holistic system of health and wellness that originated in India thousands of years ago. Historical works on Ayurveda can be found in the ancient books of wisdom known as the Vedas. It is a science of life that allows a person to live in harmony with nature and to utilize the laws of nature to create health and balance within themselves. Ayurveda is a comprehensive program that helps maintain health by using natural principles to bring the individual back into equilibrium. The program includes diet, exercise (yoga), meditation, herbs, and oils. Hydrotherapy is an essential element of Ayurveda, which includes hydration, steam, and hydrotub (bath) treatments. It not only provides a healthy daily routine, but also incorporates programs for regular periods of renewal and rejuvenation (usually four times a year). The renewal programs are similar to the European tradition of yearly "health vacations" (see Chapter 8). One hydrotherapy treatment involves Ayurvedic massage followed by a steam treatment, known as swedhana. Another, known as naysya, involves facial massage, special herbs and oils, and steam inhalation therapy. These treatments are still being done in India, just as they have been for thousands of years, and have now become popular around the world (see Chapter 8).

Ayurvedic education is available in India and other countries. Proper use of Ayurvedic treatments requires specialized training at approved Ayurvedic educational institutes. For information on educational resources for Ayurveda, please search using the keyword "Ayurveda education" on the Internet.

Colon Therapy

Colon therapy, often known as colon hydrotherapy, is a technique that introduces purified water at regulated temperatures into the colon to soften and loosen any impacted matter. This matter is then evacuated through natural peristalsis. This process is repeated a few times during a session. Colon hydrotherapy is used in combination with adequate nutrient and fluid intake and exercise. Equipment for colon therapy promotes both the safety and sanitation of this popular cleansing practice. This cleansing practice has been termed colon hydrotherapy, because natural, pure water is the main cause of the cleansing. Education and training must be done through approved educational institutes, and specialized equipment is necessary. For information on educational resources for colon therapy, please contact the International Association for Colon Hydrotherapy at www.i-act.org.

 ## SUMMARY

This chapter describes the following key common elements found in the hydrotherapy treatments presented in this textbook. Although each type of hydrotherapy treatment is unique, they are all a combination of these same basic elements. Having a familiarity with these key elements helps therapists have a better understanding of the hydrotherapy treatments taught in Chapter 7. Also, when the full potential of each element of the hydrotherapy treatment is expressed, the full potential benefit of the treatment can be attained. This is expressed in the well-known saying, "The whole is greater than the sum of its parts." The hydrotherapy treatment elements are:

- Client: Age and gender; health and wellness goals
- Therapists: Massage, estheticians, cosmetologists, fitness, bodyworkers, physical and occupational therapists
- Products: Herbs, Moor mud, essential oils, hydrosols, seaweed and algea, mineral salts, and clay (mud)
- Hydrotherapy equipment: Hydrotubs, steam, shower, hydromassage table, misting, and compresses
- Water: The "essence" of a hydrotherapy treatment
- Steps of the treatment: Pretreatment, beginning the treatment, treatment, end of the treatment, and post-treatment
- Facility and hydrotherapy treatment room: Includes the design with special features for hydrotherapy and the décor

Although it is possible for a client to receive a single hydrotherapy treatment, most hydrotherapy treatments are combined with other types of treatments, such as massage. These packages of treatments allow clients to get the maximum benefit from a session. It is usually advisable to have a series of treatments at regular intervals in order to attain the goals of a client's personal health and wellness program. Clients are also generally given a program of treatments and products to use at home between sessions at the spa or wellness center. Many simple hydrotherapy treatments can be done safely at home using a bathtub, shower, or simple steam inhalation equipment.

Historically, hydrotherapy has been a key component of most holistic health and wellness programs, and continues to be so today. Today, many clients are again interested in holistic programs that help them achieve all of their health and wellness goals. Incorporating hydrotherapy as an element of a holistic program can significantly add to the therapeutic benefits of these programs.

This chapter also gives a brief overview of the different types of hydrotherapy treatments, including hydrotub treatments, underwater hydromassage, steam therapy, Vichy shower, misting, and hot and cold compresses. It also describes the many variations for each of these treatments that can be created by using different product combinations and other treatment variables.

The chapter concludes by listing several successful hydrotherapy programs that require training from approved educational institutions, including WATSU®, Ayurveda, Kneipp therapy holistic health, Aquatic Integration, aquatic therapy, and colon therapy.

SUGGESTED READING

Harrison, J., (2007). *Aromatherapy—Therapeutic Use of Essential Oils for Esthetics.* New York: Milady Publishing.

REVIEW QUESTIONS

1. What are the common elements of hydrotherapy treatments taught in this textbook?
2. What are some of the most important health and wellness goals of clients?
3. How can hydrotherapy treatments help clients achieve all of their health and wellness goals?
4. Describe several considerations when deciding to purchase hydrotherapy equipment.
5. List several different types of hydrotherapy equipment.

6. List different types of products that can be used during various types of hydrotherapy treatments.

7. Give some examples of single hydrotherapy treatments.

8. Give some examples of combination packages of treatments that include one or more hydrotherapy treatments.

9. Explain why hydrotherapy treatments could be of value in holistic health and wellness programs that are designed to help clients achieve all of their health and wellness goals.

10. List some different types of hydrotherapy treatments that can be performed using hydrotubs, steam, and shower equipment.

11. What are some special hydrotherapy programs that require education by certified educational institutions?

Hygiene and Safety

KEY TERMS

bacteria
methicillin-resistant
   Staphylococcus
   aureus (MRSA)
virus
yeast

mold
broad-spectrum
   disinfectant
contact time (dwell
   time)
lubricant

scald protection
pressure balance

INTRODUCTION

The use of water in hydrotherapy presents some special conditions and challenges in terms of maintaining hygiene and safety. This chapter looks at hygiene and safety, taking into consideration the total environment in which hydrotherapy treatments take place. As part of their studies, professional therapists, or students being trained as professional therapists, receive formal, comprehensive education on the principles of hygiene. This chapter is intended as a supplement to that education as it applies to hydrotherapy.

MAINTAINING A GERM-FREE ENVIRONMENT

Many types of microorganisms exist—some helpful, some neutral, and some harmful. The harmful ones, known as germs, can cause infection and disease. Most of these microorganisms survive, grow, and reproduce in water environments, including water inside the

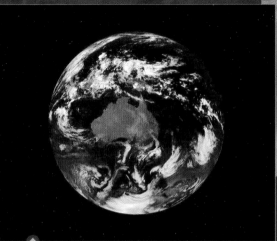

Plate 1 Hydrosphere Australia *(photo courtesy of NASA).*

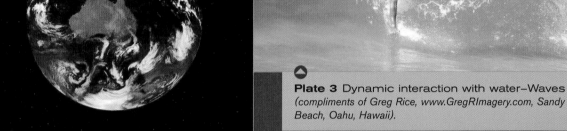

Plate 3 Dynamic interaction with water–Waves *(compliments of Greg Rice, www.GregRImagery.com, Sandy Beach, Oahu, Hawaii).*

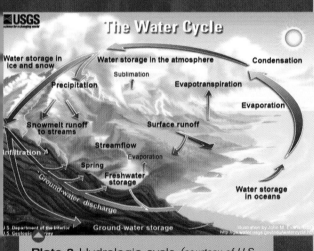

Plate 2 Hydrologic cycle *(courtesy of U.S. Department of the Interior/U.S. Geological Survey– http://ga.water.usgs.gov/edu/watercycle.html).*

Plate 4 Water Molecule.

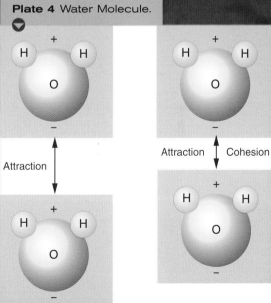

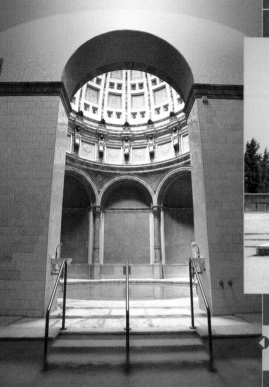

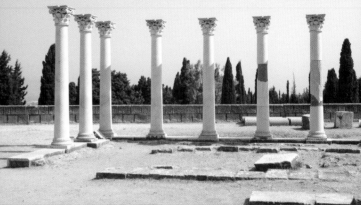

Plate 6 Ruins of Greek healing site on Island of Kos—Home of Hipprocates *(image copyright Yan Vugenfirer, 2008. Used under license from Shutterstock.com).*

Plate 5 Friedrichsbad Water Temple in Baden-Baden, Germany *(courtesy of CAMSAN, Baderbedriebe GmbH).*

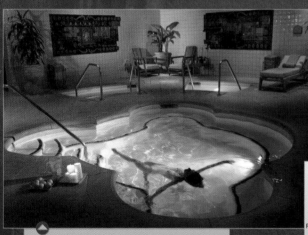

Plate 7 Hydrotherapy at Resort Spa *(courtesy of Marriott Hotel).*

Plate 8 Sources of water pollution.

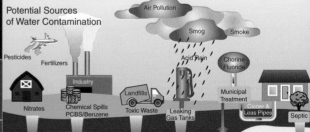

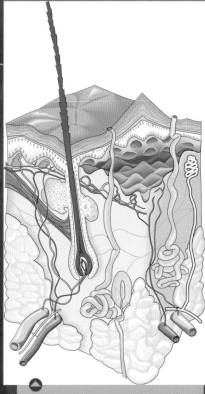

Plate 9 Skin–a fluid system.

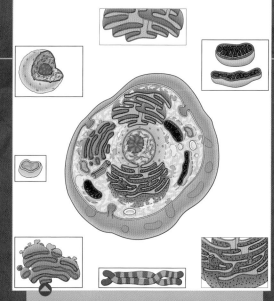

Plate 11 Human cell–a fluid system.

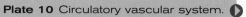

Plate 10 Circulatory vascular system.

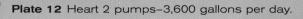

Plate 12 Heart 2 pumps–3,600 gallons per day.

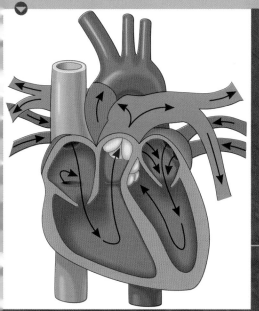

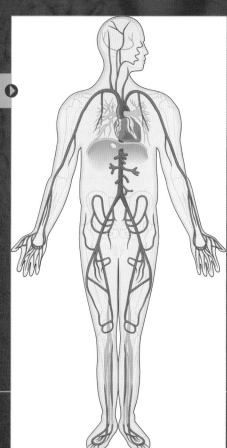

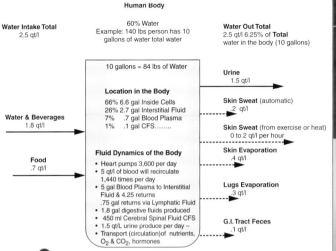

Human Body

60% Water
Example: 140 lbs person has 10 gallons of water total water

Water Intake Total
2.5 qt/l

Water Out Total
2.5 qt/l 6.25% of **Total**
water in the body (10 gallons)

10 gallons = 84 lbs of Water

Location in the Body
66% 6.6 gal Inside Cells
26% 2.7 gal Interstitial Fluid
7% .7 gal Blood Plasma
1% .1 gal CFS……..

Water & Beverages
1.8 qt/l

Food
.7 qt/l

Fluid Dynamics of the Body
- Heart pumps 3,600 per day
- 5 qt/l of blood will recirculate 1,440 times per day
- 5 gal Blood Plasma to Interstitial Fluid & 4.25 returns .75 gal returns via Lymphatic Fluid
- 1.8 gal digestive fluids produced
- 450 ml Cerebral Spinal Fluid CFS
- 1.5 qt/L urine produce per day –
- Transport (circulation) of nutrients, O_2 & CO_2, hormones

Urine
1.5 qt/l

Skin Sweat (automatic)
.2 qt/l

Skin Sweat (from exercise or heat)
0 to 2 qt/l per hour

Skin Evaporation
.4 qt/l

Lugs Evaporation
.3 qt/l

G.I. Tract Feces
.1 qt/l

Plate 13 Illustration of amount of water in the body.

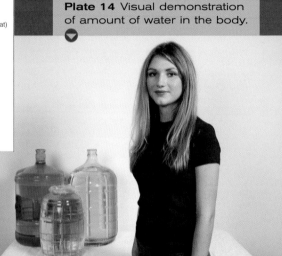

Plate 14 Visual demonstration of amount of water in the body.

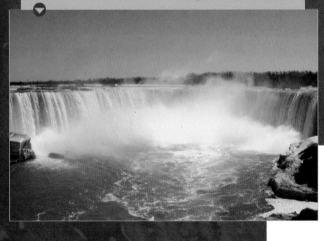

Plate 15 Flow water is energy–Niagara Falls.

Plate 16 Baby and water–Our earliest water experiences *(image copyright Zdorov Kirill Vladimirovich, 2008. Used under license by Shutterstock.com).*

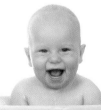

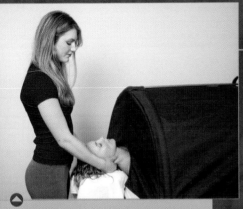

Plate 17 Massage during steam treatment.

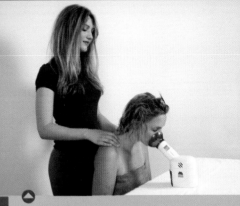

Plate 18 Steam inhalation treatment.

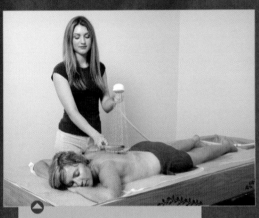

Plate 19 Handheld shower and exfoliation treatment.

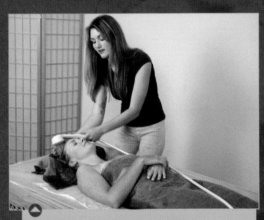

Plate 20 Handheld shower and head massage.

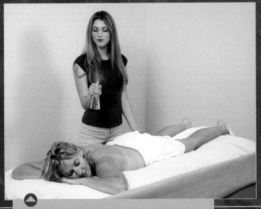

Plate 21 Misting hydrotherapy treatment–fully body.

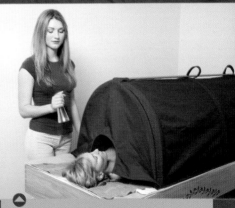

Plate 22 Misting during a steam treatment–cooling.

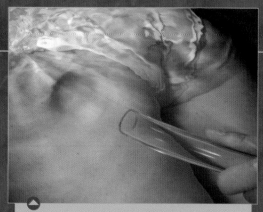

Plate 23 Hydromassage underwater cellulite treatment.

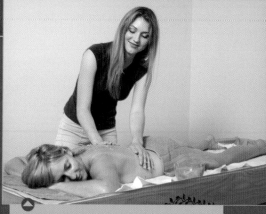

Plate 24 Wet-table and skincare product application.

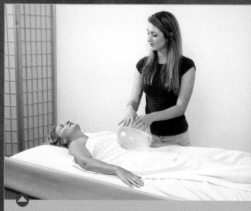

Plate 25 Dry hydromassage–stomach.

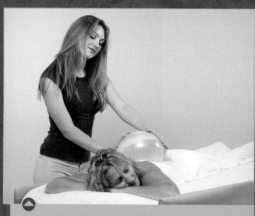

Plate 26 Dry hydromassage–back.

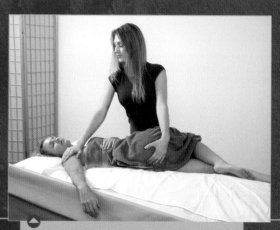

Plate 27 Hydromassage table–hip rotation.

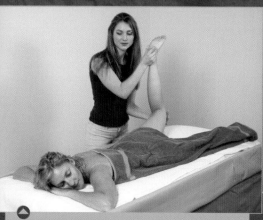

Plate 28 Hydromassage table–leg lift.

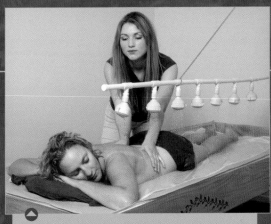

Plate 29 Vichy Shower.

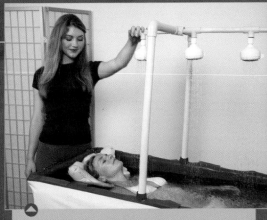

Plate 30 Vichy Shower in a hydrotub.

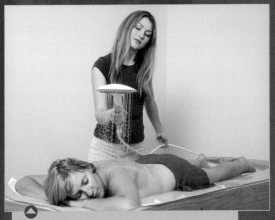

Plate 31 Handheld shower—large showerhead.

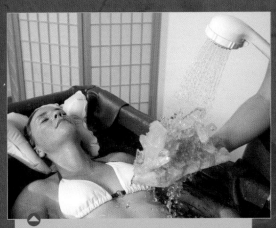

Plate 32 Energy crystal hydrotherapy treatment.

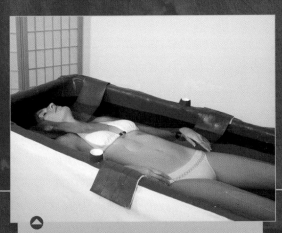

Plate 33 Hydrotub flotation treatment.

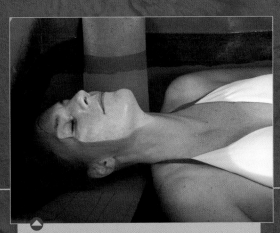

Plate 34 Hydrotub flotation treatment.

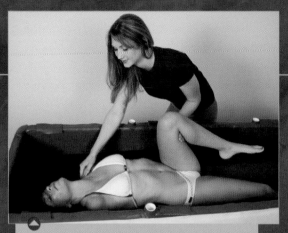

Plate 35 Hydrotub–Manipulation.

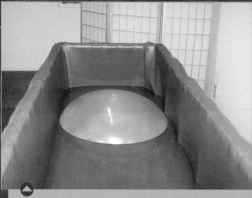

Plate 36 Hydroballoon in hydrotub.

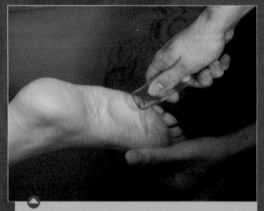

Plate 37 Hydromassage–Reflexology.

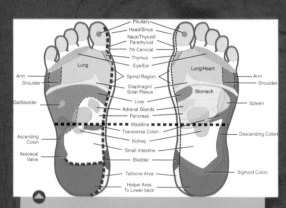

Plate 38 Reflexology chart.

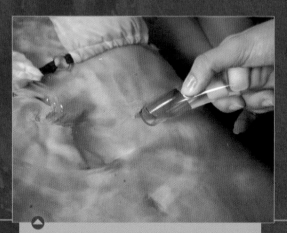

Plate 39 Hydromassage–Shiatsu.

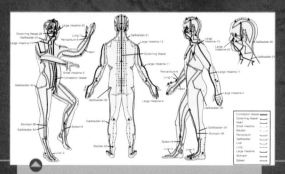

Plate 40 Shiatsu chart.

human body, water that has come from the human body, or water that has come in contact with the human body (e.g., during a hydrotherapy shower or steam treatment). Contaminated water, or water that contains germs, that comes from an infected person and ends up on hydrotherapy equipment or surfaces such as floors, can potentially infect another client or therapist who comes into contact with that water. Therefore, these germs must be removed (killed) after each treatment. What makes this process more complex in a hydrotherapy room is that these germs are relatively small and a large number of them can survive in a single drop of water.

A main hygiene concern in spas, salons, wellness, and fitness centers is maintaining a germ-free environment to prevent clients and therapists from becoming infected. By following proper hygiene procedures that meet local, state, and federal regulations and guidelines, these facilities can create optimal safety and hygienic conditions, protecting clients, therapists, and staff. The following is a review of the general principles of hygiene and safety, especially in a hydrotherapy treatment room.

DISEASE-CAUSING MICROORGANISMS

The main types of disease-causing microorganisms that can be transmitted from an infected person to another person through water (e.g., in a hydrotherapy room) are bacteria, viruses, and fungi. Even though these are microscopic organisms, it may be helpful to think of them as complex living systems that live, develop, and reproduce—size is relative. For a comparison of sizes, a small raindrop is about 500 μm in diameter, a red blood cell is 8 μm in diameter, bacteria are about 1 μm in diameter, and viruses are much smaller than bacteria. Thus, disease-causing microorganisms are of such size that they can enter into the cells of the human body. Once there, they can develop and reproduce, resulting in infection and disease. Because many of these microorganisms can survive in a single drop of water, all the water that remains in a hydrotherapy treatment room, as well as any surfaces where the water has come into contact with a client, must be disinfected.

Bacteria

Bacteria are single-cell, plantlike microorganisms. Most are helpful or even harmless, but a few can cause disease (see Figure 6–1). Once bacteria infect human body cells, they reproduce very rapidly simply

Bacteria
Single-cell, plantlike microorganisms, some of which cause disease.

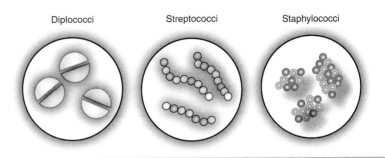

Figure 6-1 Disease-causing bacteria.

by splitting in two. Bacteria are classified by their shape—coccus, or round; bacillus, or rod shaped; and spirochetes, or spiral-shaped (see Figure 6–2). The average size of a bacterium is 1 µm, which is about one-tenth the diameter of a human cell.

Some bacteria when stained during microscopic examination turn blue; these are classified as gram positive. Bacteria that do not turn blue are classified as gram negative. This characteristic of bacteria is important to know because some chemicals used to kill bacteria work on only gram positive or only gram negative, while others kill both. Disinfectants used to clean a hydrotherapy room should kill both.

The following are some types of bacteria that are of concern to spa and wellness facilities:

- Pseudomonas: Thrive in warm, moist places.
- Staphylococcus: Can come from someone's hair, nails, or skin. Of special concern are the new strains of staphylococcus, known as MRSA **(methicillin-resistant *Staphylococcus aureus*),** that have developed a resistance to modern antibiotics and are more difficult to treat.
- Streptococcus: Can be transmitted from an infected person via water droplets from the mouth and lungs.
- Salmonella and *E. coli:* Can be transmitted via water that has come in contact with an infected person.
- Tuberculosis (TB) bacteria: Although this is not often found, it is of interest because it is the most difficult bacteria to kill. Disinfectants that kill TB bacteria are considered the most effective.

Methicillin-resistant *Staphylococcus aureus* (MRSA)
A strain of staphylococcus that has developed a resistance to modern antibiotics.

Viruses

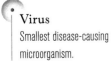

Virus
Smallest disease-causing microorganism.

A **virus** is the smallest disease-causing microorganism. Some viruses can be transmitted to a person only by direct contact with body fluids, such as blood, of an infected person (e.g., the HIV virus).

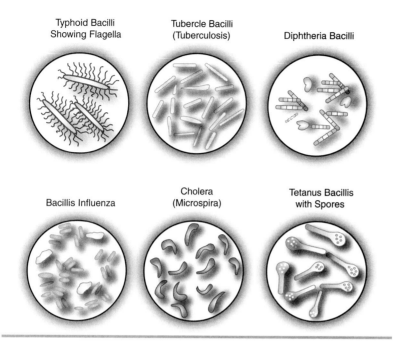

Typhoid Bacilli
Showing Flagella

Tubercle Bacilli
(Tuberculosis)

Diphtheria Bacilli

Bacillis Influenza

Cholera
(Microspira)

Tetanus Bacillis
with Spores

Figure 6–2 Groupings of bacteria.

Other viruses, such as the common cold and the influenza and herpes viruses, can be spread much more easily via microscopic water droplets from an infected person's breath or saliva. Water droplets are transferred from an infected person's mouth to his or her hands and then to surfaces, such as doorknobs or tables. When another person touches those objects, he or she may become infected. This is one reason colds and the flu are so contagious.

The following are some types of viruses that may be of concern to spa and wellness facilities:

- Cold and flu viruses
- Hepatitis
- Herpes
- HIV: This is transmitted by contact with blood or other bodily fluids from an infected person. It is not transmitted via water droplets.

Fungi

Microfungi are multicellular organisms, some of which can cause disease in human beings. There are two basic types of microfungi:

- **Yeasts** produce diseases such as ringworm, nail fungus, and athlete's foot. Spores from an infected person can be

Yeast
Microfungi that produce diseases such as ringworm, nail fungus, and athlete's foot.

transmitted to hydrotherapy equipment, floors, and surfaces in wet rooms and steam rooms. Spores are more resistant to disinfectants and are one reason why it is important to use proper grade disinfectants.

● **Molds,** which tend to grow and reproduce in warm moist conditions, can produce respiratory irritation and allergies in some individuals. It is imperative that molds not be allowed to grow in hydrotherapy treatment rooms and equipment. To help prevent the growth of molds, it is important for all areas of the hydrotherapy equipment and treatment room to be completely air dry. There should not be any areas where water accumulates, especially in hidden or hard to reach areas.

Mold
Microfungi that grows in warm, moist conditions and that can produce respiratory irritation and allergies.

HYDROTHERAPY TREATMENT ROOM HYGIENE

During a hydrotherapy treatment, a therapist brings water into contact with the client's body, primarily in the form of immersion in water, showering, or steam. In the case of a bath or shower (see Figure 6–3), the water flows over the client's body to a drain and then out of the room. In the case of steam, the water is removed from the client by a towel and/or a shower. During these treatments, water usually comes into contact with the *entire* surface area of the client's body. Thus, any microorganisms on the surface of the body can mix with the water. This water will then come into contact with the surface that the client is on, as well as with any sheets or towels the client uses. This water can also come into contact with floors and other surfaces, as in a steam room or wet room.

As mentioned earlier, water is a very effective way for disease-causing microorganisms to travel from an infected person to another individual. Whether the other individual becomes infected will depend on his or her health, the number of specific germs in the water, and other immunological variables.

Steps of Hydrotherapy Room Hygiene

Step 1: Cleaning

Immediately following a hydrotherapy treatment, after the client has left the room, any hydrotherapy equipment and surfaces in wet rooms and steam rooms must be thoroughly cleaned using suitable

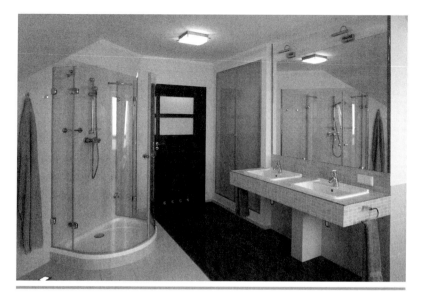

Figure 6–3 Shower facility *(image copyright Tomasz Markowski, 2008. Used under license from Shutterstock.com).*

cleaning procedures and products to remove hair, skin cells, body oils, and any other substances. Cleaning products will kill some germs, but they are *not* designed to disinfect at a level that is considered hygienic for hydrotherapy treatment rooms and equipment.

Step 2: Disinfection

Any hydrotherapy equipment and surfaces that have come into contact with water that has come into contact with the client's body must be disinfected. It is important to use a disinfectant with a proper level of efficacy for this purpose. **Broad-spectrum disinfectants** are high-grade disinfectants that are classified to kill the range of germs generally found in a hydrotherapy rooms and equipment. When used properly, these high-grade disinfectants will kill the germs that can cause infection.

BROAD-SPECTRUM DISINFECTANTS: Broad-spectrum disinfectants, especially those that kill TB bacteria, are effective in disinfecting hydrotherapy rooms and equipment. Some broad-spectrum disinfectants use mostly natural ingredients, which may have a greater appeal for use in certain spa and wellness centers. Commercial disinfectants, including all broad-spectrum disinfectants, must be registered with the EPA and will have the registration number listed on the label. The label will also state the level of efficacy—that is, which germs it kills. It will also list any

Broad-spectrum disinfectant

A high-grade disinfectant that kills the normal range of germs, that are often found in a hydrotherapy rooms and equipment.

warning for use and handling. The following is an example label (see Figure 6–4):

- Registration Number 74771-1
- Broad-Spectrum Efficacy
  Kills over 99.9% of all germs
  Bacteria (Gram + and −).
  Fungi
  TB bacteria
  HIV
- No Warning

This label gives the registration number and lists that it is broad-spectrum disinfectant. It states that this particular disinfectant kills both gram positive (gram +) and gram negative (gram −) bacteria, as well as fungi and the HIV virus. The label also indicates that this disinfectant can kill the TB bacteria, which indicates that it is a highly effective disinfectant.

   When using a disinfectant, it is essential to follow the manufacturer's directions for use. It is especially important to note how long the disinfectant must remain on the surface to be effective. This is known as **contact time** or **dwell time.**

   To find disinfectants, search the Internet for keywords "disinfectant" or "broad-spectrum disinfectant." Study the features, instructions for use, warnings, and benefits for each product. Be sure to check for EPA verification. If desired, the word "natural" could be added to the search to find potentially less-toxic disinfecting products.

Contact time (dwell time)

The time required to leave a disinfectant on a surface in order to be effective.

RECIRCULATING HYDROTHERAPY EQUIPMENT

A special concern regarding hygiene is hydrotherapy equipment that recirculates water over a part of or the entire body of a client. Examples of such equipment include a hydrotub, hot tub, or pedicure footbath. This type of equipment needs added attention in terms of cleaning and disinfection because water that comes into contact with the client's body recirculates through the pump and pumping system after the treatment. If not properly cleaned and disinfected, bacteria and other germs can rapidly grow and reproduce throughout the system. The following steps should be followed when cleaning and disinfecting recirculating equipment after a treatment:

- Research to ensure that the equipment has been designed to allow it to be safely disinfected. This should be done before buying any equipment. You should feel comfortable that the manufacturer has adequate hygiene standards and instructions to disinfect the equipment.

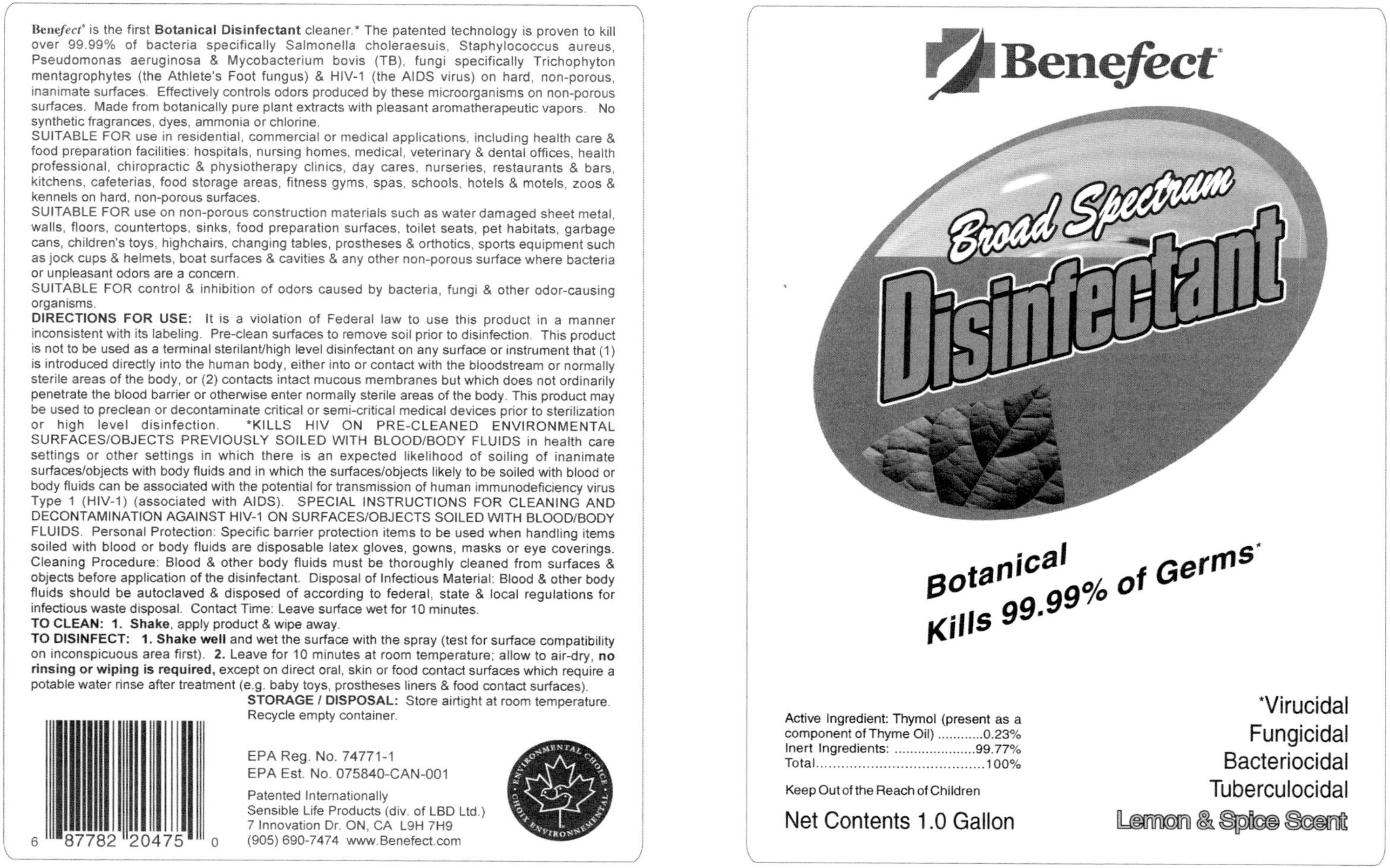

Benefect's is the first **Botanical Disinfectant** cleaner.* The patented technology is proven to kill over 99.99% of bacteria specifically Salmonella choleraesuis, Staphylococcus aureus, Pseudomonas aeruginosa & Mycobacterium bovis (TB), fungi specifically Trichophyton mentagrophytes (the Athlete's Foot fungus) & HIV-1 (the AIDS virus) on hard, non-porous, inanimate surfaces. Effectively controls odors produced by these microorganisms on non-porous surfaces. Made from botanically pure plant extracts with pleasant aromatherapeutic vapors. No synthetic fragrances, dyes, ammonia or chlorine.

SUITABLE FOR use in residential, commercial or medical applications, including health care & food preparation facilities: hospitals, nursing homes, medical, veterinary & dental offices, health professional, chiropractic & physiotherapy clinics, day cares, nurseries, restaurants & bars, kitchens, cafeterias, food storage areas, fitness gyms, spas, schools, hotels & motels, zoos & kennels on hard, non-porous surfaces.

SUITABLE FOR use on non-porous construction materials such as water damaged sheet metal, walls, floors, countertops, sinks, food preparation surfaces, toilet seats, pet habitats, garbage cans, children's toys, highchairs, changing tables, prostheses & orthotics, sports equipment such as jock cups & helmets, boat surfaces & cavities & any other non-porous surface where bacteria or unpleasant odors are a concern.

SUITABLE FOR control & inhibition of odors caused by bacteria, fungi & other odor-causing organisms.

DIRECTIONS FOR USE: It is a violation of Federal law to use this product in a manner inconsistent with its labeling. Pre-clean surfaces to remove soil prior to disinfection. This product is not to be used as a terminal sterilant/high level disinfectant on any surface or instrument that (1) is introduced directly into the human body, either into or contact with the bloodstream or normally sterile areas of the body, or (2) contacts intact mucous membranes but which does not ordinarily penetrate the blood barrier or otherwise enter normally sterile areas of the body. This product may be used to preclean or decontaminate critical or semi-critical medical devices prior to sterilization or high level disinfection. *KILLS HIV ON PRE-CLEANED ENVIRONMENTAL SURFACES/OBJECTS PREVIOUSLY SOILED WITH BLOOD/BODY FLUIDS in health care settings or other settings in which there is an expected likelihood of soiling of inanimate surfaces/objects with body fluids and in which the surfaces/objects likely to be soiled with blood or body fluids can be associated with the potential for transmission of human immunodeficiency virus Type 1 (HIV-1) (associated with AIDS). SPECIAL INSTRUCTIONS FOR CLEANING AND DECONTAMINATION AGAINST HIV-1 ON SURFACES/OBJECTS SOILED WITH BLOOD/BODY FLUIDS. Personal Protection: Specific barrier protection items to be used when handling items soiled with blood or body fluids are disposable latex gloves, gowns, masks or eye coverings. Cleaning Procedure: Blood & other body fluids must be thoroughly cleaned from surfaces & objects before application of the disinfectant. Disposal of Infectious Material: Blood & other body fluids should be autoclaved & disposed of according to federal, state & local regulations for infectious waste disposal. Contact Time: Leave surface wet for 10 minutes.

TO CLEAN: 1. Shake, apply product & wipe away.

TO DISINFECT: 1. Shake well and wet the surface with the spray (test for surface compatibility on inconspicuous area first). **2.** Leave for 10 minutes at room temperature; allow to air-dry, **no rinsing or wiping is required**, except on direct oral, skin or food contact surfaces which require a potable water rinse after treatment (e.g. baby toys, prostheses liners & food contact surfaces).

STORAGE / DISPOSAL: Store airtight at room temperature. Recycle empty container.

EPA Reg. No. 74771-1
EPA Est. No. 075840-CAN-001

Patented Internationally
Sensible Life Products (div. of LBD Ltd.)
7 Innovation Dr. ON, CA L9H 7H9
(905) 690-7474 www.Benefect.com

6 87782 20475 0

*Virucidal
Fungicidal
Bacteriocidal
Tuberculocidal

Lemon & Spice Scent

Botanical
Kills 99.99% of Germs

Active Ingredient: Thymol (present as a
component of Thyme Oil) 0.23%
Inert Ingredients: 99.77%
Total.................................100%

Keep Out of the Reach of Children

Net Contents 1.0 Gallon

Figure 6–4 Broad-spectrum disinfectant label (*courtesy of Benefect®*).

- Research to ensure that the manufacturer's instructions for cleaning and disinfecting meet local, state, and federal regulations and guidelines.
- Research to ensure that the system can be disinfected with a broad-spectrum disinfectant or that the disinfecting products recommended by the manufacturer meet the criteria of a broad-spectrum disinfectant.
- Carefully follow the equipment manufacturer's instructions for cleaning and disinfecting the system after every treatment.

A few spas and salons have had problems with clients becoming infected from exposure to contaminated water. For example, in California and a few other states that use recirculating pedicure foot baths, some clients contracted serious staphylococcus infections because the equipment was not properly disinfected between treatments.

Step 3: Drying Hydrotherapy Equipment and Room Surfaces

All hydrotherapy equipment and rooms should be wiped as dry as possible and then left to naturally air dry. Water can flow into the smallest spaces. In addition, as water condenses from steam to liquid water, as occurs in a steam room, it can remain as moisture and may not easily evaporate. It is important to ensure that water does not collect in areas where it cannot easily dry (e.g., under benches in a steam room or on hidden areas of hydrotherapy equipment). Preventing water from collecting in such areas will help eliminate the growth of any molds and bacteria in the hydrotherapy equipment and treatment room.

SAFETY IN THE HYDROTHERAPY ROOM

Client Showers Before the Hydrotherapy Treatment

It is always advised for the client to shower thoroughly before receiving a hydrotherapy treatment. This is especially important in the use of steam rooms, hot tubs, or other types of communal pools, but is also recommended before any full-body hydrotherapy treatment. This is a tradition followed at hydrotherapy centers in Europe and Japan and usually anywhere a communal pool is involved. This decreases the risk of contamination of the hydrotherapy room and equipment and is also safer for the therapist. This may not always be possible in small facilities that may use the hydrotherapy room for showering the client after a massage, steam, or some other type of treatment and that do not have a regular shower stall, but it is recommended whenever possible.

Protection from Slippery Surfaces

The use of water in hydrotherapy treatments creates some special safety issues. Water, which is a natural **lubricant,** can make footing slippery, especially when getting out of a hydrotub or walking on a wet room or steam room floor.

Lubricant
A substance that lessens friction, such as water on a hard, smooth surface.

When a client uses their hands for support on smooth, hard surfaces that have become wet, this may cause a client to slip. The possibility of a client falling due to slippery floors or equipment presents special liability concerns for a spa or wellness center, so caution must be taken to limit any accidents. One precaution is to use antislip mats on any surfaces that may become wet. Clients can also wear slippers that are designed to be slip-resistant on wet floors. In addition, a therapist should, whenever possible, assist clients as they get into or out of a hydrotub, get off or on a wet table, or enter or leave a steam room.

Another safety concern of some hydrotherapy treatments is that clients can become dizzy, may lack normal balance, or can be more likely to faint or fall. Heating treatments, such as steam room or hot hydrotub therapies, produce a natural response by the body to reduce the body's temperature. Blood flow is significantly increased to the skin to allow heat to radiate from the body. The average person has 5 qt (5 L) of blood, and usually only a small percentage (8%) of this blood flows through the skin. During a cooling response, however, the body can increase the blood flow to the skin by up to 30%. Thus, standing or sitting up immediately after a treatment can make a person feel dizzy or faint, as the body is not able to direct enough blood flow to the brain. Similarly, after some hydrotherapy treatments, the effects of buoyancy, as occurs during a flotation treatment or a relaxing hydrotub treatment, may cause the client to lose his or her normal sense of balance when standing or trying to walk. Once again, it is important for the therapist to assist the client, whenever possible, when standing or sitting up after such treatments. Assisting the client at the end of certain treatments will not only limit potential accidents but will also add a personal touch to the hydrotherapy treatment. Personalized treatments with special attention to client's needs is an important element of a total session at a spa or wellness center.

Scald Protection

All water sources in a spa or wellness center—including sinks, showers, bathtubs, and hydrotubs—should have **scald protection,** a feature that prevents the temperature from becoming scalding or uncomfortably hot. Some local and state regulations require that this feature be included, while others limit this regulation to showers. Still other regulations do not require any scald protection. However, even if there are no government regulations regarding scalding, all Vichy, Swiss, and handheld showers, as well as any custom-made systems, should have scald protection. This will protect the client in case a therapist or the client accidentally increases the water temperature to an unsafe range.

Pressure Balancing

Ideally, Vichy and Swiss showers should include a **pressure balancing** feature that prevents fluctuations in water pressure and temperature if someone else uses water elsewhere in the facility. Most professional Vichy and Swiss showers have this feature. With this feature, if someone flushes a toilet or uses a washing machine somewhere in the facility, the temperature and pressure of the water during the treatment will remain constant.

Steam Safety

When using steam therapy equipment (e.g., steam canopies, cabinets, capsules, and rooms), always make sure that steam from the steam generator does not come into direct or even close contact with the client's skin. This situation occurs more often than it should, in part because the poor design of some steam therapy equipment. It is also very important to get feedback from the client during the steam treatment. Instruct the client that he or she should tell you as soon as there is any problem or discomfort with the steam coming into contact with his or her body.

When doing inhalation therapy for the sinus areas and lungs, it is important to use safe equipment that is manufactured specifically for this purpose (Figure 7–5). Some books recommend doing this type of inhalation treatment using water at or near the boiling point in a pan or bowl next to the client, with a sheet or towel covering the client and the bowl so that the client can breathe in the steam. This is very dangerous as the pan or bowl could accidentally be tipped over, scalding the client. Always use safe equipment specifically designed for this purpose.

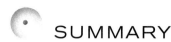

SUMMARY

Hydrotherapy treatments present some special challenges regarding safety and hygiene. During hydrotherapy treatments, water usually comes in contact with the entire surface of the client's body, and any germs on the body can be transferred to the water. This water will then come into contact with the hydrotherapy equipment and possibly with other surfaces, including floors in wet rooms. Therefore all areas of the hydrotherapy equipment and room must be cleaned and disinfected after every treatment. Because many disease-causing microorganisms (germs) survive, or even thrive, in water, the following hygiene procedures must always be followed:

- Proper cleaning to remove skin cells, body oils, or hair from equipment and other surfaces.

- A high-grade, preferably broad-spectrum, disinfectant must be used to disinfect all hydrotherapy equipment and surfaces after every treatment. Broad-spectrum disinfectants that are classified to kill TB bacteria are the most effective. Every disinfectant must be registered with the EPA, and its effectiveness, along with any warnings as to its use, should be noted on the label. Disinfectants must be used according to the directions, especially regarding the contact and dwell time.

- All surfaces of the hydrotherapy equipment and treatment room should be able to air dry and, if necessary, be wiped dry. Hidden areas where water might collect must be dried to prevent mold and other germs from growing. This is especially the case for steam rooms and wet rooms.

There are also special safety concerns regarding hydrotherapy treatments. Because water is a lubricant, it can make surfaces, such as hydrotubs and tile floors in wet rooms, slippery. This increases the risk of clients slipping while getting on or off hydrotherapy equipment or while walking on slippery floors. Some clients may feel dizzy or unbalanced after steam and hydrotub treatments due to reduced blood flow to the brain or to the relaxing effects of buoyancy. Therefore, whenever possible, it is highly recommended that therapists assist clients as they get onto (or into) and off (out of) hydrotherapy equipment or when they walk on slippery wet room floors. Slippers should also be provided to prevent clients from slipping on wet floors.

Any hydrotherapy equipment that uses recirculating water, such as a hydrotub, hot tub, or pedicure bath, must be adequately disinfected after every use. If these systems are not cleaned properly, germs will rapidly reproduce and could then come into contact with future clients. When purchasing such equipment, it is important to make sure that the equipment can be properly disinfected and comes with detailed instructions for disinfection.

Vichy, Swiss, and handheld showers should have scald protection to prevent any accidental increase in water temperature to an uncomfortable or scalding range. If possible, the equipment should also contain pressure balancing to prevent any fluctuation in water temperature and pressure during the treatment. When using steam therapy equipment, such as steam rooms, cabinets, or canopies, make sure that the steam coming directly from the steam generator cannot come into direct contact with the client's skin.

It is also recommended, whenever possible, for clients to shower thoroughly before getting any full-body hydrotherapy treatments.

SUGGESTED READINGS

Beck, M. (2006). "Sanitary and Safety Practices." In *Theory and Practice of Massage* (4th ed.). Albany, New York: Thomson Delmar Learning.

Chesky, S., Cristina, I., Rosenberg, R., (1994). *Playing It Safe: Milady's Guide to Decontamination, Sterilization, and Personal Protection*. Albany, New York: Milady Publishing.

Gerson, J. (2006). "Sanitation and Disinfection." In *Milady's Standard Fundamentals for Estheticians*. Albany, New York: Milady Publishing.

Guyton, A. C., & Hall, J. E. (2005). *Textbook of Medical Physiology* (11th ed.).

REVIEW QUESTIONS

1. Discuss the special conditions associated with hydrotherapy treatments that create special hygiene issues?
2. What are the three main categories of disease causing germs?
3. What are the three steps to follow for hygiene in hydrotherapy rooms and treatments?
4. What is the difference between cleaning and disinfecting?

5. What is broad-spectrum disinfectant?

6. What is considered to be the most difficult bacteria to kill?

7. What are the two things that can be done to help clients from slipping on wet surfaces in a hydrotherapy treatment room?

8. Why might a client feel dizzy after a heating treatment?

9. Why does hydrotherapy equipment that recirculates water over the human body require added hygiene measures?

10. Why should Vichy and Swiss shower equipment have scald protection and pressure balancing?

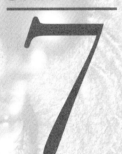

Hydrotherapy Treatments

KEY TERMS

broad-spectrum
  disinfectant

cold induced vaso-
  dilatation (VSD)

hunting response
hypothermia

INTRODUCTION

This chapter provides education on performing a variety of hydrotherapy treatments, including hydrotub, steam, and shower treatments. The training for each treatment follows a standard format, including step-by-step instructions, as well as suggestions for products and other elements that will enhance the benefits of the treatment. The treatments are divided into several general categories, including steam treatments, full-body hydrotub treatments, shower treatments, plus a few special categories. Each category begins with a general introduction that discusses aspects common to all the treatments within that category, including contraindications and other safety issues. The hydrotherapy treatments presented in each category cover a range of therapies that can be performed by therapists from different professions. These treatments can be further customized through the use of different products, length of treatment, combination with other treatments, and so forth. With the hydrotherapy treatments presented in this chapter, you will be able to formulate treatments and programs that meet the special needs of your private practice, spa, or health and wellness center. This chapter begins with a discussion of the client evaluation.

NOTE: MANY SCIENTIFIC RESEARCH STUDIES THAT HAVE BEEN DONE ON HYDROTHERAPY FOR EACH OF THE MAIN CATEGORIES ARE PRESENTED IN DETAIL IN THE ON-LINE COMPANION.

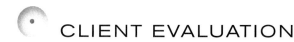

CLIENT EVALUATION

All therapy programs involve an initial client evaluation to determine the client's health and wellness issues and goals. Based on this information, which should include all relevant information regarding the client's medical history, you can recommend a treatment program, which may range from a single treatment to a series of treatments or a permanent program that is part of a larger total health and wellness program. Client evaluations are a key element of any therapy program and an essential element of a hydrotherapy program. The following are some suggestions for the client interview (see Chapter 5).

Client Feedback on Health and Wellness Goals

During the interview, you should ask the client about his or her health and wellness goals for each area in the following list. You can use the Health and Wellness Goals form (see Table 7–1) to take notes regarding your client's key health and wellness goals, as well as any additional relevant information. This form also includes a place for you to note the different hydrotherapy treatments that can be recommended as part of a treatment program regarding each goal.

> **NOTE:** THE HEALTH AND WELLNESS GOALS FORM IS AVAILABLE ON THE ON-LINE COMPANION FOR THIS TEXTBOOK ALONG WITH SEVERAL EXAMPLES OF CLIENT INTERVIEWS.

Health and Wellness Goals

- Daily wellness
- Appearance and beauty
- Fitness
- Healthy aging
- Prevention
- Enhancement
- Symptoms
- Rehabilitation
- Major medical

Using the information from the form and the client interview, you can recommend hydrotherapy treatments and programs that address the client's health and wellness goals. Different hydrotherapy

Table 7–1 Health and Wellness Goals: Hydrotherapy Treatment Program

Name: _____   Date: _____

Daily Wellness

_____

Hydrotherapy Treatments and Programs

_____

Appearance and Beauty

_____

Hydrotherapy Treatments and Programs

_____

Fitness

_____

Hydrotherapy Treatments and Programs

_____

Healthy Aging

_____

Hydrotherapy Treatments and Programs

_____

Table 7–1 Health and Wellness Goals: Hydrotherapy Treatment Program (*continued*)

Prevention

Hydrotherapy Treatments and Programs

_____

Enhancement

Hydrotherapy Treatments and Programs

_____

Symptoms

Hydrotherapy Treatments and Programs

_____

Rehabilitation

Hydrotherapy Treatments and Programs

_____

Major Medical

Hydrotherapy Treatments and Programs (physician approval)

_____

treatments and programs, usually in combination with other types of treatments, can be used, depending on your client's goals.

Clients often are not as familiar with hydrotherapy as they are with massage and esthetic programs. Therefore, the client interview, evaluation, and recommendations regarding hydrotherapy treatments and programs are especially important to explain the benefits of a hydrotherapy program, rather than having clients depend on information from brochures. In general, clients know what improvements they want, but they are looking for professional advice from trained therapists regarding the programs they should include.

Client Feedback on Previous Experience with Hydrotherapy

It is also recommended that you ask for feedback from any clients who have had previous experience with hydrotherapy or other important experiences with water.

- *Any previous experience with hydrotub, steam, or shower treatments:* This could have been anywhere, with or without a therapist. Did they enjoy the treatments? Did they find anything uncomfortable about the treatments—for example did they find the water or steam temperature too hot in a steam room, hot tub, or hydrotub? Some people may have had great experiences, while others may have had negative experiences, usually with getting too hot or too cold. Find out whether your client has any special concerns.

- *The client's relationship with water in natural settings:* Many people have experienced a profound sense of well-being from being in the ocean, a lake, or river. Many have spent time at natural hot springs. Based on these experiences, they may have a deep connection with water and an appreciation for its transforming powers. Some clients, however, may have a fear of water. Still others may have no real sense of connection with water, one way or the other. You may find it helpful knowing whether a client really appreciates water or has any anxiety relating to water.

- *Any special modesty issues:* For many hydrotherapy treatments, clients can be draped similar to the way they may be draped during massage or full-body esthetic treatments. However, there can be some special challenges with draping during certain hydrotherapy treatments. Client comfort is what is most important. If necessary, a client can wear a bathing suit or some other form of special spa clothing during a treatment.

BASIC TREATMENT FORMAT

Each hydrotherapy treatment taught in this chapter is explained following the same format. This treatment format consists of the following elements.

Description and Benefits

This section provides a general explanation of the treatment. It also describes benefits that a client can expect from the treatment. In addition, by knowing from the client interview what are the client's health and wellness goals, the benefits of a specific hydrotherapy treatment can be discussed with the client in relationship to those goals.

Equipment

This section describes the hydrotherapy equipment that is used in the treatment. Depending on the treatment, there may be different options, as there are usually several different types of hydrotherapy systems that can be used for a specific treatment. Specific manufacturers of hydrotherapy equipment will not be listed, as they are constantly changing and it may not be possible to include all of them. However, resources for locating specific types of hydrotherapy can be found in the Hydrotherapy Equipment Resource Guide in Appendix B. This resource guide provides information on how to locate company Web sites; lists of trade magazines and trade shows in the spa, esthetic, and massage industries; and other resources useful for locating hydrotherapy equipment.

Products

This section suggests natural products that can be used with the treatment. Refer to Chapter 5 for the general categories of natural products that are suitable for use with hydrotherapy treatments. As with equipment, this section will list types of products, but it will not provide specific manufacturers. See the Hydrotherapy Product Resource Guide in Appendix C for information on finding products for use with hydrotherapy treatments.

Steps of the Treatment

1. *Pretreatment:* This step deals with anything that needs to be done before the treatment begins or before the client enters the room—for example, filling a hydrotub or turning on a steam generator.

2. *Beginning the treatment:* These steps need to be done from the time the client enters the room to the time the actual treatment begins—for example, the client getting into a hydrotub.

3. *Treatment:* These are step-by-step procedures for performing the main part of the hydrotherapy treatment.

4. *End of the treatment:* This is what must be done from the time the main part of the treatment ends to the time the client leaves the treatment room—for example, getting out of the hydrotub, drying, and so forth.

5. *Post-treatment:* Regarding the client, this step can include resting after the treatment or perhaps drinking water or herbal teas. The therapist would suggest this as part of the total treatment. For the therapist, post-treatment includes cleaning and disinfecting the room and hydrotherapy equipment and making the treatment room ready for the next client.

Additional Suggestions

The following types of suggestions will be provided, when necessary, for a specific hydrotherapy treatment:

- Reminders of contraindications or safety concerns
- Tips on treatment variations—for example, different techniques and products
- Special suggestions regarding clients, such as doing treatments on older/elderly or overweight clients
- Suggestions on combining this treatment with another treatment or including this treatment in a series of treatments over an extended period of time

HYDROTHERAPY TREATMENTS: GENERAL PRINCIPLES AND SPECIFIC TREATMENTS

A description of the components of a treatment that are common to all the hydrotherapy treatments within a specific category is provided in each section. This information is not repeated for each specific treatment. Following the description of the common elements for a particular category, instructions are provided for performing specific hydrotherapy treatments within that category.

Steam Therapy

COMMON ELEMENTS OF STEAM THERAPY

Dynamic Water Principles

The following list describes how water is used in steam therapy treatments. After the water has been transformed into steam, it is brought into contact with the client's body to produce various health and wellness transformations and benefits.

1. Heat is added to water in the liquid form, bringing the water to the boiling point (212°F/100°C) and converting it to water in the gas (vapor) state. The greater the amount of heat added to the water, the greater the amount of steam generated and the quicker the water will come to a boil.

2. The steam expands and rises to fill the space in the steam cabinet, capsule, canopy, or steam room. Because steam rises so quickly, the temperature at the higher areas of the space will be hotter than it is in the lower areas.

3. As the steam cools, it condenses back into the liquid state, releasing heat. The steam will condense on the client's skin and on the canopy, capsule, or cabinet. In the small space of a steam cabinet, capsule, or canopy, only about 1 qt (1 L) of water is necessary for approximately a 30-minute steam treatment. A much greater amount of water is necessary to heat a steam room, depending on the size of the room. Energy—usually electricity or gas—is required to heat the water to generate the steam.

4. Heat exchange will occur between the steam and the client's body in the steam cabinet, capsule, canopy, or steam room. The greater the temperature created by the steam, the greater (quicker) will be the heat exchange (heating) of the client's skin and core body temperature. As water condenses on the skin, the level of moisture on the skin will increase.

Steam Temperature: Hotter Is Not Necessarily Better

NOTE: FOR CONVERSION FROM FAHRENHEIT TO CENTIGRADE, SEE FAHRENHEIT AND CENTIGRADE CONVERSION IN APPENDIX A.

The temperature of the space in a steam canopy, capsule, cabinet, or room is usually between 105°F (40.5°C) and 122°F (50°C).

The humidity in the space is 100%, which negates any cooling effect from the body sweating, as sweat cannot evaporate in 100% humidity. As mentioned earlier, the temperature of the space will be hotter at higher areas in the system than at lower areas, because steam rises very quickly.

The same temperature is not suitable for all clients. Clients who are more sensitive to heat need the steam temperature to be lower than average—perhaps as low as 105°F (40.5°C)—in order to feel comfortable. These clients will often give feedback that they do not like being in a steam room because they find it to be too hot. Remember: A temperature of 105°F (40.5°C) with 100% humidity is actually very hot, as the body cannot cool off by sweating. However, other clients, due to their unique body type, need a higher temperature before they can experience the full effects of a steam treatment. For these clients, a temperature of about 122°F (50°C) may be required. For most people, a temperature of 105°F (40.5°C) to 115°F (46.1°C) is a comfortable range.

> **NOTE:** SOME BOOKS SUGGEST STEAM TEMPERATURES THAT ARE MUCH HIGHER THAN 122°F (50°C). PLEASE NOTE THAT IN A STEAM ROOM AT 100% HUMIDITY, THIS IS *VERY* HOT. FOR SAFETY REASONS, THIS TEMPERATURE SHOULD BE THE UPPER LIMIT. GERMANY HAS PROBABLY THE MOST ADVANCED TECHNOLOGY IN THE BUILDING AND USE OF STEAMS ROOMS. AN AUTHORITATIVE GERMAN TEXT ON STEAM AND HYDROTHERAPY RECOMMENDS A STEAM ROOM TEMPERATURE BETWEEN 104°F (40°C) AND 116°F (47°C), ALTHOUGH THERE ARE A FEW STEAM ROOMS IN GERMANY WITH TEMPERATURES AS HIGH AS 122°F (50°C).[1]

For some full-body skin care treatments, the purpose of the steam treatment may be to heat the skin as quickly as possible, but not for very long (e.g., for about 10 minutes). For this type of treatment, you would want the temperature in the higher range. If, on the other hand, the purpose of the treatment is mainly relaxation, you may want to keep the temperature lower, as you do not want the client to heat too quickly and become uncomfortable and you want the treatment to last longer.

Length of Treatment

A normal steam treatment lasts between 25 and 30 minutes, which is usually sufficient enough to comfortably increase the client's skin and core body temperature and to allow the body to sweat profusely. In general, after about 25 to 30 minutes, most clients will begin to feel overheated and uncomfortable. If you find that a client feels uncomfortable after 15 or 20 minutes, you should set the steam temperature for that client at a lower-than-average setting. These clients will often state that they do not like steam treatments because they find the steam to be too hot. If, however, a client feels that he or she did not get heated enough during 25 to 30 minutes, then the temperature could be set higher. You should record each client's temperature preference so that future treatments can be set at the desired temperature.

Client feedback regarding length of treatment is very important. If at anytime during a treatment the client states that he or she is feeling uncomfortably hot, the treatment should be ended or the steam temperature decreased. If the temperature is decreased and the treatment continues, cool towels or misting should be applied to the client's head and/or neck. If the client stills feels uncomfortable, the treatment should be stopped immediately, and he or she should be allowed to cool down before moving.

Anatomy and Physiology During Treatment

The following are the main transformations that take place in a client's anatomy and physiology during a steam therapy treatment:

- The skin—including the epidermis, dermis, and subcutaneous layers—will increase in temperature due to heat exchange from the steam. These layers will heat more quickly and to a higher temperature than will the body's core temperature, because these outer layers are in direct contact with the steam. The fat in the subcutaneous layer has an insulating effect that keeps the core body temperature from heating up too quickly.

- The temperature of the core body, which includes the systems of the body other than the skin, will increase in temperature according to the temperature of the steam and the duration of the treatment.

- As the temperature of the cells in the skin and core of the body increases, the metabolic activity of these cells will increase. An increase in temperature of the cells by 1°C will increase the cell's metabolic activity by 12%.

- As the metabolic activity of the cells throughout the body increases, circulation to the cells will increase, providing the necessary oxygen and nutrients for the cells.

- The volume of blood circulating to the skin will increase as the body tries to cool itself by radiating greater amounts of heat from the skin to the environment. Normally the blood flow to the skin is a small percentage—about 8% of the 5 qt (5 L) of blood in the body. However, when the body is overheated, blood flow in the skin can increase to 30% of total blood volume.

- The hypothalamus, in the brain, will sense an increase in the core body temperature and will stimulate the sweat glands. These glands will produce sweat, reaching a rate that can exceed 1 qt (1 L) per hour. For people who have acclimatized to hotter environments, the rate of sweating can exceed 2 qt (2 L) per hour. An additional benefit of sweating is that it allows for detoxification of the body through the removal of toxins contained in the sweat.

- The rate of osmosis between the cells and the interstitial fluid and between the interstitial fluid and the capillaries will increase.

- The rate of diffusion of substances in the blood plasma, interstitial fluid, and cellular fluid will increase. Products on the skin—especially those that are fat (lipid) soluble—will also diffuse (be absorbed) more quickly into the skin.

Immediate and Long-Term Benefits

Steam therapy treatments produce multiple immediate and long-term benefits for clients. Steam therapy treatments cause significant sweating and detoxification, a temporary increase in cellular metabolism, and greater circulation to the cells. There is also a significant increase in blood flow to the skin. In addition, steam therapy treatments, when done properly, produce deep and unique states of relaxation, making these treatments a powerful form of relaxation therapy. Steam therapy, when used effectively for relaxation, can help balance higher levels of stress and tension.

As a result of these different effects, steam therapy treatment can provide a wide range of immediate and long-term benefits in all areas of health and wellness, including daily wellness, appearance, fitness, healthful aging, and prevention. Clients have also reported such benefits as increased creativity, emotional balance, as well as spiritual experiences. Steam therapy has proven effective in dealing with a range of symptoms, including pain and trauma from former and recent injuries and rehabilitation of injuries, complications from overuse of parts of the body, and other physical issues.

Equipment: Different Types and Special Features

There are several types of steam therapy equipment available for full-body steam treatments and for steam inhalation therapy:

General Types of Full-Body Steam Equipment

- Steam canopies allow treatments on a massage table or other treatment table. Some of these canopies are portable, while others are permanently attached to the massage or treatment table. One advantage of this system is that the client is lying down during treatment, which allows for greater client relaxation. Another is that the therapist can easily massage the client's head, neck, and shoulders before, during, or after treatment. The temperature and products used can also be personalized for each client. Steam cabinets allow the client to sit during steam treatments. These systems usually do not need to be permanently installed. The temperature and products used during the treatment can be personalized for each client, and the client's head can be outside the steam cabinet during treatment.

- Some steam capsules allow for one or two people to sit inside the enclosed area. These systems are usually not permanently installed and can be moved when needed. The temperature and products used can be personalized for each client. The client's entire body is inside the capsule.

- Steam rooms are usually large enough to accommodate several people at one time, depending on the size of the room. Steam rooms are often used in large spa, wellness, and fitness centers. The temperature cannot be easily changed, but clients can sit at higher or lower levels in the steam room to control the temperature.

- Steam inhalation equipment is readily available and inexpensive for inhalation therapy. Some equipment has better features than others, so it is important to thoroughly research the options available.

NOTE: WORKING WITH ANY TYPE OF STEAM THERAPY EQUIPMENT REQUIRES PROPER TRAINING IN THE USE OF THAT SPECIFIC PIECE OF EQUIPMENT. STEAM THERAPY EQUIPMENT MEANS WORKING WITH STEAM AND BOILING WATER, AND CAUTION MUST ALWAYS BE USED. ONE POTENTIAL RISK FOR CLIENTS WITH SOME STEAM

THERAPY EQUIPMENT IS THE CLIENT'S SKIN COMING INTO DIRECT
CONTACT WITH THE STEAM.

Products

Certain natural products can be added to the steam being generated
during a steam treatment. Some products can also be applied to the
client's skin before the steam treatment begins. Both approaches can
produce effective interaction between the product and the client's skin.

- *Products added to the steam:* Most steam equipment
  includes a feature that allows products to be added directly
  to the steam being generated—either by placing the product
  directly in the steam or by having the steam come into contact and mix with the product. Examples of products mixed
  with steam include essential oils, herbs, and mineral salts.
  These products then come into contact with the client's
  skin or are inhaled and absorbed by the bloodstream in the
  lungs. The surface of area of the lungs for absorption of air
  and other molecular substances is approximately 750 ft^2. It
  is important to understand that products mixed with steam
  and inhaled can be absorbed into the blood, so caution must
  be used when introducing products into the steam.

- *Products placed on the client's skin and hair:* Products that
  have a therapeutic value for the skin and hair can also be
  used during steam treatments, depending on the goal of
  the treatment. The increased temperature of the skin will
  increase the rate of absorption of products. Note, however,
  that water-soluble products may be washed off by water as
  it condenses on the skin. Many skin care products are oil-
  based and are thus not very water-soluble. These oil-based
  products are also more easily absorbed by the skin.

- *Products for inhalation therapy:* Some essential oils, such
  as eucalyptus oil, are known to have therapeutic value
  when used for inhalation therapy. Also, a small amount
  of sea salt is often used during inhalation therapy. Steam
  used alone can be very beneficial, even without any additional products added.

Contraindications

Steam treatments can produce dramatic changes in the functioning
of the human physiology. There is a significant increase in cardiac
output, which can go from a normal of rate 1.25 gal/min to as high as

3 gal/min. There is also an increase in the heart rate and a significant increase in blood flow to the skin. All of this places greater demands on the circulatory system. Although this increase is usually not a problem for normal, healthy individuals, it can be contraindicated for people with certain conditions.

Steam therapy treatment is contraindicated for clients with the following conditions:

- *Clients with major medical conditions:* If your client has *any* major medical condition for which he or she is receiving medical supervision and care, you should have the client check with his or her doctor for permission before giving a steam treatment.

- *Clients who have cardiovascular health issues are a major concern:* These people are usually under medical supervision and are taking medication. For the client's safety, people with such conditions should not receive steam therapy treatments. If there is any doubt, don't do the steam treatment unless the client has permission from his or her physician.

- *Women who are pregnant*

- *Clients with recent cuts that are still healing, current skin infections, and other active skin conditions such as psoriasis*

Safety Considerations

Avoid overheating a client to the point that he or she becomes uncomfortably hot or shows other signs of discomfort, such as dizziness or disorientation. Because steam therapy treatments can produce very fast, dramatic changes in physiology, the client should be regularly monitored during a steam treatment to ensure that he or she is comfortable.

At the end of a steam treatment, allow the client several minutes to cool down before sitting up, standing, or walking. Then, when possible, assist the client with sitting up, standing, or walking. Remember, as much as 30% of blood may now be flowing though the skin, which means that as the client stands or walks, there may not be enough blood flow to the brain, making it difficult for the client to walk.

Another major safety issue is the fact that steam rooms can become very slippery. Be sure to aid clients as they leave the steam room, as they may become dizzy and fall on the slick floor as they try to stand up and move.

Special Considerations

Pretreatment

- Turn on the equipment's steam generator in advance so that it is ready to produce steam at the same time that steam treatment is ready to begin.

- If possible, have the client relax between the time he or she enters the spa or wellness center and the time of the steam treatment.

- Offer the client some herbal tea or water before the treatment, because the client can lose more than 1 qt (1 L) of water during the treatment. However, do not have him or her drink too much, as this will increase the need for a visit to the bathroom during treatment. Clients will mainly become rehydrated after the treatment.

Beginning the Treatment

- Follow similar draping procedures that you would for a massage or full-body esthetics treatment. Another option is to have your client wear a bathing suit or disposable spa items during treatment.

- Always assist the client when getting into or out of the steam therapy equipment.

Treatment

- Check on the client at regular intervals or stay with him or her during the entire treatment. A client should not be left alone for long periods of time or for the entire treatment.

- After 10 to 15 minutes, the client will begin to start feeling mildly overheated. At this point, you can place a small, cool towel on your client's face and/or neck. An alternative is to use a misting bottle to spray the client's face and neck (aim slightly above the head). You can also add few drops of essential oils or hydrosols to the water in spray bottle.

- Occasionally massage the face, neck, and possibly the shoulders—if the steam equipment allows. In-depth massage on parts of the body can be done during steam treatments on a massage table with a steam canopy.

End of the Treatment

- At the end of a full-body steam treatment, turn off the steam being generated and allow the temperature inside the steam cabinet, capsule, or canopy to return to a comfortable level.
- Allow the client as much time as possible before he or she moves from the steam equipment.
- Always assist the client with sitting up, standing, or walking immediately after the steam treatment.

Post-Treatment

If possible, it is good to have the client rest as long as possible after the treatment. The client should be kept warm and allowed to rest in a quiet area. This can greatly enhance the total beneficial effects of the treatment.

Additional Suggestions

Combining Steam Therapy with Other Treatments

Steam therapy treatments can be used in combination with (as part of a "package" for) most types of massage and full-body skin care treatments, and even with some facial treatments.

Series of Steam Therapy Treatments

Steam therapy treatments can be an essential component of ongoing programs that require a series of treatments at regular intervals. For example, steam therapy treatments given at regular intervals have proven to be very helpful in detoxification and weight-management programs. In another example, skin care rejuvenation programs could include steam treatments at regular intervals. Likewise, inhalation therapy, which helps deal with our constant exposure to air pollution, requires a series of treatments in order to produce the desired benefits of a prevention program.

Relaxation Steam Therapy

STEAM THERAPY TREATMENTS

DESCRIPTION AND BENEFITS

The main benefit of this treatment is to provide deep relaxation for the client. Steam therapy treatments done with the intention of relaxation can produce profound states of relaxation that are unique to steam treatments (see Figure 7–1). Relaxation therapy is a powerful therapeutic tool that is beneficial for all health and wellness goals. It can help balance the effects of the overstimulated, stressful aspects of modern life. The side effects of higher levels of stress, tension, and anxiety include psychosomatic symptoms and related diseases. Relaxation therapy is a nondrug, effective treatment modality for stress management. Aromatherapy, soothing body products, and music can be combined with steam treatments to enhance experiences of relaxation and decrease feelings of stress, tension, and anxiety.

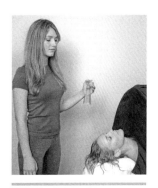

Figure 7–1 Relaxation treatment.

EQUIPMENT

Steam cabinet, capsule, canopy, or room

PRODUCTS

Aromatherapy using essential oil and/or hydrosols, Essential oils combined with oils such as jojoba that are applied to the skin

STEPS OF THE TREATMENT

1. *Pretreatment:* Preheat the water so that it is ready to produce steam when the treatment is ready to begin. The steam temperature for relaxation treatment should be in a normal range. You do not want the client to heat up too quickly or get overheated.

2. *Beginning the treatment:* Make sure the client is comfortable. If this is the client's first steam treatment, explain about the nature of the treatment, including the experience and the benefits.

3. *Treatment:* The treatment can be between 25 and 35 minutes, depending on scheduling considerations. Because the goal of this treatment is relaxation, the client should always feel comfortable and not overheated.

Optional—Aromatherapy: Most steam systems include a feature for using essential oils for aromatherapy. Use an essential oil that the client enjoys and that produces a relaxing effect. Essential oils can also be added to massage oils and placed on the client's body before the treatment begins.

Optional—Massage: Steam cabinet and steam canopy equipment allows you some access to the client's head, neck, and shoulders, which could be massaged during the steam treatment. Most clients find this very relaxing.

Cooling the Client: After about 10 minutes, or when the client begins to feel hot, ask your client if you can mist their head and face with water or put a cool towel on the forehead. This produces a soothing effect and may help the client feel less overheated.

Client Body Position: If the steam equipment system allows, the client can change positions during treatment to remain relaxed throughout the treatment.

4. *End of the treatment:* Turn off the steam and allow the client several minutes to gradually cool down. Assist the client from the steam equipment system if possible.

5. *Post-treatment:* The client should rest for a period of time after the steam treatment, usually in another room. The client should also drink water to rehydrate before leaving.

ADDITIONAL SUGGESTIONS

With the use of the steam canopy system that allows you to give a steam treatment with the client laying on the massage table, it is possible during relaxation steam treatment to give the client instructions on correct, normal breathing. For these instructions, please see the Breathing Treatment in the Hydrotub section.

Exfoliation Treatment

DESCRIPTION AND BENEFITS

Full-body steam therapy is an excellent way to prepare the skin for exfoliation treatments as it not only allows a product to be absorbed by the skin, but it also increases circulation to the area and increases the metabolic rate of the cells (see Figure 7–2 and Plate 19). The heat from the steam also helps break the bonds that keep surface skin cells attached. This makes it easier to remove the dead skin cells by a combination of friction and exfoliation products. The effects of the exfoliation will be deeper, more even, and longer lasting. Clients also benefit from the relaxation of a personalized steam treatment.

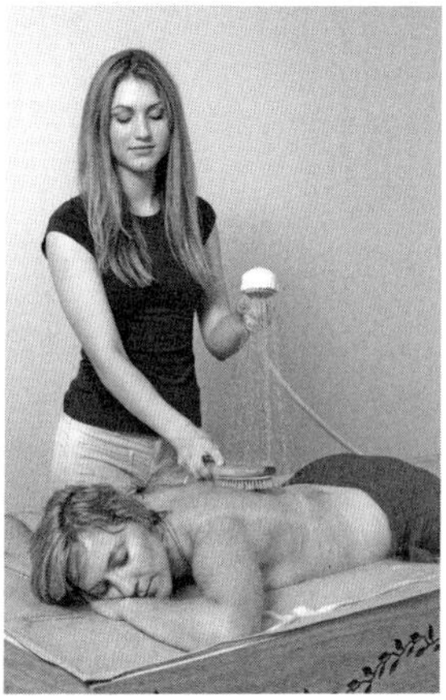

EQUIPMENT

Steam canopy for treatments on a massage table or steam cabinet, capsule, or steam room

Figure 7–2 Exfoliation treatment.

PRODUCTS

Some exfoliation products are placed on the skin before treatment to help loosen the surface skin cells. Others are placed on the skin before friction is applied, providing greater friction when removing the cells by rubbing with a dry brush or exfoliation glove.

STEPS OF THE TREATMENT

1. *Pretreatment:* Preheat the system so it is ready to produce steam when the treatment is ready to begin. The temperature of the steam treatment should be in a normal range, as the purpose of the treatment is to increase the temperature of the skin.

2. *Beginning the treatment:* Make sure that your client is comfortable to make the treatment as relaxing as possible. Apply any exfoliation products to the skin at this time.

3. *Treatment:* The steam treatment should last about 25 minutes. If time is a factor, the treatment can be as short as 10 minutes, as the main purpose is to heat the skin. For a 10-minute steam treatment, the temperature should probably be set higher.

Cooling the Client: After about 10 minutes, ask your client if you can mist their head and face with water or put a cool towel on the forehead. This produces a soothing effect and will help your client feel less overheated.

Client Body Position: As a preparation for exfoliation, it is important that the entire surface of the client's skin be exposed to steam. In some steam equipment systems, such as a steam canopy or steam room, it may be necessary for your client to change positions during the treatment.

4. *End of the treatment:* Assist your client from the steam equipment system to the table that is to be used for exfoliation. If the steam treatment was done using a steam canopy on a massage or esthetic table, you may be able to continue the treatment on the same table.

5. *Post-treatment:* The steam treatment is followed by an exfoliation treatment.

ADDITIONAL SUGGESTIONS

As mentioned above, steam therapy can be used with many full-body skin care treatments, including cellulite, body-masks, and as an alternative to body-wraps.

Steam Therapy for Massage Preparation

DESCRIPTION AND BENEFITS

This treatment combines steam therapy followed by a massage (see Figure 7–3 and Plate 17). When performed properly, a steam therapy treatment can be deeply relaxing for the client. The client will then be more relaxed at the start of the massage treatment, which is a beneficial state for receiving massage therapy. Steam therapy will also increase general circulation throughout the body and to the cells of the body. Finally, increasing the temperature of the skin and the core body will make it easier to stretch the connective tissue matrix, including the muscles, ligaments, tendons, joints, and the total body fascial matrix. Thus, steam therapy can be a very effective preparation for most types of massage treatments, including those dealing with muscle tension, sports injuries, back pain, arthritis, and related conditions.

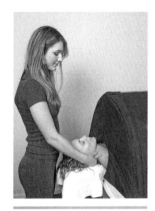

Figure 7–3 Steam therapy as preparation for massage.

EQUIPMENT

Steam cabinet, capsule, canopy, or steam room

PRODUCTS

Aromatherapy can be used during this steam treatment. Oils, such as jojoba, can be placed on the client during the steam treatment and be absorbed into the skin prior to massage. Products that provide relief from joint stiffness and pain, such as some types of tiger balms or special organic muds, could be placed on joints before the steam treatment.

STEPS OF THE TREATMENT

1. *Pretreatment:* Preheat the water so it is producing steam when the steam treatment is ready to begin. Have the client drink about 8 oz of water before the treatment to balance water loss due to sweating. If possible, have the client rest before beginning the treatment. The steam temperature should be in the normal range. However, if time is an issue and only about 15 minutes are available for the steam treatment, the temperature could be in the warmer range.

2. *Beginning the treatment:* Make sure the client is comfortable. If this is the client's first steam treatment, explain about the nature of the treatment, including the experience and the benefits.

3.   *Treatment:* The length of the treatment should be 25 to 30 minutes.

     Optional–Massage: Some steam equipment system allows you to massage the client's head, neck, and shoulders during the treatment. This can be form of premassage before the final massage therapy. It can also be effective in treating some forms of neck and shoulder problems.

4.   *End of the treatment:* Turn off the steam and gradually allow your client to cool down for several minutes. Assist your client from the steam equipment system to the massage table. If the steam treatment was done using a steam canopy on a massage table, you may be able to continue with the massage treatment on the same table.

5.   *Post-treatment:* After the combined steam and massage treatment, the client should rest as long as possible and drink water or other natural beverages to rehydrate.

ADDITIONAL SUGGESTIONS

When combining steam therapy with massage, the steam therapy is usually done before the massage. However, it is also possible to do the massage first, followed by steam therapy.

Steam Therapy for Detoxification

DESCRIPTION AND BENEFITS

Steamy therapy takes advantage of the body's natural cooling mechanism of producing sweat when the body's core temperature increases. The body can produce more than 1 qt (1 L) of sweat per hour. This sweat is used not only for cooling the body but also for natural purification and detoxification through the removal of toxins in the sweat. Detoxification is a hydrotherapy treatment that promotes benefits for all of a client's health and wellness goals. While the client is detoxifying, he or she also benefits from the profound state of relaxation created during a steam treatment. In the ancient hydrotherapy tradition of Ayurveda from India, the steam treatment called swedhana, which is still being used today, is an essential part of a total program for the purification and balancing of the physiology.

EQUIPMENT

Steam cabinet, capsule, canopy, or steam room

PRODUCTS

Aromatherapy can be used during the steam treatment to enhance relaxation or detoxification. During this treatment, other products, such as massage oils, are generally not placed on the skin, as the main purpose of the treatment is produce a high rate of sweat for detoxification. If you use special products for detoxification, you may be able to combine them with this steam treatment.

STEPS OF THE TREATMENT

1. *Pretreatment:* Preheat the system so it is ready to produce steam when the treatment is ready to begin. The client should drink a glass of water or a natural beverage before the treatment begins.

2. *Beginning the treatment:* The steam temperature for a detoxification treatment should be in the normal range. Of course, it can be adjusted to meet any special needs of the client.

3. *Treatment:* The length of the treatment should be 25 to 30 minutes. Because the purpose of this treatment is for detoxification

through sweating, it is important that the client has a full treatment. Check the client throughout the treatment to be sure he or she is comfortable. Do not overheat the client by setting the temperature too high.

Cooling the Client: After about 10 minutes, ask your client if you can mist the head and face with water or put a cool towel on the forehead. This produces a soothing effect and may help your client feel less overheated. If the client is feeling overheated after 10 or 15 minutes, the temperature inside the steam cabinet, capsule, canopy, or steam room is too high; adjust it accordingly.

Client Body Position: If the steam equipment system allows the client to lie down—for example, in a steam canopy or steam room—the client does not need to change positions, though they are free to do so if it makes them more comfortable.

4. *End of the treatment:* Turn off the steam and allow the client several minutes to gradually cool down. Assist the client from the steam equipment system.

5. *Post-treatment:* To get the full benefit of the treatment, it is important for the client to rest after the treatment for as long as possible. The client should stay warm, possibly covered by a sheet or blanket. Give the client water or some other natural beverage to rehydrate.

ADDITIONAL SUGGESTIONS

Encourage your client to drink extra water at home after the session is over to continue rehydrating. More than 1 qt (1 L) of water can be lost from the body during a steam treatment. A loss of this much water in sweat will create a 2.5% level of dehydration of the total of approximately 10 gal of water in the body.

Steam Therapy for Full-Body Skin Care

DESCRIPTION AND BENEFITS

In this skin care treatment, a product is applied to the body, followed by a steam therapy treatment (see Figure 7–4 and Plate 24). The heating, moisturizing effect of a full-body steam treatment enhances the interaction between the skin and the product, thus promoting greater absorption of the product by the skin. There is also an increase in blood flow to the skin and in the metabolic activity of the skin cells. The rates of diffusion and osmosis, as part of cellular circulation, will also increase.

EQUIPMENT

Steam cabinet, capsule, canopy, or steam room

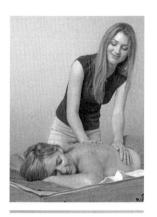

Figure 7–4 Skin care treatment.

PRODUCTS

Some examples of products to use during the full-body treatment are seaweed creams, Moor mud, clay, natural oil products (e.g., jojoba), mineral-based products, and products that are a combination of several natural products.

Full-body skin care treatments are becoming more popular. Professional estheticians are very knowledgeable about the many full-body skin care products available and choose products that they feel will work best to produce the desired outcome of the treatment. With some types of steam equipment, for example, a steam canopy, it is also possible to apply products to the face and have the face gently heated by the steam. Also becoming popular is the use of freshly blended natural items, such avocado and papaya, that are applied to the skin before the steam treatment begins.

Information is also available in the Hydrotherapy Product Resource Guide in Appendix C.

STEPS OF THE TREATMENT

1. *Pretreatment:* Preheat the water so that it is ready to produce steam when the treatment is ready to begin. The steam temperature should be in a normal range.

2. *Beginning the treatment:* Apply the product to the skin before beginning the steam treatment.

3. *Treatment:* The duration of the treatment can be about 25 minutes. The goal of this treatment is to heat the skin for increased product absorption. If the treatment needs to be shorter, the steam temperature should probably be higher. With some steam equipment system, it may be possible to massage the product into certain areas of the skin during the treatment.

    Client Body Position: If the steam equipment system allows, the client can change positions throughout this treatment to ensure that the steam comes into contact with the entire surface of the skin that contains product.

4. *End of the treatment:* Turn off the steam and allow the client to cool down gradually for several minutes. The client can be rinsed off with a handheld shower on a wet table, or the client can take a normal shower, depending on the goal of the treatment and if rinsing the body after the treatment is desirable. Assist the client from the steam equipment system to another table or room if necessary to continue the skin care treatment.

5. *Post-treatment:* If possible, allow the client to rest after the treatment. Provide water or a natural beverage to rehydrate.

ADDITIONAL SUGGESTIONS

Many skin care programs are using full-body steam treatments in place of body wrapping. It can be more effective and comfortable for the client. Skin care is a daily program as well as a lifetime program. Steam therapy combined with skin care products and treatments can become part of a series of treatments done at regular intervals.

Enhancement Steam Therapy Treatments

DESCRIPTION AND BENEFITS

In the traditions of the Native Americans, the Mayans, and other ancient cultures, various uses of steam, herbs, chanting, prayer, and other elements were used in purification rituals, both for physical purification and for the psychic or spiritual purification. Some of the effects from these rituals include enhanced spiritual awareness and renewal, greater connection with higher aspects of nature's intelligence, and greater creative and intuitive insights. These rituals were often done as a group performance. Although it is not possible to exactly re-create these sessions at a spa or wellness center, it is possible to introduce some element of them into special steam therapy treatments that use herbs, music, and aromatherapy along with a special theme or intention for the session. These treatments can produce similar experiences as mentioned above. Steam therapy treatments, especially those done on systems in which the client is lying down, can be profoundly relaxing. Combining this deep relaxation with the enhancing elements mentioned here can produce some extraordinary experiences.

EQUIPMENT

Steam canopy, capsule, cabinet, or steam room

PRODUCTS

Essential oils and herbs known for enhancing relaxation or for heightening consciousness can be used. Music that enhances relaxation, that contains soothing chanting, or that enlivens consciousness can be played during treatment. An important element of such treatments is establishing the intention of the treatment and maintaining a deep level of relaxation and sacred atmosphere during the entire session.

STEPS OF THE TREATMENT

1. *Pretreatment:* Preheat the system so it is ready to produce steam when the treatment is ready to begin. Turn on soothing music so it is playing when the client enters the room.

2. *Beginning the treatment:* Maintain the intention and atmosphere of the treatment during the entire session.

3. *Treatment:* The duration of the treatment can be 25 to 35 minutes. The steam temperature should be in a comfortable range. The client should not get overheated during the session. Stay with the client or check on him or her at regular intervals to ensure that they are comfortable. If possible, massage the client's face, neck, and shoulders at times during the treatment.

4. *End of the treatment:* Turn off the steam and give the client several minutes to gradually cool down.

5. *Post-treatment:* Assist the client from the steam equipment and to the next treatment or the resting area. A longer resting period is especially beneficial after this type of treatment. Also offer the client water, a natural beverage, or herbal tea to rehydrate.

ADDITIONAL SUGGESTION

A massage treatment could follow the steam session.

Inhalation Steam Therapy

DESCRIPTION AND BENEFITS

Today, everyone is exposed to greater air pollution—some people more so than others. During winter months, humidity levels can be very low and the temperatures very cold. Steam inhalation is a simple and easy treatment that can produce multiple benefits, including cleansing, hydrating, relaxing, and detoxifying effects for the entire respiratory system. This is a treatment that can be given in any treatment room and can also be recommended for the client to do at home. This is a simple treatment that any client will find very beneficial and is an immediate way to offer a quality hydrotherapy treatment.

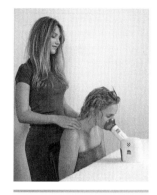

Figure 7–5 Inhalation treatment.

EQUIPMENT

Several types of simple inhalation therapy equipment systems are on the market today. Most have an option that allows products, such as essential oils (e.g., eucalyptus), to be added to the steam being inhaled. Because inhalation equipment varies in terms of features and quality, careful research is recommended. (See the Hydrotherapy Equipment Resource Guide in Appendix B.) Please note that there is one brand of steam inhalation equipment that is highly recommended in the appendix.

Inhalation therapy can also be part of a full-body steam treatment. During steam treatments that take place in steam rooms or steam capsules, the client will automatically be inhaling steam. When using steam canopies or cabinets, it is possible to adjust a towel over the client so he or she can inhale the steam (see Figure 7–5 and Plate 18).

PRODUCTS

Different steam inhalation equipment allows products to be mixed with the steam in different ways. Products are not necessary for this treatment, but it is possible to include the use of some essential oils, such as eucalyptus, that have a traditional use for inhalation therapy. Also, adding a small amount of natural sea salt to the steam being inhaled can be beneficial. Remember that substances mixed with steam can enter the bloodstream in the lungs, so only use products and product combinations that are recommended for inhalation treatments.

STEPS OF THE TREATMENT

1. *Pretreatment:* Preheat the system so it is ready to produce steam when the treatment is ready to begin.

2. *Beginning the treatment:* Have the client sit comfortably and begin the treatment.

3. *Treatment:* The duration can be about 10 minutes, depending on the goal of the treatment. Check with your client throughout the treatment to ensure that he or she is comfortable with the amount and temperature of the steam. Adjust the temperature accordingly.

4. *End of the treatment:* Turn off the steam and dry the client's face with a towel. If possible, massage the client's face after the treatment.

5. *Post-treatment:* Always carefully clean and disinfect the steam inhalation equipment. (See Chapter 6 for more information on hygiene.)

ADDITIONAL SUGGESTIONS

- Combine inhalation treatments with a facial massage before, during, or after the treatment. Emphasis should be on the sinus areas. Most massage therapists have basic training in facial massage techniques.

- Steam therapy can be very beneficial following the infectious stage of a cold or flu. It can also help after exposure to severe cold or high levels of air pollution. It is also useful when included as an element of a total health and wellness program with other treatments at regular intervals. This can also include the use of inhalation treatments as part of a client's home program.

Hydrotub Treatments

COMMON ELEMENTS OF HYDROTUB TREATMENTS

Dynamic Water Principles

The following list describes the basic principles of the behavior of water that are fundamental to hydrotub hydrotherapy treatments. Therapists transform the water in various ways to be used during the hydrotub treatment and then the client is brought into contact with the water by immersion in the hydrotub.

- In hydrotub treatments, water is used in the liquid form, although there will be greater evaporation of water into the gas state from the water in the bath, especially if it is in a hotter range.

- Heat exchange occurs because the client's body is in direct contact with water. This contact produces very rapid heat exchange between the water and the body. If the water temperature is hotter than the client's body, then the temperature of the skin and core body will increase. If the water temperature is cooler, then the temperature of the skin and core body will decrease. The rate of heat exchange between the water and the body is more than 20 times greater than the rate of heat exchange between the body and the air temperature. Whereas a person will feel comfortable when the air temperature is 70°F (21.1°C), that same person will feel very cold in water of the same temperature.

- The water principle of buoyancy is an important aspect of most hydrotub treatments. Buoyancy reduces the effects of gravity on the body by about 95%, so the body is almost weightless. Reducing gravity on the body brings about feelings of profound relaxation as well as producing favorable conditions for working on the body in a gravity-free environment.

- The solvent property of water allows water-soluble products to be dissolved in the bath water. Sea salts and other mineral salts dissolve quickly in water and have known therapeutic effects. Various herbal and seaweed products also dissolve in water. Some products that do not dissolve in water, such as certain mud and clay products, can still be mixed into the water for use during treatment. Likewise, some oils, such as essential oils, will not dissolve in water but can be mixed into the water for short periods before they separate and float to the water's surface. Hydrotub baths give you the opportunity to be creative in producing a variety of combinations of natural products, such as mineral salts, herbs, essential oils, clays, muds, and oils, for creating special effects during the treatment.

● In some hydrotubs, water jets, air jets, or a hydrowand can produce water pressure against the client's body to create a deep massaging effect. Water pressure directed to the client's body will create a pumping effect (pressure) on the body's fluid systems. By using a hydrowand, you can apply direct pressure to specific areas of the body or create hydromassage strokes in specific directions. This offers a very unique and effective technique of massaging the client's body underwater.

Water Temperature

The temperature of the bath water will depend on the goal of the treatment.

● *Neutral range:* This neutral water temperature range is generally between 95°F (35°C) and 98°F (36.6°C). In water at this temperature, a client will feel comfortable, without getting hot or cold. The client should be able to remain comfortable in the water for normal or extended periods of time. In this neutral range, the core body temperature should stay constant at approximately 98.6°F (37°C).

NOTE: THE NEUTRAL TEMPERATURE RANGE WILL BE SLIGHTLY DIFFERENT FOR DIFFERENT CLIENTS, SO IT IS ALWAYS IMPORTANT TO ASK CLIENTS WHETHER THEY ARE COMFORTABLE. ADJUST THE TEMPERATURE AS NEEDED.

● *Hotter range:* In this range, the water temperature is approximately 99°F (37.2°C) or above and usually no greater than 104°F (40°C). The hotter the water temperature, the more quickly the skin and core temperatures will increase. Water temperatures above the neutral range will feel comfortable and relaxing at first, but will eventually make the client feel overheated as the core body temperature rises. Water conducts heat 20 times greater than air, and at a temperature as high as 104°F (40°C) there will be a significant heat exchange between the hotter water and the skin and core temperature of the body (approximately 98.6°F [37°C]), There are known health risks using water temperatures higher than 104°F (40°C). The U.S. Consumer Product Safety Commission (CPSC), in release # 79-071, states that "hot tub water temperatures should never exceed 104°F." The release also states that "extremely hot water during hot tub use can threaten life. Soaking in a hot tub with water heated to 106°F, for example, can raise human body temperature to the point of heat strokes (or impairment of the body's ability to regulate its internal temperature). These conditions can be fatal even to fully healthy adults." All hot tub manufactures follow these guidelines set the upper limit on hot tubs at 104°F (40°C). The Japanese have a long tradition of home baths at temperatures of approximately 108°F (42.2°C). Several thousand deaths each year are associated with fainting and cardiovascular problems created during these baths, usually unsupervised and alone, in water at such high temperatures. Although healthy individuals are usually fine in water as high as 104°F (40°C), it is always recommended to check on the client during the treatment to ensure that he or she is comfortable. Once again, the recommendation regarding the water temperature is the same as the CPSC, a temperature of no higher than 104°F (40°C).

- *Cooler range:* The cooler range of water temperature for hydrotubs is usually below 95°F (37.2°C), but no lower than about 89°F (40°C). It is possible for someone to be in water in this temperature range, especially if the water is cooled gradually, and not feel chilled for some time. At the cooler temperatures, there is heat exchange from the client's body to the water as the skin and core body temperature decrease. Using water in this range can help cool the body when it has been overheated for long periods of time in hot weather, sporting events, or other activities.

- *Cold range:* Some spa and wellness facilities provide a cold pool that is often kept at about room temperature—from 68°F (20°C) to 72°F (22.2°C). People often use this pool as a cold plunge or brief cold bath, usually after heating treatments, such as steam treatments. A cold plunge usually lasts fewer than 60 seconds. Even though there is minimal heat exchange due to the short exposure, the cold water will produce dramatic changes in the client's physiology (see the next section for more information).

- *Additional Note: In addition to controlling temperature, water pressure can also be controlled.* Water pressure from a hydrowand or hydrojet should be in a comfortable range. As can be seen from photos of treatments using hydromassage, the use of pressure produces a deep massaging effect that can be very comfortable for the client. The pressure from a hydrowand can usually be controlled by a valve or by increasing or decreasing the distance of the hydrowand from the client's body. As always, client feedback is very important, as what is comfortable for one client may not be comfortable for another.

Length of the Treatment

The length of the treatment depends on the therapeutic goal and the temperature of the water.

- Hydrotub treatments in a neutral temperature range can be for short, medium, or longer periods of time. A relaxing hydrotub or bath treatment could be 30 minutes or longer. Some flotation treatments last more than 60 minutes.

- Hotter hydrotub treatments, which have water temperature in the 99°F (38°C) to 104°F (40°C) range, will be shorter in length. In general, the hotter the water, the shorter the treatment. It is essential during these treatments to get client feedback to make sure he or she is comfortable. As explained earlier, the CPSC considers 104°F to be the maximum safe water temperature for adults and recommends that sessions at that temperature not exceed 15 minutes. Note: This recommendation is for people using hot tubs unsupervised. In a spa or wellness setting, the duration can be longer as long as the client is carefully monitored. Still, when the water temperature is 104°F (40°C), the supervised treatment does not generally exceed 20 minutes.

- The duration of hydrotub and bath treatments that use water at a temperature less than 95°F (34°C) is determined by the goal of the treatment, the temperature of the water, and the client's comfort. Treatments in the colder range are usually shorter than treatments in the neutral or warmer range, as clients can quickly become uncomfortable (hypothermia).

- A cold water plunge, in which the water temperature is usually in the range of 68°F (20°C) to 72°F (22.2°C), are usually for a very short duration following a heating treatment. Plunges into icy cold water are usually not available at spa and wellness centers, as this would require cooling water to keep it at this lower temperature. In addition, icy plunges can be very shocking to the body, which could pose potential health risks for some individuals.

Anatomy and Physiology During a Hydrotub Treatment

When a person gets into water that is hotter or cooler than the client's own body temperature, the sensations of hot or cold can be very intense. These sensations of hot and cold will gradually become less intense as an adaptation to the sensory input of hot and cold develops. At hotter and colder temperatures, the client may have a strong conscious motivation to exit the water; this is protective mechanism of the body. To make exposure to cooler or warmer water—for example, in a range of 90°F (32.2°C) to 104°F (40°C)—more comfortable, you may want to begin with the water temperature closer to body temperature and then gradually increase or decrease it as needed.

- *Exposure to neutral-temperature water:* When the client is immersed in neutral-temperature water, he or she will likely experience a sense of relaxation, which is enhanced by feelings of weightlessness (buoyancy).

- *Exposure to hot water:* When a client is immersed in water that is at a higher temperature than the core body temperature, there will be a heat exchange with the skin and the core body temperature will increase. This increase will initiate a cooling response in the body in an attempt to bring the core body temperature back to normal. This automatic response includes an increase of circulation to the skin by as much as 30% of the total blood flow and a stimulation of the sweat glands to produce sweat. Under normal circumstances, this response would allow heat to leave the body as radiant heat and as evaporation of sweat from the skin. Because the body is immersed in water that is hotter than the core body temperature, however, the body absorbs radiant heat from the water and even though sweating occurs, no heat is lost as the sweat cannot evaporate.

- *Exposure to cool water:* When a client is immersed in cool water, heat will be lost from the body and the skin, and the core body temperature will decrease. To attempt to return the core body temperature to normal, the body will create a significant reduction of blood flow to the skin, goose bumps will appear on the skin, and a person may begin to shiver involuntarily. There will also be a strong conscious desire to exit the water and get warm. In general, the colder the water, the more dramatic the change. As with heat, sensations of cold are processed by the hypothalamus in the brain.

- *Exposure to cold water:* When a client gets into very cold water, the sensation of cold will produce an immediate heating response by the body. Even if the exposure to cold water is so short that there is no time for cooling of the core body temperature, the strong sensation of cold produced by cold receptors in the skin will initiate an immediate heating response. There are 10 times more cold receptors in the skin than heat receptors, so the skin is very sensitive to cold. The body's response to the sensation of cold water will produce a strong conscious motivation to exit the water, decrease blood flow to the skin, goose bumps, and involuntary shivering. The response is not produced by a decrease in core temperature but by the strong sensations of cold on the skin. Even though immersion in cold water is uncomfortable, brief exposure to cold water (e.g., 15–60 seconds) is sometimes used as a hydrotherapy modality, especially following a heating treatment, such as a hot hydrotub bath or steam treatment. This brief exposure to cold water produces a stimulating reaction that most people find refreshing and enlivening and that lasts long after the treatment is over. It also serves as a balancing element to the heating treatment.

- *Buoyancy:* When the human body is immersed in water, buoyancy will remove most of the effects of gravity. This significantly reduces any muscle activity necessary to maintain normal movements and posture. Sensations of floating can produce feelings of relaxation. The degree of reduction of gravity on the body, the ability to float, and the amount of freedom of movement will vary according to the equipment being used. In hydrotubs with special design features, it is possible for the therapist to work with the body in a gravity-free state. When the body is in this gravity-free environment, vascular resistance is decreased, which makes it easier for the heart to pump blood.

- *Hydro-pressure massage:* Underwater hydro-pressure massage done on the body in a gravity-free environment is usually very comfortable and relaxing for the client. Using this technique, a therapist can produce a significant massaging effect on the skin, muscles, organs, vascular system, cells, and total fascial matrix of the body. The gravity-free environment, along with, the heat of the water, and the degree of the hydropressure combine to create a special, very therapeutic form of massage that can be controlled by the therapist using a hydrowand. Hydrojets found in hydrotubs and hot tubs can produce similar effects but cannot be controlled in the same manner as a hydrowand. Home hydrotubs and hot tubs have become very popular for home use.

Equipment

Hydrotub equipment ranges from a simple bathtub to hydrotubs with advanced features, including computerized hydrojet functions. Regardless of the equipment used, it is possible to provide clients with a wide range of highly beneficial hydrotub treatments.

Chapter 5 discusses the different types of hydrotubs and other hydrotherapy equipment that can be used for full-body immersion. The chapter includes an analysis of the various features of the equipment as well as resources for locating it. Hydrotubs used for hydrotherapy treatments can be as simple as a bathtub or as complex as some of the more elaborate pieces of equipment on the market. Essentially, a hydrotub is any type of bathtub that can be used for therapeutic hydrotherapy treatments. The following is a brief summary of hydrotub equipment.

Simple Bathtubs

You don't need expensive hydrotubs to provide great hydrotub treatments. Simple bathtubs, without water- or air-powered jets, are suitable for relaxation treatments. Various product combinations and aromatherapy can be used. Simple bathtubs are less expensive and easier to install, clean, and maintain than more complex hydrotubs. A longer bathtub is recommended so the client can immerse his or her entire body. Bathtubs can be modified to have a higher overflow drain, which allows the water to be at a higher level than in a normal bathtub.

Hydrotubs

A wide range of hydrotubs in a variety of sizes and styles are available today. Simple models include only a few water- or air-powered jets. More developed hydrotubs include advanced technical features, such as multiple water or air jets. They may also include a hydrowand that therapists can use to perform underwater massage directly on specific parts of the client's body. Additional features include music, color, light, or aromatherapy features. Some hydrotubs have computerized programs that allow therapists to select different patterns of automatic hydromassage from the water or air jets. Some hydrotubs also include automatic cleaning systems. Hydrotubs have a wide price range and are very expensive at the high end. Because client comfort is always a key consideration, longer, wider hydrotubs are generally recommended.

See the Hydrotherapy Equipment Resource Guide in Appendix B for more information.

Products

Products that can be used during hydrotub treatments are also discussed in Chapter 5. It is interesting to note that when it comes to the use of natural products in hydrotherapy, there is no limit to the possible product combinations. Therapists can use their education, creativity, intuitive skill, and experience with herbs, essential oils, minerals, salts, and clay products to produce combinations that achieve unique synergistic effects. Therapists can then customize these blends according to the needs of a particular client. It is as if all the products of nature are available and then water becomes the medium in which we can mix these products together to create special synergistic blends which then come into contact with the client's body. With the possible addition of the energies of crystals color light therapy, music, and sound vibration, the potential of water to produce health and wellness transformation is truly remarkable. The following is a list of natural products and other elements that are commonly used in hydrotub treatments:

- Mineral salts: Sea salt and Dead Sea salts
- Moor muds: From organic plant sources that have been aged through time
- Seaweed products
- Herbal products
- Essential oils: For aromatherapy
- Hydrosols: Water-soluble flower extracts that dissolve in water
- Music or natural sounds: The sound of ocean waves, dolphins, whales, chanting, or primordial sounds.
- Colored light therapy
- Crystals and gemstones

Contraindications

The contraindications for hydrotub treatments with hot water and cold water are the basically the same as for steam and shower treatments.

- *Clients with major medical conditions:* If your client has *any* major medical condition for which he or she is receiving medical supervision and care, you should have the client check with his or her doctor for permission before giving a hydrotub treatment, especially heating or cooling treatments.

- *People who have cardiovascular conditions:* These people are usually under medical supervision and are taking medication. For the client's safety, people with such conditions should not receive heating or cooling hydrotub treatments.
- *Women who are pregnant*
- *Clients with recent cuts that are still healing or skin infections:* If there is any doubt, have your client get approval from a doctor. Even if your client has a doctor's permission, you should also feel comfortable giving the treatment.
- Most clients, even those with medical problems, can get a relaxing hydrotub treatment using a neutral water temperature that does not increase or decrease the core temperature of the body, except for those with skin problems mentioned above.

Safety Considerations

- Avoid overheating a client to the point that he or she becomes uncomfortably hot or shows other signs of discomfort, such as dizziness or disorientation. Clients should be monitored during the hydrotub treatment.
- If the client has had a hot hydrotub treatment, if possible, allow him or her to cool down before standing or walking.
- When possible, assist the client with sitting up, standing, or walking at the end of the treatment, especially if the treatment included hot water.
- Be cautious of slippery hydrotherapy equipment and wet floors.

Steps of the Treatment

Pretreatment

- Fill the hydrotub with water at the appropriate temperature so that it is ready when the client is ready for the treatment. If the water temperature is going to be in the hotter or cooler range, it is possible to begin the treatment with the water in a neutral range and then gradually heat or cool the water to the desired temperature. This will allow the body to slowly adapt to the hotter and cooler water.

● Add any natural products to the water. Products can also be added during the treatment.

Beginning the Treatment

● Follow the same procedures for draping that you would for a massage or full-body esthetics treatment. Another option is to have your client wear a bathing suit or disposable spa item.

● Assist the client getting into the hydrotub, if possible, especially if the client has any special needs.

Treatment

Special considerations will depend on the type of the treatment. However, it is recommended that you check on your client during the treatment. A client should not be left alone for long periods of time or for the entire treatment.

End of the Treatment

● Hydrotbub treatments are generally very relaxing, so gently tell the client that the treatment is finished.

● Wait a few minutes and then assist the client from the hydrotub, especially if it has been a heating treatment.

● The client should be allowed to rest quietly after the treatment or assisted to another room if the client has another treatment following the hydrotub treatment.

Post-Treatment

● The hydrotub must be cleaned after each use. If there is water on the floor or other surfaces from the treatment, they should be dried.

● The hydrotub must be disinfected after each use. Special procedures should be followed if water was recirculated through water jets or through a hydrowand. (See Chapter 6 for more information on hygiene and safety.)

Additional Suggestions

Combining Hydrotub Treatments with Other Treatments

● Hydrotub treatments can be combined with most massage and esthetic treatments, usually before these other treatments.

● Because hydrotub treatments can be very relaxing, it makes them a perfect part of a half-day or a whole-day package.

Series of Hydrotub Treatments

Hydrotub therapy, especially as part of a combination of treatments, can be very effective in programs that require a series of sessions. These can include weight management, stress management, detoxification, and skin care. Some spa and wellness centers have developed ongoing holistic health and wellness programs that provide treatments, including hydrotherapy treatments, at regular intervals. For example, Ayurvedic health and wellness programs include rejuvenating programs that are done four times a year, at the change of each season.

Home Program

Clients can be given instructions to do treatments at home in their own bathtub.

Relaxation Hydrotherapy

DESCRIPTION AND BENEFITS

Relaxation therapy is a very powerful therapeutic modality that helps bring balance to the constant overstimulation of our nervous system, especially the sympathetic nervous system, by the stress and demands of modern life. A hydrotub treatment is a deeply relaxing treatment that can be part of a relaxation therapy package or a relaxation treatment by itself (see Figure 7–6). There are many variations for using hydrotherapy as a relaxation treatment. Combining hydrotherapy with natural products, music, aromatherapy, variations in water temperature, or other elements adds unique elements to the relaxation experience. A relaxing, simple bath treatment is a very popular treatment with clients and is very easy to perform. The Japanese are masters of the relaxing bath, with a continuous tradition that dates back more than a thousand years.

EQUIPMENT

Simple bathtub, hydrotub

PRODUCTS

Virtually any combination of herbs, essential oils, oils, mineral salts, seaweeds, and algae can be used. Therapists can use their knowledge

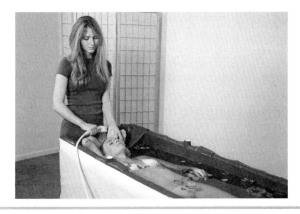

Figure 7–6 Relaxation treatment.

and intuition to create combinations that enhance relaxation, including music and light therapy.

STEPS OF THE TREATMENT

1. *Pretreatment:* Water should be added to the tub so it is ready for the client. The temperature should be in the neutral range—between about 95°F (36°C) to 98°F (38°C)—and should be comfortably warm. The client should not become overheated during the treatment. Products can be added to the bath water at this stage (or during the treatment).

2. *Beginning the treatment:* Assist the client into the hydrotub. The client should feel as if he or she is getting personal attention to all aspects of the treatment, as if he or she is receiving a royal relaxation treatment.

3. *Treatment:* The duration of the treatment can be from 25 to 45 minutes, depending on scheduling considerations. Because the water is neutral in temperature, the client can remain comfortable in the water for long periods of time. The therapist should check on the client, without disturbing him or her, during the treatment.

    Optional—Hydropressure: If available, a water or air jet could be used during treatment. Because the goal of a relaxing treatment is to create a quiet, relaxed state, gentle hydropressure is recommended.

    Optional—Massage: The therapist may perform a light massage of the client's head, neck, and shoulders during the bath. If so, the massage should be gentle and should contribute to the client's relaxed state.

4. *End of the treatment:* Provide the client with a towel and assist him or her from the hydrotub.

5. *Post-treatment:* The client should rest for as long as possible before leaving the spa or wellness center. The client should also be given water or herbal tea for hydration. This type of treatment will often be followed by another treatment.

ADDITIONAL SUGGESTIONS

The relaxation treatment combines very well with most other treatments, especially as preparation for a massage, skin care treatment, or a hair styling session.

Detoxification

DESCRIPTION AND BENEFITS

Detoxification in a hydrotub is based on the principle of water that is hotter than the body's core temperature coming into direct contact with the body. Because the heat exchange between the water and the body is more than 20 times greater than the heat exchange between the body and air, the water will quickly heat the human body, which is approximately 60% water. Heating the body with hot water dramatically increases the activity of the approximately 3 million eccrine sweat glands, which, in turn, can produce up to or more than 1 qt (1 L) of sweat per hour. Even when the body is underwater, sweat glands will still produce sweat. However, because the sweat cannot evaporate in the water, it will not produce any cooling effect. Clients will not only feel relaxed after the treatment, but will also notice both the short-term and long-term benefits of detoxification.

EQUIPMENT

Bathtub, hydrotub, hot tub

PRODUCTS

Products that promote relaxation and detoxification, such as certain essential oils sea salt or Epsom salt, can be added to the bath water. However, these products are not essential for detoxification, as it is the production of sweat by the sweat glands that is key to the treatment.

STEPS OF THE TREATMENT

1. *Pretreatment:* Fill the tub with water of the appropriate temperature. For most clients, a water temperature close to, but no hotter than, 104°F (40°C) should feel comfortable. However, some clients may prefer the water slightly cooler than this. Make a note of any client preference for water temperature for any future treatments.

2. *Beginning the treatment:* The client may prefer the water to be cooler at first with hot water added to gradually increase the

water temperature. This can be more comfortable for the client, rather than entering water that is around 104°F (40°C).

3. *Treatment:* The length of the treatment should be about 15 to 20 minutes. It is important not to overheat too quickly. It is also recommended to use a misting bottle or a cool small towel on the client's forehead to keep him or her comfortable as the body temperature rises.

4. *End of the treatment:* Because the client has been overheated, it is essential to assist him or her from the tub, as some clients may feel dizzy as they stand up.

5. *Post-treatment:* After any heating treatment, it is recommended that the client lie down and rest. Many spas and wellness centers have a resting room or area where a client can relax after a treatment. Encourage the client to drink extra water after the session to rehydrate.

ADDITIONAL SUGGESTIONS

- The detoxification hydrotub treatment can be combined with massage and part of combined detoxification and relaxation treatment.

- Detoxification hydrotub treatments can also be helpful with weight-management programs, in that they promote detoxification and increase cellular metabolism.

Full-Body Skin Care

DESCRIPTION AND BENEFITS

Hydrotub sessions provide an excellent way to perform various skin care treatments (see Figure 7–7). Products can be dissolved or mixed into the water, which then comes into contact with the client's skin. With hydrotub treatments, the temperature of the water can be controlled. Hotter water increases the rate of diffusion of products, as well as increasing the metabolic rate of skin cells and the circulation of blood to the skin. In addition, products that are not water soluble and will not easily wash off, can be applied to the client's skin before entering the tub. During these treatments, the client can soak for the necessary length of time to allow for maximum product interaction with the skin.

EQUIPMENT

Bathtub, hydrotub

PRODUCTS

Estheticians receive training in the use of different skin care products that produce a wide range of benefits for the skin. Many of these products are designed to be used in bath sessions. Skin care trade magazines, continuing education, special training, and trade shows provide information about the available products and how best to use them. Many natural

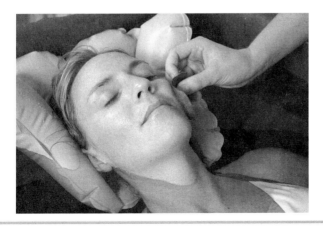

Figure 7–7 Full-body skin care treatment.

products, such as jojoba, aloe vera, and avocado, are known for their skin care properties and can be used to produce a therapeutic effect on the skin during a hydrotub treatment.

See the Hydrotherapy Product Resource Guide in Appendix C.

STEPS OF THE TREATMENT

1. *Pretreatment:* The temperature should be in the warmer range, from about 99°F (37.2°C) to 104°F (40°C). It should be comfortably warm and should not make the client overheated. This warmer water temperature will increase the client's skin and core body temperature. Products can be added to the bath water either before the client enters the tub or during the treatment. Some products should be applied to the client's skin before the client enters the water.

2. *Beginning the treatment:* The length of the treatment should be 15 to 20 minutes.

3. *Treatment:* This is a heating treatment, and thus the client may feel overheated. To cool the client, a misting bottle can be used. It is also possible to offer the client something cool or cold to drink. It is important to check on the client during the treatment to make sure he or she is feeling comfortable. It may be possible to massage some products into the skin during the hydrotub treatment, as this will enhance the interaction of the product with the skin.

4. *End of the treatment:* Assist the client from the hydrotub, especially if the treatment has increased the core body temperature.

5. *Post-treatment:* The client should rest after the treatment for as long as possible. The client should also be offered water, herbal tea, or some type of hydrating beverage.

ADDITIONAL SUGGESTIONS

- This treatment works very well in combination with other skin treatments, such as facials, or simply as part of a relaxing day at the spa.

- This treatment can be very effective as part of total skin care program in which the client receives a series of treatments on a regular schedule.

Preparation for Massage Treatments

DESCRIPTION AND BENEFITS

A hydrotub treatment can be a great preparation for a massage (see Figure 7–8). Hydrotub treatments are deeply relaxing, which also reduces muscle tension. In addition, heating the core body temperature makes the muscles, tendons, and ligaments more flexible. The total fascial matrix becomes especially more flexible, which allows it to rotate and stretch more easily during the massage.

EQUIPMENT

Bathtub, hydrotub, hot tub

PRODUCTS

Because the primary goal of this treatment is to increase the core body temperature and to produce relaxation, aromatherapy products that promote relaxation can be added to the water. Oils, such as jojoba oil, can be applied to the skin before the treatment as they will not easily wash off and the heat will increase the absorption of the skin. Products such as special creams for joint pain can also be applied before the treatment. Mineral salts, such as sea salts and Epsom salts, can also be added.

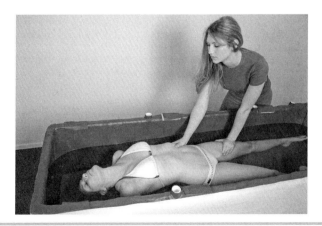

Figure 7–8 Hydrotub therapy as preparation for massage.

STEPS OF THE TREATMENT

1. *Pretreatment:* The water temperature can be in the warmer range—up to 104°F (40°C). Although the goal is to heat the core body temperature, the client should remain comfortable and should not feel overheated during or after the treatment.

2. *Beginning the treatment:* Assist the client into the hydrotub.

3. *Treatment:* The length of the treatment should be 15 to 20 minutes. It is important to monitor the client during the treatment and cool him or her with misting or a cool cloth as needed.

4. *End of the treatment:* Assist the client from the hydrotub and to the room where the massage will be performed.

5. *Post-treatment:* Clean and disinfect the hydrotub and prepare the room for the next treatment.

ADDITIONAL SUGGESTION

If the design of the hydrotub permits, some massage of the neck, shoulders, or face can be done during the hydrotub treatment.

Hydrotub Massage and Bodywork

DESCRIPTION AND BENEFITS

Some hydrotubs allow massage therapists and bodyworkers to use massage and other types of bodywork on clients while in the hydrotub. These treatments include massage, range-of-motion movements, assisted stretching, and hydromassage. The main difference between doing these treatments in a hydrotub as compared to a massage table, is that the client is in a gravity-free environment in which the body can be heated and additional hydromassage can be included. Bodywork treatments in a hydrotub can be especially helpful with sports injuries, acute and chronic injuries from accidents, general structural problems associated with aging, and situations in which a client is very sensitive to touch or pressure. The additional relaxation associated with hydrotub treatments can also be very beneficial.

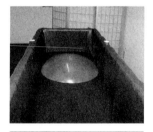

Figure 7–9
Hydroballoon.

A new hydrotub technology uses large balloons called hydroballoons that can hold as much as 15 gal of water. These hydroballoons are filled with water while the client is in the water. The client can then lie on the mostly submerged hydroballoon for support. The hydroballoon can be used for assisted stretching or as a form of traction and has many other uses. Figure 7–9 (Plate 36) shows a mostly submerged hydroballoon without a client in the hydrotub. Figure 7–10 (Plate 35) shows a client lying on a hydroballoon while being worked on by a therapist.

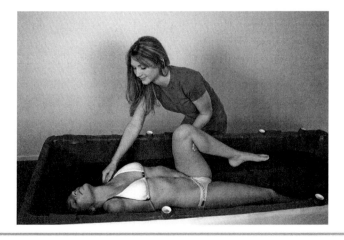

Figure 7–10 Bodywork treatment.

EQUIPMENT

The best types of hydrotubs for these treatments are those that are as long as possible and that allow maximum access to the client. There is also the option of using hydroballoons.

PRODUCTS

Products that promote relaxation and reduce muscle tension and joint pain could be applied before the treatment.

STEPS OF THE TREATMENT

1. *Pretreatment:* The water temperature should be in the neutral to warm range. If the goal is to heat the client's core body temperature in order to increase the ability of the body to stretch and rotate, the water should be in the warm to hot range, from 100°F (37.8°C) to 104°F (40°C).

2. *Beginning the treatment:* Assist the client into the hydrotub, especially if he or she is having difficulty in moving.

3. *Treatment:* The duration of the treatment can be from 15 to 30 minutes, depending on the goal of the treatment and the temperature of the water.

    Optional—Massage: It may be possible to massage a client while he or she is in the hydrotub, though this is much more limited than performing massage on a table. In general, massage in the hydrotub is used to treat specific problem areas of the body and is not used for a total body massage.

    Optional—Assisted Stretching and Rotating: The reduced gravity, relaxation, and warmth offered by a hydrotub make it possible to do standard assisted stretching movements and to assist in moving limbs through various range of motion movements. Some of the treatments can be enhanced by the use of hydroballoons.

    Optional—Hydromassage: If the hydrotub has a hydrowand feature, hydromassage can be done on specific areas of the body. Hydromassage can greatly enhance circulation to the affected areas. It can also provide a unique hydromassage of different muscles and joints and can be very effective at reducing adhesions between muscle cells (fibers).

4. *End of the Treatment:* Allow the client as much time to relax as possible before asking the client to leave the hydrotub. Assist the

client from the hydrotub. Some clients may feel dizzy as they stand after being overheated.

5. *Post-treatment:* After any heating treatment, it is good to have the client rest after the treatment. Many spas and wellness centers have a resting room or area where a client can relax. The treatment may also be followed by massage and bodywork on a regular massage table.

ADDITIONAL SUGGESTION

Bodywork treatments normally require several sessions over an extended period of time.

Flotation Hydrotherapy

DESCRIPTION AND BENEFITS

Flotation therapy is based on the water principle of buoyancy. When someone is immersed in water, the principle of buoyancy reduces the effects of gravity on the body. In a flotation treatment, the body is completely horizontal and the client floats in the water. See Figures 7–11 (Plate 34) and Figure 7–12 (Plate 33). The water temperature stays constant in the neutral range, which does not produce a heating or cooling effect on the client. In general, the goal of the treatment is to produce a profound sense of relaxation. Clients often report unique experiences during flotation, such as personal or creative insights, a feeling of connection with nature, and spiritual awakening. Flotation treatments can be very effective as part of ongoing stress-management programs.

EQUIPMENT

- *Hydrotub flotation:* Some hydrotubs are longer than the human body and include features to aid with flotation. These features provide enough support to keep the client from sinking while also allowing a complete feeling of floating. This allows significant reduction of sensory deprivation, because the client's ears are underwater; in addition, the light in the room should be minimal. Although the tub may restrict clients from extending their arms out to the side, most of the benefits of flotation therapy are possible.

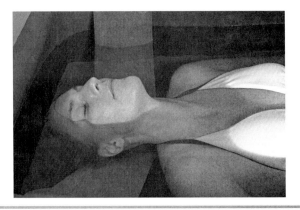

Figure 7–11 Flotation.

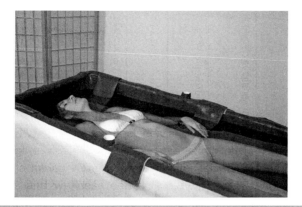

Figure 7–12 Flotation treatment.

Music and aromatherapy are possible additional features. An advantage to this system is that new (fresh) water is used for each treatment and is drained after the treatment.

- *Flotation tanks:* In flotation tanks, the water surface is large enough for the client to float with arms and legs extended without touching the sides of the tank. Sea salt and other mineral salts are added to the water to make it more buoyant so that the body floats effortlessly in the water. Most flotation tanks are enclosed to reduce the input of sound and light as much as possible. The purity and hygiene of the water is maintained in much the same way as in a hot tub—with filters and chemically treated water. Flotation tank equipment systems come with directions for use by clients, as well as maintenance and cleaning instructions.

For more information, see the Hydrotherapy Equipment Resource Guide in Appendix B.

PRODUCTS

Products are not used in flotation tanks. However, it is possible to use products, especially those that promote relaxation, in hydrotubs that allow flotation.

STEPS OF THE TREATMENT

1. *Pretreatment:* For treatments in a hydrotub that allow for flotation, preheat the water to about 95°F (35°C). Products can be added at this time. For treatments done in a flotation tank, follow the manufacturer's instructions; some flotation tanks as well as some

hydrotubs also have features for music, aromatherapy, and color light therapy.

2. *Treatment:* The length of the treatment is usually either 45 minutes, 1 hour, 1 hour 15 minutes, or 1 hour and 30 minutes.

   Flotation tank treatments: During flotation tank treatments, contact is not possible between the therapist and the client. Sometimes, clients may feel claustrophobic and may want to end the treatment sooner than planned. Other clients may have negative emotions, such as anxiety, fear, or sadness, surface. Therefore, it is important that the client knows the therapist is always available in case there are any problems.

   Hydrotub treatments: In hydrotub flotation treatment, the therapist is more involved in the treatment. The therapist should check on the client at regular intervals to see that everything appears normal. However, the therapist should not disturb the client; instead, the therapist should visually confirm that the client seems comfortable.

   Water temperature: After about 20 minutes, the therapist should check the water temperature to ensure that it is still at a comfortable level. An ideal temperature range is from 95°F (35°C) to 98°F (36.6°C). The client must know to tell the therapist if the water becomes too cool or warm.

3. *End of the treatment:* Gently end the session and give the client a few minutes before asking the client to exit the system. Assist the client from the hydrotub or floatation tank. Clients may be very unsteady after a long flotation session.

4. *Post-treatment:* Because of the deeply relaxing nature of flotation treatments, clients should have as much time as possible to rest and adjust before engaging in normal activity. Offer the client water or a natural beverage after the treatment.

ADDITIONAL SUGGESTION

Because of the unique and profound states of relaxation that are produced, a series of flotation treatments can be a valuable part of a wellness program, especially a stress-management program.

Breathing Therapy During a Hydrotub Session

DESCRIPTION AND BENEFITS

Proper breathing is essential to our overall wellness. A breathing therapy program can promote general wellness and also help clients stay more relaxed throughout the day, especially in stressful, demanding, or pressure situations. Breathing therapy combines deep relaxation with instructions on correct breathing during a hydrotub session. When a client is relaxed in a hydrotub, there is decreased muscle tension and breathing can be more relaxed and effortless. While the client is deeply relaxed, verbal instructions on proper breathing can be given. Training seminars for normal, relaxed breathing are often used as part of stress-management programs.

The basic elements of proper normal breathing are well known. Yet, many people do not breathe correctly, either due to stress, muscle tension, or just poor breathing habits. Because the elements of normal breathing are relatively simple and natural, it is easy to guide clients though a session on normal breathing while they are getting a relaxing hydrotub treatment.

EQUIPMENT

Bathtub, hydrotub

PRODUCTS

Products that increase relaxation and a sense of well-being, such as certain essential oils for aromatherapy, can be added to the water in the hydrotub.

STEPS OF THE TREATMENT

1. *Pretreatment:* Preheat the water in the neutral range—between about 95°F (36°C) and 98°F (38°C). The water temperature should be comfortably warm, and the client should not become heated or cold during the treatment. Products can be added to the bath water before the client enters the tub and/or during the treatment. Relaxing music can also be played during the session but at a low level.

2. *Beginning the treatment:* Assist the client into the hydrotub. The atmosphere of the room should be very relaxed.

3. *Treatment:* The duration of the treatment can be from 25 to 45 minutes, depending on scheduling considerations. Because the client is not being heated or cooled, he or she can remain comfortable in the water for longer periods of time.

Normal Natural Breathing Instructions: When the client is completely relaxed and comfortable, guide the client through the basic principles of proper breathing:

- Breathe from the diaphragm in slow, relaxed, easy rhythms.

- Take relaxed, full breaths.

- Breathe through the nose. Avoid breathing from the upper chest or sucking air in through the nose. Breathing should be coming from a natural contraction and relaxation of the diaphragm. The client should breathe in this manner for several minutes. After a short break, he or she should repeat this technique for several more minutes.

Optional—Visualization: As the client practices normal breathing during the treatment, have him or her visualize using proper breathing techniques in daily life situations—both normal and stressful (for example during rush hour traffic). When the client is not in treatment, he or she can remember the experience of proper breathing and apply it in daily life. Developing a deep association between proper breathing experienced during the treatment and proper breathing during the day can have significant benefits for daily health and wellness.

4. *End of the treatment:* Assist the client from the hydrotub.

ADDITIONAL SUGGESTIONS

Several additional resources on the principles of correct breathing are available. One popular resource is Dr. Andrew Wile's *Mindbody Tool Kit* (see Suggested Readings at the end of this chapter).

Crystal Energy Hydrotub Therapy

DESCRIPTION AND BENEFITS

Just as water can be transformed by adding heat, pressure, or natural products, the energy of water can be transformed with the use of natural quartz crystals and other gemstones. The use of crystals has an ancient tradition as part of energy work. Because of the special synergy that crystals have with water, they have long been used to transform the energy of water. Water that has been transformed by crystals is then used to transform the energy of the client (see Figure 7–13 and Plate 32). Many therapists are trained in energy work and using crystals for multiple energetic benefits. The use of crystals with water can enhance these effects.

EQUIPMENT

Bathtub, hydrotub (a longer, deeper hydrotub is preferred for this treatment), quartz crystal (the crystal in Figure 7–13 can also be seen in Figure 10–3)

PRODUCTS

Products that a therapist feels may increase relaxation or enhance the effects of crystal energy in the water

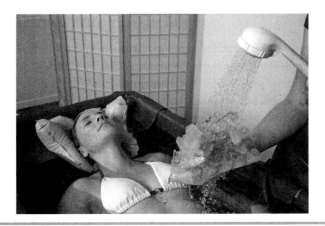

Figure 7–13 Crystal energy water treatment.

STEPS OF THE TREATMENT

1. *Pretreatment:* If a hydrotub is being used, preheat the water in the neutral range, between about 95°F (36°C) and 98°F (38°C). The water temperature should be comfortably warm; the client should not become overheated or cold during the treatment. Fill the hydrotub to a height of about 4 to 6 inches.

2. *Beginning the treatment:* Assist the client into the hydrotub. The atmosphere should be very relaxed.

3. *Treatment:* The duration of the treatment can be from 25 to 45 minutes, depending on scheduling considerations. As the client is not being heated (or cooled), he or she can remain comfortable in the water for a long period of time.

   Water Flowing over Crystal: As the client lies in the tub, begin to add water to the hydrotub so that it flows over the crystals. Continue to add water until the water is at the optimal level for a relaxing treatment. As the client relaxes in the crystal-enhanced water, you may choose to add other elements to the treatment, such as massage, misting, or music, to enhance the effects of the treatment. This treatment can be adjusted to each therapist's unique approach to energy work. If it is not possible to have water flow over the crystals while the client is in the hydrotub, as described previously, this could be done before the client gets into the hydrotub.

4. *End of the treatment:* Gently end the treatment. Assist the client from the hydrotub.

5. *Post-treatment:* The client should rest as long as possible after the treatment. Provide the client with drinking water or a natural beverage.

ADDITIONAL SUGGESTIONS

- Other gemstones can be used, according to their traditional purposes.

- Crystals and gems can also be placed in a container that allows water to flow over them into the hydrotub. A handheld shower could also be used to create flowing water over the crystals that are in a container directly onto the client in a hydrotub or on a wet table.

Color Light Therapy in Hydrotub Treatments

DESCRIPTION AND BENEFITS

In the same way that water can be transformed by crystals, it can also be transformed by using different colors of light. Different colors of light can be passed through water to the client's body. It is possible that the water is enhanced by the light or the light is enhanced by passing through water. Either way, when the enhanced light and water come into contact with the client's body, it can transform the client's physical, mental, emotional, and spiritual energy.

EQUIPMENT

Hydrotub with a built-in color light therapy system; or a separate color light therapy system that can be used during a hydrotub treatment

PRODUCTS

Products that increase relaxation or enhance the effects of color light energy in the water.

STEPS OF THE TREATMENT

1. *Pretreatment:* Preheat the water in the neutral range, between about 95°F (36°C) and 98°F (38°C). The temperature should be comfortably warm and should not overheat the client.

2. *Beginning the treatment:* Assist the client into the hydrotub. The atmosphere should be very relaxed.

3. *Treatment:* The duration of the treatment can be from 25 to 45 minutes, depending on scheduling considerations. Because the client is not being heated or cooled, he or she can remain comfortable in the water for longer periods of time.

   Color light therapy: Shine the color light through the water to specific areas of the client's body—for example, to the chakra areas or along the shiatsu energy meridian lines and points (Figure 7–18). The light could also be moved along the body to stimulate energy flow through the body.

   NOTE: SOME COLOR LIGHT THERAPY EQUIPMENT CAN BE USED IN THIS WAY, WHILE OTHER SYSTEMS ARE FIXED INTO THE HYDROTUB.

4. *End of the treatment:* Gently end the treatment. Assist the client from the hydrotub.

5. *Post-treatment:* The client should rest as long as possible after the treatment.

ADDITIONAL SUGGESTIONS

Many therapists, especially those doing energy work, have some training in the use of color light therapy and are knowledgeable about which colors are associated with which physical, mental, emotional, and spiritual elements (see Table 7–2). There are also several books available on this topic (see Suggested Readings at the end of this chapter).

Table 7–2 Color Light Therapy			
Red	**Orange**	**Yellow**	**Green**
energy, enthusiasm, passion, vitality	joyfulness, warmth, happiness	mental energy and creativity, focus, concentration	balanced thoughts and feelings, healing
Turquoise	**Blue**	**Violet**	**Magenta**
refreshing, cooling, soothing	calming, relaxing, deep inner peace, serenity	spiritual healing, intuition, meditation, spiritual awareness	compassion, awareness of spiritual self, letting go

Lymphatic Hydromassage Therapy

DESCRIPTION AND BENEFITS

Hydromassage, by using a hydrowand in a hydrotub, is an effective way to promote lymphatic circulation. The hydropressure stimulates the flow of lymphatic fluid through the lymphatic vascular system by adding a gentle pressure on the surface of the body. By using the hydrowand, the therapist can cover most of the body while also focusing on specific areas of the lymphatic vascular system. This treatment can also be part of skin care treatments, general circulatory treatments, or any treatment program that benefits from improved lymphatic circulation.

Many therapists have had training in lymphatic massage. Lymphatic massage in a hydrotub, using hydropressure, offers another modality for this type of massage (see Figure 7–14).

EQUIPMENT

Hydrotub with hydrowand

PRODUCTS

Products are usually not an essential part of a lymphatic hydromassage treatment.

STEPS OF THE TREATMENT

1. *Pretreatment:* Add water to the hydrotub so that it is ready for the client at the beginning of the treatment. The temperature should be in the neutral to warm range, between 96°F (36°C) and 101°F (38°C).

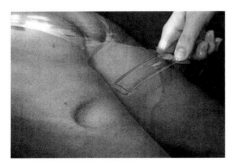

Figure 7–14 Lymphatic hydromassage treatment.

The temperature should be comfortably warm and should not overheat the client.

2. *Beginning the treatment:* The length of the treatment can be 20 to 30 minutes or longer, depending on scheduling and other considerations.

3. *Treatment:* Hydropressure from the hydrowand should be directed along the skin in the direction of the heart. Lymphatic vessels have valves that prevent backflow of lymphatic fluid, and the natural flow of fluid in these vessels is in the direction of the heart. In areas with high concentrations of lymph nodes—for example, in the groin area or the armpits—the hydropressure can be held for longer periods of time. When possible, it is also good to use small circular motions in these areas. The amount of water pressure can be controlled by increasing or decreasing the distance between the surface of the body and the hydrowand. Some hydrowands have the ability to adjust the pressure. The hydrowand makes it easier to cover most of the body, including the head, in hydrotubs that are long enough. Therapists can also use their hands to perform massage when they are not using the hydrowand. (Refer to Figure 4–17 to see the area of the skin that can be covered by the hydrowand.)

   The skin has a large number of lymphatic vascular capillaries. Most others areas of the body also have some lymphatic capillaries for lymph drainage. By using a light hydropressure to slowly cover most of the area of the body that can be massaged with a hydrowand, it is possible to stimulate a significant level of the lymphatic circulation.

4. *End of the treatment:* Allow the client a few minutes to rest before helping him or her to move from the hydrotub.

ADDITIONAL SUGGESTIONS

- It is recommended that therapists study the anatomy and physiology of the lymphatic circulation system. This information can be found in textbooks used for therapists' professional basic training or in other basic textbooks on anatomy and physiology. Even if the intention of a hydrowand treatment is not to massage the lymphatic system, there will still be a massaging effect on the system, so it is good to review the anatomy and physiology of the lymphatic system.

- A recommended resource for more in-depth training on lymphatic massage can be found in *Therapeutic Massage*, by Mark Beck.

Reflexology Hydromassage

DESCRIPTION AND BENEFITS

A unique way to perform reflexology is to use hydrowand pressure massage on the client's feet or hands while they are underwater (see Figure 7–15 and Plate 37). Therapists may also want to combine manual reflexology massage with the hydropressure massage. A reflexology chart is illustrated in Figure 7–16 and Plate 38.

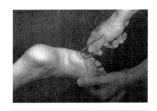

Figure 7–15
Reflexology hydro-massage treatment.

EQUIPMENT

Hydrotub with a hydrowand, special footbaths

The hydrotub or footbath should allow the therapist access to the feet for performing a hydropressure reflexology treatment.

PRODUCTS

Although it is not necessary to use any product for this treatment, the addition of mineral salts, essential oils, and seaweed and herbal preparations to the water can enhance the treatment.

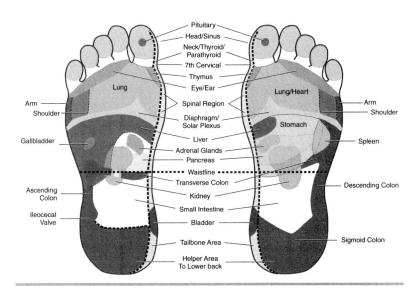

Figure 7–16 Reflexology chart.

STEPS OF THE TREATMENT

1. *Pretreatment:* Add water to the tub so that it is ready for the client. The temperature should be in the neutral to warm range, between 98°F (36°C) and 102°F (38.9°C). The temperature should be warm enough to increase the temperature of the feet and/or hands, which will also increase circulation and metabolic activity.

2. *Beginning the treatment:* If the treatment is done in a hydrotub, assist the client into the hydrotub and give the client a few minutes to relax before beginning the treatment.

3. *Treatment:* The length of the treatment can be 20 to 25 minutes. Hydropressure from the hydrowand should be moved slowly and systematically over the different reflexology zones of the hand and/or feet. Both straight and circular motions can be used and pressure can be applied to specific spots for longer periods of time. The hydrowand can be used as an extension of the therapist's hand. Traditional manual reflexology can be used along with the hydromassage.

   Contrast reflexology bath: The temperature of the water can be varied, especially in small footbaths. If a hose for hydrotherapy is part of the hydrotub, it may be possible to alternate pouring cold water on the feet for about 15 to 60 seconds and then placing the feet back into the warm water. This contrast between cold and warm water produces a stimulating effect.

4. *End of the treatment:* Dry the client's hands and feet. As an added option, apply a moisturizing product to the hands and/or feet.

5. *Post-treatment:* It is very important that the equipment used to recirculate the water be properly cleaned and disinfected. (See Chapter 6 for more information on hygiene.) A **broad-spectrum disinfectant,** or an approved disinfectant supplied by the manufacturer, should be used to clean the recirculating equipment and the hydrotub or footbath.

Broad-spectrum disinfectant
A high-grade disinfectant that kills the normal range of germs. Recommended for use in hydrotherapy rooms and equipment.

ADDITIONAL SUGGESTIONS

This is a great treatment to have as part of a combination of treatments. It can also be given in a regular series of treatments over time—for example, once every month. Most massage therapists have had training in reflexology. Courses and books that cover the basics of reflexology are also available.

Hydrotub Hydromassage Shiatsu

DESCRIPTION AND BENEFITS

Shiatsu hydromassage using a hydrowand in a hydrotub provides another modality for shiatsu massage. Promoting a balanced flow of energy along the body's meridian lines is the primary goal of shiatsu massage. The hydropressure from the hydrowand provides a deep, comfortable pressure that can easily be directed along the meridian lines and to specific points along those lines (see Figure 7–17). A shiatsu chart is illustrated in Figure 7–18 and Plate 40.

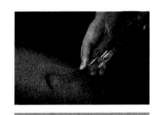

Figure 7–17 Shiatsu hydromassage treatment.

> **NOTE:** THIS TREATMENT IS INCLUDED AS AN OPTION FOR THERA- PISTS WHO ALREADY HAVE SOME FORM OF CERTIFIED TRAINING IN SHIATSU MASSAGE.

EQUIPMENT

Hydrotub with a hydrowand. A longer hydrotub is particularly useful in this treatment.

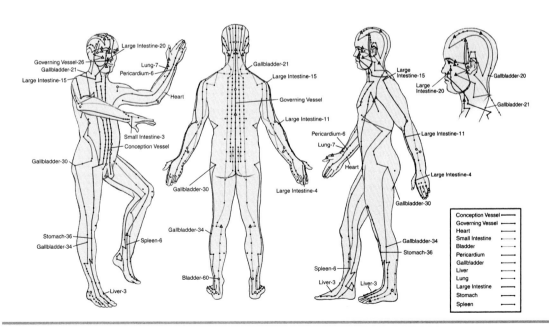

Figure 7–18 Shiatsu chart.

PRODUCTS

Although products are not an essential component of this treatment, aromatherapy can be used for its soothing and relaxing qualities. Also, a therapist may want to add a product that he or she feels will benefit the treatment.

STEPS OF THE TREATMENT

1. *Pretreatment:* Add water to the hydrotub so that it is ready for the client. The temperature should be in the neutral to warm range, between about 96°F (36°C) and 101°F (38°C). The temperature should be comfortably warm; because this is not a heating treatment, the client should not get overheated.

2. *Beginning the treatment:* Assist the client into the hydrotub. Allow him or her to relax for a few minutes before beginning the treatment.

3. *Treatment:* The treatment can last about 30 minutes or longer, depending on scheduling and other considerations. The hydropressure from the hydrowand should be directed along the meridian lines, in the same manner that a therapist would use his or her hands to give a traditional shiatsu treatment. The hydrowand, and the pressure it generates, becomes an extension of the therapist's hands. The pressure can be held at specific points along the meridian lines when needed. The hydrowand makes it easier to cover most of the body, including the head in hydrotubs that are long enough. For points on the head that cannot be reached by the hydrowand, normal hand and finger pressure can be used.

4. *End of the treatment:* Allow the client a few minutes to rest before helping him or her from the hydrotub.

5. *Post-treatmet:* All steps should be followed for properly disinfecting the hydrotub and the recirculating hydrowand system.

ADDITIONAL SUGGESTIONS

- This treatment can be given by itself or can be part of a total package of treatment. This treatment can also be part of a series of treatments at scheduled intervals.

- The same basic techniques described in this treatment can be done on the body's pressure points (see the pressure points chart in Figure 7–19).

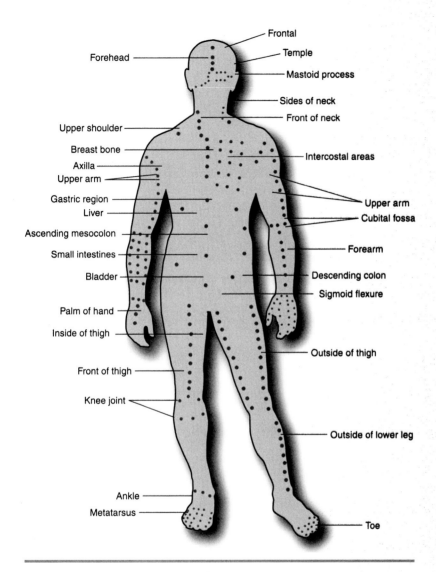

Figure 7–19 Pressure points chart.

Cellulite Hydromassage

DESCRIPTION AND BENEFITS

Using the hydrowand for cellulite massage is an excellent way to massage areas of the body showing signs of cellulite. The hydrowand produces a deep massage of the dermis and subcutaneous layers of the skin, which not only increases circulation but also massages the connective matrixes that keep the adipocytes (fat cells) in alignment (see Figure 7–20 and Plate 23). Setting the water temperature in the warmer range will heat the skin cells and connective matrix, thus increasing the cells' metabolic activity and the flexibility of the connective matrix.

EQUIPMENT

Hydrotub with a hydrowand. A longer hydrotub is recommended.

PRODUCTS

Many products have been created for use in the treatment of cellulite. Some of these products that do not easily rinse off with water can be used during this treatment. The increased skin temperature, as well as the pressure of the water from the hydromassage, will increase the ability of the skin to absorb these products.

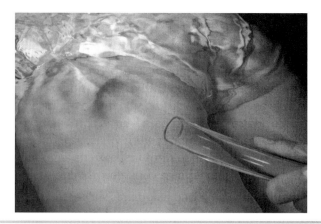

Figure 7–20 Cellulite hydromassage treatment.

STEPS OF THE TREATMENT

1. *Pretreatment:* Add water to the tub so that it is ready for the client. The temperature should be in the warm range—between 99°F (37.2°C) and 104°F (40°C). The temperature should be warm enough to increase the skin temperature. This will increase circulation to the skin and will make the matrix that holds the adipocytes (fat cells) in alignment more flexible and more stretchable.

2. *Beginning the treatment:* Cellulite creams or other products for the skin can be placed on the skin before the treatment begins.

3. *Treatment:* The treatment can be 20 to 30 minutes. The hydrowand should be moved slowly and systematically over the areas of the body with cellulite. Both straight and circular motions can be used. Therapists can also apply manual massage along with the hydropressure massage. The hydrowand essentially becomes an extension of the therapist's hands.

4. *End of the treatment:* Certain cellulite creams are designed to be applied to the skin after treatment. See the Hydrotherapy Product Resource Guide in Appendix C.

5. *Post-treatment:* A broad-spectrum disinfectant should be used to properly clean and disinfect the recirculating equipment used in the hydrowand. (See Chapter 6 for more information on hygiene.)

ADDITIONAL SUGGESTIONS

- For cellulite treatments to be effective, they are normally done as a series of treatments at regular intervals.

- The hydrotub cellulite treatment could also be done before certain types of cellulite treatments that use manual or mechanical massage.

Cellular/Vascular Hydromassage

DESCRIPTION AND BENEFITS

The human body is composed of approximately 100 trillion cells. Each cell exists in a fluid environment and depends on continual circulation of nutrients and oxygen, as well as the removal of by-products (e.g., carbon dioxide and lactic acid) from cellular metabolism. The cardiovascular system, including the lymphatic vascular system, brings circulation to all the cells of the body. Hydromassage can be done on the cells and the vascular system of the body. Because the pressure from a hydrowand is firm but gentle and the massage is done underwater, it is ideal for cellular and vascular massage (see Figure 7–21 and Plate 39). This type of massage can stimulate circulation to the cells, within the cells, and within the vascular system. Hydromassage can also promote cellular and vascular alignment. When doing this massage, the therapist should view the body as a dynamic, fluid cellular system, as described in Chapter 3.

When we perform any massage and apply pressure to the body, we are applying pressure to the cells and vascular system of that area of the body. In this treatment, we are putting our attention on the cells and vascular system at the cellular level, rather than on the muscle or fascial system level. Hydromassage of the cells and vascular system at the cellular level offers tremendous possibilities for wellness at the cellular level.

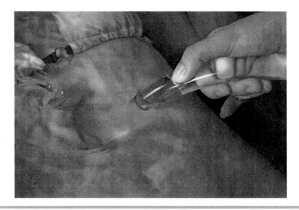

Figure 7–21 Cellular and vascular hydromassage treatment.

EQUIPMENT

Hydrotub with a hydrowand

PRODUCTS

Products are not an essential element of this treatment, but the therapist can add products if he or she wishes.

STEPS OF THE TREATMENT

1. *Pretreatment:* Add water to the tub so that it is ready for the client. The temperature should be in the neutral to warm range—between 96°F (36°C) and 101°F (38°C). The temperature should be comfortably warm and should not overheat the client.

2. *Beginning the treatment:* Assist the client into the hydrotub. Allow the client a few minutes to relax before beginning the treatment.

3. *Treatment:* The treatment can last 20 to 30 minutes or longer. Hydropressure should be applied systematically over most of the body. Straight-line strokes can be used along with holding the pressure on specific areas for longer periods of time. Circular motion can also be used on some areas, such as the stomach. The strokes of the hydrowand should be slow and flowing. It is helpful to visualize that you are massaging the cells as well as the complex vascular system (blood vessels) of the body.

4. *End of the treatment:* Let the client rest a few minutes before assisting him or her from the hydrotub.

5. *Post-treatment:* A broad-spectrum disinfectant should be used to properly clean and disinfect the hydrotub and recirculating equipment used in the hydrowand. (See Chapter 6 for more information on hygiene.)

ADDITIONAL SUGGESTIONS

Therapists should review information on the anatomy and physiology of the vascular system and of the cells of the body. Teaching Exercise 3-3 is a simple but effective way to get a feeling of working with cells in a fluid environment.

Hydrotherapy Shower Treatments

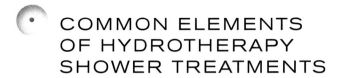

COMMON ELEMENTS OF HYDROTHERAPY SHOWER TREATMENTS

Dynamic Water Principles

- Water in the liquid form is used for hydrotherapy shower treatments. During a shower treatment, there is also a considerable amount of water that evaporates into the gas (vapor) state, thus increasing the level of humidity around the client.

- Water pressure produces a flow of water through multiple showerheads in a Vichy or Swiss shower or though a single showerhead in a handheld or regular shower. This results in fine streams of water coming into contact with the client's body and producing pressure on the skin. Water pressure from Vichy and Swiss and handheld showers usually varies from light to medium. The pressure can be strong enough to stimulate circulation of both the blood and the lymphatic fluid, especially in the area of the skin.

- There will be some heat exchange between the water and the client's body. This heat exchange will vary, depending on the temperature of the water.

- Turbulent water flow, such as that found at a waterfall, has been associated with an increase in negative ions, which is known to produce a fresh, invigorating feeling. The flow of water through multiple showerheads in a Vichy or Swiss shower creates turbulence similar that found in a waterfall. This increase in negative ions during the shower may partly explain the clean, fresh, invigorating feeling provided during these treatments.

Temperature

During a Vichy or Swiss shower, or a handheld shower, the water temperature is generally in the warm range—between 100°F (37.7°C) and 108°F (40°C). This range of temperatures produces a state of relaxation for the client. Vichy and Swiss showers usually last for about 10 minutes, which means the client's body does not usually have time to overheat. It is possible to alternate periods of warm water with brief periods (about 45 seconds) of cold water to add a stimulating and invigorating element along with the relaxing effects of the Vichy and Swiss showers.

Length of Treatment

The duration of hydrotherapy shower treatments, especially Vichy and Swiss showers, is about 10 minutes, which is generally long enough to create the desired effect. The length of this treatment is limited by the fact that there is a high flow rate of water—up to 10 gal/min—which requires a significant amount of hot water. Many spa and wellness centers have a limited amount of hot water for all the various water needs, and thus these types of showers must be kept relatively short.

Anatomy and Physiology

The main physiological change during shower treatments is a slight increase in skin and body temperature. This type of treatment is usually not long enough for a significant change in temperature. However, if the shower will be followed by another treatment, such as skin care, the water temperature can be set in the higher range to increase the skin temperature. The water pressure of the shower can be strong enough to stimulate both blood and lymph circulation. The greater the water pressure, the greater the effect will be on the circulation.

Vichy and Swiss showers produce a spray over large areas of the body at the same time. The skin is very sensitive to the sensory input of the pressure and temperature of a shower spray. Vichy, Swiss, and handheld showers all create unique patterns of sensory stimulation, which produces anything from a special feeling of relaxation to a sense of well-being to euphoric feelings. Some of this effect may be enhanced by the abundance of negative ions from the shower. When these shower treatments include alternations between hot and cold, they can lead to feelings of being deeply relaxing and yet stimulated at the same time.

Shower treatments are a form of hydromassage that produces a wonderful sensation of a water massage, which is similar to and yet very different from a normal massage. Research has shown that the experience of a relaxing massage stimulates the hypothalamus to produce the hormone oxytocin. An increase in oxytocin has been correlated with a great feeling of connection with others, emotional security, and comfort. This may be one explanation for the beautiful feelings produced by a Vichy, Swiss, or even a handheld shower.

Immediate and Long-Term Benefits

The immediate benefit of a Vichy, Swiss, or handheld shower treatment is the feeling of being deeply relaxed, refreshed, and enlivened (stimulated), all at the same time. The added benefit of a handheld shower is the nurturing experience of being showered and rinsed while lying relaxed on a treatment table. This adds much more of a personal element to a treatment than simply allowing a client to take a standard shower.

One longer-term benefit of these treatments is the balance they create between the sympathetic and parasympathetic nervous systems, which are the stimulating and relaxing autonomic controls of the body. Most people today are overstimulated and overstressed. Hydrotherapy shower treatments help balance this overstimulation with states of deep relaxation. In addition, the stimulating effect on the circulation of blood and the lymphatic system is beneficial to the overall health of the skin.

Equipment

Several companies manufacture and sell Vichy, Swiss, and handheld showers as well as wet table systems. Refer to the Hydrotherapy Equipment Resource Guide in Appendix B for suggestions on researching this type of equipment.

Following are some points to consider regarding hydrotherapy shower equipment:

- All shower systems, including Vichy, Swiss, and handheld, should have scald protection and pressure-balancing features. This protects the client from being scalded by extreme fluctuations in water temperature.
- The system should be easy to clean and disinfect.
- The system should be designed for client comfort. This will enhance the client's feeling of relaxation and wellness, which is one of the main goals of the treatment. This feature is especially true regarding wet tables. The more comfortable the client is, the more beneficial the treatment will be for the client.

NOTE: SOME WET TABLES ARE VERY POORLY DESIGNED IN TERMS OF CLIENT COMFORT. IF POSSIBLE, RECEIVE A TREATMENT ON A SYSTEM THAT YOU ARE CONSIDERING PURCHASING AND IF POSSIBLE, COMPARE SEVERAL DIFFERENT SYSTEMS.

- If you cannot afford to build a wet room, look for Vichy shower systems that do not require one.
- Some Vichy and Swiss shower systems are multipurpose, allowing both massage and steam therapy treatments. These features can increase the number of treatment options in a hydrotherapy treatment room.

Products

In general, products are not applied to the body immediately before or during shower treatments, as these treatments will rinse any product from the body. However, certain oil-based or natural oil products that do not easily wash off can be used. Aromatherapy or misting with water mixed with essential oils or hydrosols can be a positive additional feature during these treatments.

Contraindications

- Because the water temperature is normally kept at a comfortable level and the water pressure is generally light, the main contraindications are skin infections, recent cuts, or breaks in the skin.
- Any type of cardiovascular problem is contraindicated for a contrast Vichy or Swiss shower that alternates hot water with cold water. This includes Raynaud's Syndrome and cold sensitivities.
- It is very important for the therapist to feel comfortable doing any treatment on a client. If there is any doubt about the client's medical condition as related to a special shower treatment, it best not to do the treatment. The client can always take a normal shower at the spa or wellness center or take a shower at home.

Safety Considerations

- As mentioned above, all shower equipment should have scald-protection and, if possible, pressure-balancing features. Scald protection is essential to ensure that the therapist cannot accidentally increase the water temperature above scalding during a treatment. Pressure-balancing features keep the water from fluctuating if water is being used elsewhere in the facility.
- Wet tables and wet room floors can be slippery, especially when they are wet. Always help a client from the table and when walking on wet floors. Also, provide the client with slip-resistant slippers.

Special Considerations

- Follow similar draping procedures that you would for a massage or full-body esthetics treatment. Shower treatments are more challenging when it comes to draping, because you want as much of the body exposed to the shower spray as possible, but you also do not want the client to get cold. Be creative!

- It is recommended to use lightweight towels or sheets for draping during shower treatments, as they will get very wet. Lightweight items wash and dry more quickly and are easier to work with, especially once they get wet.

- Instead of draping, clients can wear a bathing suit or disposable spa items, depending on modesty issues.

- It is very important to keep clients warm during shower treatments. They must not get cold or chilled during any shower treatment, especially a handheld shower. This may require a creative use of towels. Perhaps most important, it is necessary to clearly communicate to clients that they should tell you as soon as they get cold or chilled. Clients will often get cold and not tell you, which can ruin the treatment for them and they may never return to the spa. This is one of the most common, yet easily avoided, complaints regarding shower and hydrotherapy treatments in general.

End of the Treatment

- Most clients are very relaxed after a hydrotherapy shower treatment. Always try to create a comfortable transition between the end of the hydrotherapy shower treatment and the next step.

- Assist the client from a wet table or wet-room after a shower treatment.

Post-Treatment

If this treatment is not followed by another treatment, allow the clients to rest as long as possible and enjoy the wonderful feelings they are experiencing as a result of these special shower treatments.

Always clean and disinfect any part of the system, including the wet-room floor that comes into contact with water from the client's body. (Refer to Chapter 6 for more information on hygiene.)

Additional Suggestions

Vichy and Swiss showers, as well as some handheld showers, are great treatments at the end of a combination package. These treatments are also valuable as part of an ongoing wellness program that includes relaxation treatments being done at regular intervals.

SHOWER HYDROTHERAPY TREATMENTS

Vichy Shower

DESCRIPTION AND BENEFITS

A Vichy shower is a horizontal shower treatment using multiple shower-heads that spray the client who is lying on a wet table (see Figure 7–22 and Plate 29). There are many variations to this treatment, but the overall effect has been described as being both deeply relaxing and stimulating. The main elements of the treatment that can be controlled are the length of the treatment, the temperature of the water, the pressure of the water, the movement of the water on the body, and massage of the client's body. This treatment can also be used to rinse products from the body, but the primary benefit is the unique states of relaxation that are produced.

EQUIPMENT

- *Horizontal shower with multiple showerheads:* These Vichy shower systems normally contain anywhere from five to seven showerheads.

- *Wet table:* Clients lie on the wet table during the treatment. This usually requires that the treatment is done in a wet room with a floor drain.

- *Special systems:* Some Vichy equipment systems have an enclosed capsule or canopy that covers the client. This elimi-nates the need for a wet room. It also allows normal treatment rooms to be used, depending on the size of the room and the availability of plumbing lines.

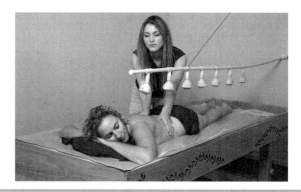

Figure 7–22 Vichy shower treatment.

PRODUCTS

Because this treatment produces a powerful rinsing effect, products are not usually placed on the client's body during treatment. However, if a massage is done during the shower, massage oils can be used.

STEPS OF THE TREATMENT

1. *Pretreatment:* The room should be ready, including all necessary towels.

2. *Beginning the treatment:* Assist the client onto the wet table, and prepare him or her for the shower.

    Draping the Client: Drape the client in such a way that as much of the body can come into direct contact with the water as possible.

    NOTE: BECAUSE MUCH OF THE CLIENT'S BODY IS UNCOVERED DURING THIS TREATMENT, IT IS IMPORTANT TO ENSURE THAT HE OR SHE DOES NOT GET CHILLED. THE CLIENT CAN BE KEPT WARM BY STARTING THE TREATMENT AS SOON AS THE CLIENT IS ON THE WET TABLE AND THEN COVERING THE CLIENT WITH A DRY TOWEL IMMEDIATELY AFTER THE WATER IS TURNED OFF.

    Follow the manufacturer's instructions to ensure that the water that initially comes into contact with the client is at a comfortable temperature. You may want to run water through the handheld shower until the appropriate water temperature is reached before turning on the Vichy shower. Be sure to ask the client for feedback and adjust the water temperature as needed.

3. *Treatment:* The treatment duration normally lasts about 10 minutes, though it can be longer. These showers use a considerable amount of water, both hot and cold, which can be a limiting factor on the length of treatment. The water temperature should be in a comfortably warm range.

    Optional—Contrasting Warm with Cold Water: One treatment option is to decrease the temperature to a colder setting (usually the coldest setting) for 30 to 45 seconds and then return the temperature back to normal. This could be done about five times during a 10-minute treatment. Many clients find that this contrast produces a positive effect both during and after the treatment. However, some clients find it very uncomfortable and instead prefer a constant comfortable temperature. It is important to note client preferences and record this for future treatments. This option should also be practiced in a training session before performing it on clients.

The water pressure from the showerheads is normally set to a firm pressure. During the treatment, it is possible to decrease or increase water pressure simply by controlling the valve that turns the water on and off. This option is not often used during Vichy showers.

Optional—Hydromassage: The showerheads of the Vichy shower system are connected to one pipe that can be moved from side to side during treatment. Some systems allow the showerheads to be rotated—the pipe remains in one position while the showerheads move in a semicircular motion. This movement of the showerheads causes the spray from the showerheads to produce a hydromassage of moving water across the larger surface areas of the client's body.

Optional—Manual Massage: The traditional Vichy shower treatment, as performed in Vichy, France, includes a normal massage from two therapists while the water showers the client on the wet table. The massage, which lasts 6 to 7 minutes on each side of the body, starts at the feet and moves to the head. The massage therapists use very quick, medium-pressure effleurage strokes and cross strokes on the arms and legs and a combination of effleurage stokes and circular strokes on the stomach, chest, back, and buttocks. The head massage is a combination of straight and circular strokes. Because this is a very brief massage that covers nearly the entire body, there is time for only a few strokes on each area. It is usually not possible to have two massage therapists performing the Vichy shower at most facilities, so one therapist normally does the treatment.

NOTE: THE VICHY SHOWER TREATMENTS GIVEN IN VICHY, FRANCE, USES A LOW FLOW RATE OF WATER FROM MULTIPLE SHOWERHEADS. THE FOCUS IS ON PROVIDING A CONTINUAL FLOW OF WARM WATER OVER THE ENTIRE BODY WHILE THE CLIENT IS BEING MASSAGED, RATHER THAN ON USING MEDIUM TO STRONG WATER PRESSURE FROM THE SHOWERHEADS.

4. *End of the treatment:* After turning off the water, make sure the client is quickly covered with a towel or sheet to keep him or her warm. Allow the client to relax for a few minutes before assisting him or her from the wet table. Wet tables and wet room floors can be slippery, especially when wet, so always assist the client.

5. *Post-treatment:* Have the client rest for as long as possible after the treatment. The wet table and any surfaces, such as a wet room floor, must be properly cleaned and disinfected, preferably with a broad-spectrum disinfectant. (See Chapter 6 for more information on hygiene.)

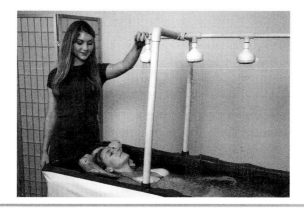

Figure 7–23 Hydrotub with Vichy shower.

ADDITIONAL SUGGESTIONS

- A Vichy shower can also be done as part of a hydrotub treatment if the hydrotub includes this feature (see Figure 7–23 and Plate 30).

- The Vichy shower treatment is a great way to end any combination of treatments.

Swiss Shower

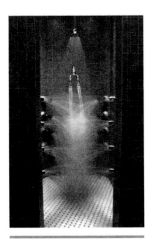

Figure 7-24 Swiss shower treatment *(courtesy of Broadmoor Resort, Colorado Springs, CO).*

DESCRIPTION AND BENEFITS

A Swiss shower is a vertical shower treatment that uses multiple shower-heads (see Figure 7-24). The client stands in an enclosed shower stall. A Swiss shower system usually has between 12 and 15 showerheads that are located to produce a spray that hits most of the body—front, side, and back. These shower systems often offer additional showerhead(s) directly above the client's head. A Swiss shower is often given at the end of other treatments, and produces feelings of being relaxed and invigorated at the same time. It is similar to a Vichy shower, except that the client is standing. It is also used to rinse off any product.

EQUIPMENT

Swiss shower equipment system: This system usually has between 12 and 15 showerheads that are designed to cover most of the client's body. Some come with an additional showerhead directly above the client's head. In some systems, the temperature and water pressure controls are inside the shower stall and are controlled by the client. In other systems, the temperature and water pressure controls are out-side the water stall and are controlled by the therapist. The equipment should always have scald-protection and pressure-balancing features.

Before offering Swiss or Vichy shower treatments at your wellness center of spa, it is a good idea to run the shower at a temperature of about 98°F (40°C) to find out how long this temperature can be main-tained before water runs out. This provides you with an idea of how much hot water capacity you have in your facility. You should also check to see how long it takes for your water heating system to produce enough hot water for another full shower treatment. In addition, many spas and wellness centers have multiple uses for hot water. Swiss and Vichy showers require a large volume of water. Thus, it is important to know whether there is enough hot water for all these uses. Running a Swiss or Vichy shower when a washer or other equipment is also run-ning may decrease water flow to the shower and/or lead to a change in temperature. This is easy to check by running the washing machine and the shower (Vichy, Swiss, or handheld) at the same time. Even with a pressure-balancing feature, some showers cannot adjust adequately in this situation.

PRODUCTS

Because this treatment produces a powerful rinsing effect, products are not normally placed on the client's body during this treatment.

STEPS OF THE TREATMENT

1. *Pre-Treatment:* Prepare the Swiss shower for the treatment, including making sure there are nonslip mats on the floor (if available).

2. *Beginning the Treatment:* The water is first turned on and once the temperature is correct, the client enters the shower. Assist the client to the shower if the client is coming from another treatment.

3. *Treatment:* The treatment usually lasts about 10 minutes, though it can be longer. These showers use a considerable amount of hot water, which may be a limiting factor on duration of treatment. With most systems, the client controls the water temperature and pressure from inside the shower stall, and thus he or she is able to keep the temperature comfortably warm. In other systems, the water temperature and pressure controls are outside the shower stall, allowing the therapist to control these features. Either way, the temperature is normally in a warm, comfortable range—neither too hot nor too cold.

    Optional—Alternating Temperature: Whether the controls are inside or outside the shower stall, one treatment option is to decrease the temperature to a colder setting for 30 to 45 seconds and then return the temperature to normal. This could be done about five times during a 10-minute treatment (see instructions for the Vichy shower treatment).

    The water pressure is usually firm. During the treatment, it is possible to decrease or increase water pressure simply by controlling the valve that turns the water on and off.

4. *End of the treatment:* Turn off the water and provide a towel for the client to dry off. Assist the client when walking on wet floors. If possible, provide slip-resistant slippers.

5. *Post-treatment:* If this is the last treatment, it is important for the client to rest as long as possible after the treatment and enjoy the wonderful effects of this special shower treatment.

    The shower stall must be cleaned and disinfected after the treatment. It is possible for fungal spores from the feet of an infected person, for example, someone with athlete's foot, to come into contact with someone else who will use the shower stall.

ADDITIONAL SUGGESTION

Like the Vichy shower, the Swiss shower is a great way to end a longer session at the spa or wellness center. Also, because this treatment is very relaxing, it can be offered as part of an ongoing stress-management and wellness program.

Handheld Shower

DESCRIPTION AND BENEFITS

A handheld shower system includes a handheld shower with a hose long enough to reach across the entire length of the client on a wet table plus a mixing valve to control water temperature and pressure. Many spas and wellness centers cannot afford a Vichy or Swiss vertical or horizontal shower system, but many can afford a handheld shower system. Handheld showers can be used very effectively for relaxation therapy. A handheld shower can be used to give a client a hydromassage with one showerhead rather than multiple showerheads (see Figure 7–25 and Plate 20), as from a Vichy or Swiss shower. This type of hydromassage, which is controlled by the therapist, can produce experiences similar to those from a Vichy or Swiss shower. A handheld shower has far more applications that just for rinsing off a client.

It is possible to use a much larger handheld shower that can cover a larger area of the body (see Figure 7–26 and Plate 31). This could essentially be used as a mini–Vichy shower.

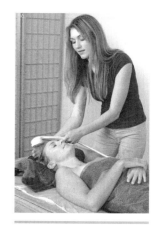

Figure 7–25 Handheld shower treatment.

EQUIPMENT

A handheld shower system includes a handheld shower, a hose long enough to reach across the entire wet table, and a mixing valve to control the water temperature. It is a good idea for the handheld shower system to have scald protection. Normally, it is necessary to use a wet table in wet room, although some handheld shower systems will work in a normal treatment room using special wet tables.

PRODUCTS

Generally, a handheld shower is used to rinse products off the body. However, during some treatments, for example hair and scalp treatments, products are added during the treatment and rinsed off at the end of the treatment.

STEPS OF THE TREATMENT

1. *Pretreatment:* A handheld shower treatment is usually given in combination with another treatment, so the client will already be on a wet table.

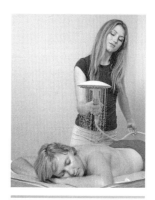

Figure 7–26 Large handheld shower.

2. *Beginning the treatment:* Before using the handheld shower on the client, turn it on and run water to the drain, not on the client, until the water reaches a comfortable temperature. Normally, the therapist determines the water temperature by running the water over his or her hand. It is also possible use a temperature gauge to measure the temperature for greater precision.

3. *Treatment:* Once the water reaches the correct temperature, bring the water into contact with the client's body. Immediately check with the client to see if temperature is comfortable.

   Optional–Personal Shower (Rinsing) Treatment: Use the hand-held shower to cleanse and rinse products from the client's body and/or head at the end of the treatment.

   Optional–Hydromassage Treatment: Use the handheld shower to massage the client's body. This can be done by massaging as much of the client's body as possible, both front and back, by using the water pressure from the showerhead. It can also be used to focus on a specific area of the body–for example, an area of joint or muscle discomfort. The handheld shower can also be used as a hydromassage for the head. When performing hydromassage, it is usually possible to control the pressure of the water, depending on the purpose of the treatment.

   Draping the Client: Keeping the client properly draped and warm during a handheld shower treatment requires some creativity and practice. For wet table treatments, use lightweight towels, as they do not absorb as much water and they also dry more quickly.

4. *End of the treatment:* Turn off the water and provide a towel for the client to dry off. Assist the client from the table and when walking on wet floors. If possible, provide slip-resistant slippers.

5. *Post-treatment:* If this is the last treatment, it is important for the client to rest as long as possible after the treatment. The wet table must be cleaned and disinfected as well as the floor and any other surfaces the water has come in contact with.

ADDITIONAL SUGGESTIONS

Handheld showers should include scald protection to prevent accidentally scalding a client.

Handheld Shower for Hair and Scalp Hydromassage

DESCRIPTION AND BENEFITS

A handheld shower for hair and scalp hydromassage is one of the best, most pleasing hydrotherapy treatments available. It is easily done, requiring only a handheld shower, and some product. (see Figure 7–27 and Plate 20). Most clients enjoy having their head, hair, and scalp massaged, and the water flowing from the handheld shower dramatically enhances the effects. There are many variations and options for this treatment, depending in part on who is performing the treatment—for example, a massage therapist, cosmetologist, or esthetician.

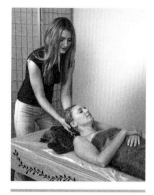

Figure 7–27
Hydrotherapy hair and scalp treatment.

EQUIPMENT

Handheld shower for use on a wet table. There are some wet table systems that do not require a wet room.

PRODUCTS

- Massage therapists often use products, such as massage oils, that enhance the effects of massage on the head, hair, and scalp.
- Estheticians will generally use products that have benefits for the skin.
- Cosmetologists will generally use products that benefit the hair and scalp. They may also use a product in preparation for a hair cut or styling treatment.

STEPS OF THE TREATMENT

1. *Pretreatment:* A handheld shower treatment is usually given in combination with another treatment, so the client will already be on a wet table.

2. *Beginning the treatment:* Before using the handheld shower on the client, turn it on and run water to the drain, not on the client, until the water reaches a comfortable temperature.

3. *Treatment:* Once the water reaches the correct temperature, bring the water into contact with the client's hair and scalp. The length of the treatment can be as long as possible, depending on the

goal of the treatment and scheduling considerations. Clients usually prefer as much time as is reasonable for this treatment. The treatment is a combination of applying the product, massaging by hand, and doing a hydromassage with a handheld shower. This treatment is deeply relaxing, which means it is also deeply therapeutic.

4. *End of the treatment:* Turn off the water and provide a towel for the client to dry off or the therapist can use the towel to dry the hair. Assist the client from the table and when walking on wet floors. If possible, provide slip-resistant slippers.

5. *Post-treatment:* If this is the last treatment, it is important for the client to rest as long as possible after the treatment. The wet table must be cleaned and disinfected as well as the floor and any other surfaces the water has come in contact with.

ADDITIONAL SUGGESTIONS

This treatment is one of the simplest, yet most client-pleasing, of all hydrotherapy treatments available. It offers treatment options to a wide range of therapists and works very well in combination with other treatments as part of a total package.

Hydromassage Table

HYDROMASSAGE TABLE

The hydromassage table has a water-based design that supports the unique fluid and the structural elements of the human body in a way that allows for special treatment options. The human body is a dynamic, fluid system that is 60% water (liquid), 20% fat (liquid), and 20% solid structural elements including mainly proteins, crystallized mineral matrix (bone), and carbohydrates (glycogen) (see Chapter 3). The fluid support that the hydromassage table provides for the human body, which is approximately 80% liquid, allows a therapist additional treatment options that can be used along with traditional massage as well as some new treatment options. The following are the special features of the hydromassage table:

- The hydromassage table naturally molds to support the unique shape of each client. Each human body has its own unique shape, length, width, and weight. The human body is a curved system and some of these curved surfaces—for example, the lower back and the backside of the neck—are deeply curved. The hydromassage table contours to each curved surface of the body providing a special, complete support. In addition, the hydromassage table can provide comfortable support for virtually any size (weight) client, which is especially important as many of our clients are getting larger.

- The hydromassage table is heated and remains at a constant temperature of between 95°F (35°C) and 99°F (37.2°C), although the temperature could be set higher or lower. The heated table promotes relaxation and prevents heat loss from the client's body, regardless of the room temperature.

- The fluid motion of the hydromassage table allows the therapist to move, stretch, and rotate the client's body as one integrated system, without restrictions due to gravity that is normally experienced on a traditional massage table. This feature creates special opportunities for working with the total integrated structural system of the body, or for focusing on the fascial system, or the craniosacral system, as well as the vascular and cellular systems.

- The hydromassage table allows the therapist to produce various wave motions that clients find very relaxing and comforting.

Benefits

- *Relaxation therapy:* The combination of unique support, warmth, and fluid motion of the hydromassage table produces immediate and profound relaxation for the client.

- *Special massage therapy application:* As mentioned above, the hydromassage table offers unique opportunities for working with the integrated structural elements of the body, allowing the body to be stretched, rotated, and moved in ways that have special therapeutic applications.

- *Overweight clients:* Water contours and supports the unique shape of any object, including the human body. The hydromassage table offers special support and comfort for overweight or obese clients.

- *Client comfort:* The hydromassage table offers special support and comfort for clients who have painful body conditions and who find it difficult to lie on traditional massage tables. It is also of value for elderly clients, who are often more fragile.

- *Massage with clothes on*: Most of the benefits described above can be enjoyed by clients with clothes-on. This is a great way to give treatments to clients who would only feel comfortable getting a treatment clothed. The benefits from these treatments can be very therapeutic.

- *Traditional massage techniques:* Most types of massage therapy techniques can be done on the hydromassage table. The table fully supports the client but remains relatively stable, even with the greater fluid motion for the client on the table.

Equipment

Hydromassage tables, designed for use by massage therapists as well as other therapists are relatively new. Refer to the Hydrotherapy Equipment Resource Guide in Appendix B for different equipment options. The following are a few key design features of the hydromassage table:

- The water in the table is heated, and there is a temperature control option.

- The volume of water in the water mattress is enough to allow any size client to lie comfortably and be fully supported on the hydromassage table.

- The table should be able to be adjusted to the therapist's desired height. However, once water is in the table, it will be too heavy to adjust without removing the water.

NOTE: SOME TABLES HAVE HYDRAULIC LIFT SYSTEMS THAT ALLOW THE TABLE HEIGHT TO BE ADJUSTED AT ANY TIME DURING THE TREATMENT.

NOTE: SOME TYPES OF HYDROMASSAGE TABLES ARE MORE ROBOTIC IN DESIGN AND CREATE MECHANICALLY INDUCED MOTION AND PRESSURE THAT THEN HAS A MASSAGING EFFECT ON THE CLIENT. THESE TABLES ARE NORMALLY DESIGNED FOR USE WITH-OUT A THERAPIST. THE USE OF THESE TYPES OF HYDROMASSAGE TABLES ARE NOT DISCUSSED IN THIS TEXTBOOK, AS THE FOCUS IS ON HYDROTHERAPY TRAINING AND TREATMENTS FOR THERAPISTS.

MANUAL HYDROMASSAGE TABLE TECHNIQUES

The wave motion, buoyancy, and warmth of a hydromassage table, when combined with massage and other modalities, such as aroma therapy and music, produce unique and profound relaxation for the client. Relaxation therapy is a very therapeutic, natural, non-drug approach to healing the effects of modern life, which can often be stressful and overstimulated. The states of relaxation produced by the proper use of the hydromassage table are profound and unique.

The following is a description of a series of techniques/movements that a therapist can perform on a client that work well with the hydromassage table. These techniques are similar to techniques used in traditional massage, and can be used in a series, as presented below, or each technique can be used separately in combination with other bodywork techniques. These techniques take advantage of the fluid, buoyant, heated nature of the table, which works synergistically with the fluid, dynamic, heated properties of the human body. It is recommended to practice this series of techniques so that they become familiar, automatic, and natural. The benefit of using these techniques on the hydromassage table, whether individually or in a series, is that it takes full advantage of the special fluid properties of the table.

Techniques with the Client in the Supine Position (face up)

These rotations and stretches can be done once or multiple times (1 to 10 times) with even pressure. They can also be done in a wavelike rhythm. With each repetition, the client's body relaxes a little more, allowing increased stretching. The last press, twist, or pull of each technique can be held for about 15 seconds in the fully stretched and/or rotated position.

Shoulder Press

This creates wave motion (energy) in the table that then is transferred to the client's body, either in the form of a sensation of the wave motion or physical energy of the wave motion.

With both hands, press on both shoulders to create a gentle wave motion (see Figure 7–28). Begin with creating about 10 wave motions over 20 seconds. It is possible to vary pressure in creating the wave as well as the frequency of the waves.

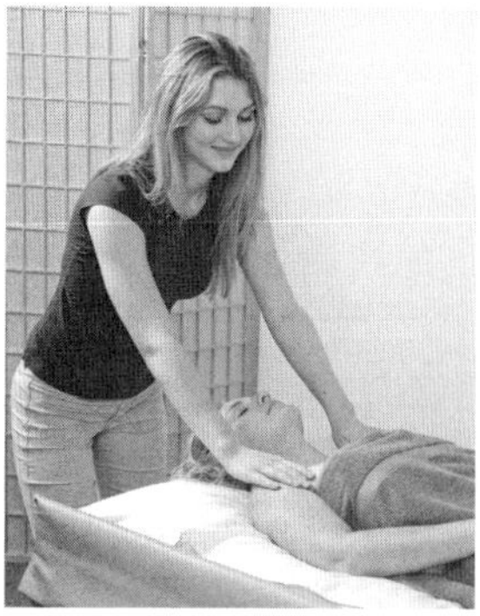

Head and Neck Stretch

This allows gentle stretching of the upper spine, with a greater effect towards the head end.

- Using both hands, lift the head slightly and pull the head toward you creating a gently stretching effect (see Figure 7–29).
- At the end of the stretch, rotate the head clockwise (to the right) and then back to the center and then counterclockwise (to the left) and then back to center. Both the stretching and rotating can be done from 1 to 10 times.

Hip and Lower Spine Stretch

This movement creates a deep stretching of the lower back and spine (see Figure 7–30).

- Face the side of the client's body.
- Place one hand under the knee joint and lift the leg to bring the knee toward the head end of the body. Stable: The other hand is under the lower back.
- Press the leg as far as it will comfortably move. The angle of the knee can either be straight toward the head end of the body or at various angles to the right or left of the head end.

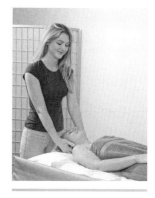

Figure 7–28
Wave motion.

Figure 7–29 Neck stretch.

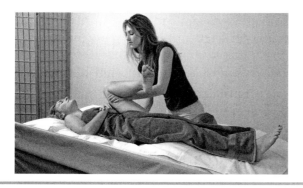

Figure 7–30 Spine rotation.

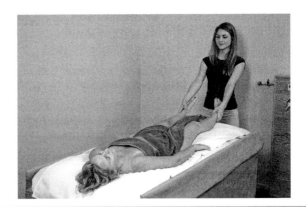

Figure 7–31 Leg pull.

Leg Pull

This movement produces a stretching motion on the entire structural system of the body, which relieves some of the compression on the structural system caused by supporting the weight of the body.

Grab both ankles and pull toward you. This stretch can be varied vary by pulling with more force on one leg and then with more force on the other leg (see Figure 7–31).

Arm Pull

This movement stretches both the structural system of the body and muscles of the upper body.

Grab both wrists and pull toward you. This stretch can be varied by pulling with more force on one arm and then with more force on the other arm (see Figure 7–32). Because the arms are more sensitive to being pulled and stretched than the legs, you should ask the client for feedback to determine what is comfortable.

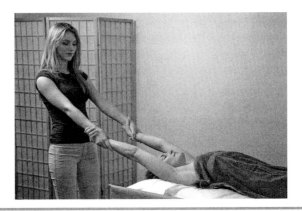

Figure 7–32 Arm pull.

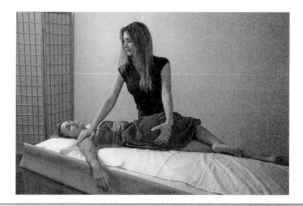

Figure 7–33 Hip rotation.

Hip Rotation

This movement allows a deep rotational stretch of the lower spine.

- Place one hand on the side of the body at hip level.
- Rotate the hip and spine by pushing up and forward. Stable: The other hand is placed on the shoulder on the same side of body to keep the upper body from rotating (see Figure 7–33 and Plate 27).

Techniques with Client in the Prone Position (face down)

These rotations and stretches can be also be done once or multiple times (1 to 10 times) with even pressure. They can also be done in a wavelike rhythm. With each repetition, the client's body relaxes a little more, allowing increased stretching. The last press, twist, or pull of each technique can be held for about 15 seconds in the fully stretched and/or rotated position.

Rotation and Pressing on the Lower Back (Lumbar Sacral Area)

This movement focuses on relaxing the muscles of the lower back and gently stretching the lower back.

- Place one hand on the lower back, in the area of junction of the lumbar and the sacral vertebrae (see Figure 7–34). The other hand can be placed higher on the lower back.
- While pressing down, create a rotating circular motion. The amount of pressure and the circular motion can be varied. It should feel as if you are rotating and rocking the lower back area. The pressure should be firm but comfortable and once again, in a wave-like motion.

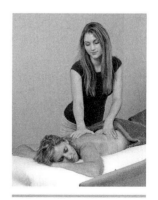

Figure 7–34 Sacral area rotation.

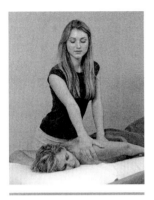

Figure 7–35 Shoulder stretch.

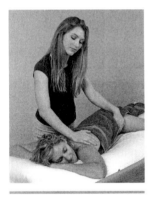

Figure 7–36 Hip and spine rotation.

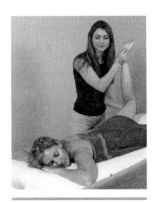

Figure 7–37 Lower spine stretch.

Shoulder Stretch and Spine Rotation

This movement allows a stretching of the upper shoulder area and the upper spine.

With one hand under the shoulder, lift the shoulder. Stable: The other hand is on the upper hip on the same side of the body (see Figure 7–35).

Rotation of Hip and Spine

This motion creates a rotation and stretching of the lower to upper spine.

Place one hand on the side of the body below the hip. Lift and pull the hip toward you. For greater stretching, you can also pull the hip slightly in the direction of the feet. Stable: The other hand is placed on the shoulder on the same side (see Figure 7–36).

Leg Lift and Rotation for Lower Spine Stretch

This movement produces a stretching of the hip joint and lower spine, an area that most of the compressive forces of the weight of the body impact each day.

Place one hand under the knee and lift the leg. To create additional stretching of the lower spine, rotate the leg as it is lifted. The other hand is placed on the ankle of the same leg (see Figure 7–37 and Plate 28).

Leg Pull

This movement creates a gentle stretching force on the structural system of the body, with more of an effect on the lower body.

Grab both ankles and pull toward you. This stretch can be varied by pulling with more force on one leg and then with more force on the other leg (see Figure 7–38).

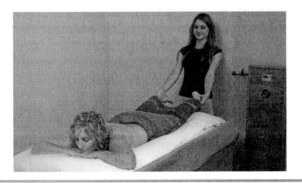

Figure 7–38 Leg pull.

Arm Pull

This movement creates a gentle stretching force on the structural system of the body, with more of an effect on the upper body.

Grab both wrists and pull toward you. This stretch can be varied by pulling with more force on one arm and then with more force on the other arm (see Figure 7–39). Because the arms are more sensitive to stretching and pulling than are the legs, ask for client feedback to determine what is comfortable.

The following are some examples of treatments that can be done on the hydromassage table.

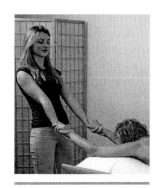

Figure 7–39 Arm pull.

Relaxation "Wave" Therapy Treatment

This treatment combines gentle massage and touch with relaxing wave motions. Relaxing massage modalities are best for this treatment, as the main goal of this treatment is relaxation.

Wave motion: A wave motion can be created by pressing on the client's body with medium pressure, usually using both hands, about every 2 seconds. It is usually best to begin with the shoulders. This pressure will create a wave movement that flows from the client's shoulders to the feet. When the wave motion reaches the feet, it will return with less energy toward the head. This wave motion will create a very soothing, calming effect on the client. Experiment with the amount of pressure and the timing. Continue this motion for 2 or 3 minutes. As the wave motion returns to the head end, it will create a subtle massaging effect on the entire backside (or front side) of the client's body. With your left hand, lift the back of the head a few inches and create a few wave motions by pressing on the right shoulder with the right hand. Then, with the left hand, pull the head toward you, creating a gentle stretch on the neck (cervical) vertebra. The wave motion will add to the stretching effect. By pressing down on almost any part of the body, a gentle wave motion can be created. However, it is easier to create this motion from the shoulders and/or the legs.

Myofascial Therapy

This brief section on the use myofascial therapy on the hydromassage table is to demonstrate the potential of combining these two therapeutic approaches. The goal of this treatment is to improve the alignment and structural flexibility of the fascial matrix of the body by combining traditional myofascial techniques and the use of the hydromassage table. By gently stretching and rotating the body, combined with the fluid motion and heat of the hydromassage table, the therapist can stretch and rotate the fascial matrix to improve its alignment and flexibility. The following hydromassage techniques can be combined with manual myofacial techniques and passive stretches as needed.

Supine Shoulder Press: Begin a wave motion by pressing on the client's shoulders with medium pressure, usually using both hands. Do this for 2 to 3 minutes. As the wave motion returns to the head, it will create a subtle massaging effect on the entire backside of the client's body.

Along with the use of other myofascial techniques, include the shoulder stretch and spine rotation through the hip rotation with the client in the supine position.

Client in the Prone Position: Have the client lie on his or her stomach. Some clients will feel comfortable with the head turned to the side; others will feel more comfortable with the head looking down in the face cradle. Follow the same sequence as you did with the client in the prone position, combining myofascial techniques with the series of hydromassage manual techniques. Start with rotation and pressing on the lumbar sacral area and end with the arm pull with the client in the supine position.

Massage on the Hydromassage Table

Most massage techniques can also be performed on the hydromassage table. Although the client's body is stable and supported on the hydromassage table, there will be some movement of the whole body when pressure is placed on a specific part of the body. This movement is generally very minimal, unless the therapist intentionally wants to generate a greater wave motion. The advantage of the table's fluid nature is that the body can stretch and rotate as one system, and the stretching and rotating is felt throughout the entire body. The water mattress is heated, which produces a sense of warmth and comfort, even in a treatment room at a cooler temperature.

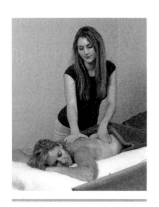

Figure 7–40
Hydromassage table.

NOTE: THE HYDROMASSAGE TABLE IS NOT A WATERBED. HOWEVER, IT DOES HAVE MANY OF THE SAME PRINCIPLES. ONE MAIN DIFFERENCE BETWEEN THIS TABLE AND A WATERBED IS THAT WATERBEDS ARE MUCH LARGER–SOMETIMES VERY LARGE. THE MATTRESS SIZE FOR THE HYDROMASSAGE TABLE IS MUCH SMALLER; THEREFORE IT IS MORE STABLE AND ALLOWS THE THERAPIST ACCESS TO ALL PARTS OF THE CLIENT'S BODY, SIMILAR TO ANY MASSAGE TABLE. (SEE FIGURE 7–40).

Hydrotherapy Misting

COMMON ELEMENTS OF HYDROTHERAPY MISTING

Misting is a simple, inexpensive form of hydrotherapy that has many practical uses. It is normally used in combination with other treatments, including other types of hydrotherapy treatments.

Misting Water Principles

- A single spray of mist consists of a large number of water droplets that are much smaller than a raindrop. A small raindrop is about 500 micrometers in diameter and is spherical in shape. Forcing water under pressure through a small opening breaks the surface tension of the water, creating a spray of mist water droplets as small as 5 micrometers.

- The smaller water droplets from a mist spray evaporate very quickly, which creates a soothing and cooling effect.

- Water-soluble products, such as hydrosols, will dissolve evenly in each small droplet of mist.

- Products that do not dissolve in water, such as essential oils, can be temporarily mixed in the water used to create a misting spray by shaking the bottle just before spraying.

Anatomy and Physiology During Misting

- The small mist droplets that land on the skin, or that are close to the skin, evaporate very quickly. This evaporation removes heat from the body and from air surrounding the body, producing a cooling effect.

- Water that stays on the body but that does not evaporate produces water moisture on the skin.

- A misting spray can be used to apply water-soluble and oil-based products to the body. Some of these products have an effect directly on the surface of the skin. Other products, such as oil-based products, can be absorbed into the skin, especially if the product is massaged into the skin. Misting is an excellent form of aromatherapy, using a wide variety of hydrosols and essential oils.

Equipment

Misting bottles, which come in many sizes and shapes, are very inexpensive and are available in most drug stores. Test different bottles to find the type that produces a mist spray that meets your needs.

Products

- Products that dissolve in water work well with misting. Hydrosols (the water-soluble essence of flowers and plants) can be used for aromatherapy. Other products, such as mineral salts, herbal solutions, and other substances, can also be used, depending on the treatment. Some oils, such as essential oils, can be temporarily mixed with the water in the misting bottle by shaking the bottle.
- Bottled spring water, filtered water, or distilled water that has the chlorine removed is recommended for use in misting treatments.

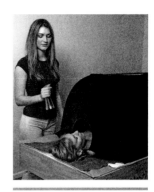

Figure 7–41 Misting face treatment.

Misting Treatments

Description and Benefits

Misting is used as an additional component of other treatments as a way to produce a soothing, cooling effect for the client. Many hydrotherapy treatments heat the client's body. The soothing, cooling gentle mist is a special touch that can enhance a client's total hydrotherapy experience. See Figures 7–41 (Plate 22) and 7–42 (Plate 21) for illustrations of misting treatments.

How to Mist: Create a spray of mist about 10 inches above the client's body and allow the spray of mist to come into contact with the body by gravity. Some of the water will evaporate before it falls on the client, creating a cooling effect around the body while also releasing aroma from any products in the water. Do not spray directly onto the client's face. If you are misting other areas of the body to increase moisture on the skin, the mist can be spayed directly on the skin.

Misting can also be personalized by dissolving or mixing natural products, such as lavender hydrosol, into the water used to produce the mist. You may want to have your clients choose their own products, depending on what they find most enjoyable.

Equipment

Misting bottle: Misting bottles are readily available and inexpensive, and come in different sizes, shapes, and colors.

Products

Hydrosols (the water-soluble portion of essential oils) can be added to water that is used for misting. Hydrosols bring the essence of the flower and other plant essences into a water mist on and around the client. See Appendix C.

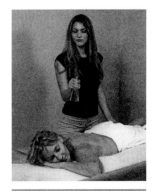

Figure 7–42 Misting treatment.

Steps of the Treatment

1. *Pretreatment:* Fill the bottle with room-temperature water for the treatment. You will learn from experience how much water to use. You may want to add a natural product to the water in the misting bottle, although this is not necessary. Misting with only water works well for cooling.

2. *Treatment:* Misting is often used as an additional element during other types of treatments. The following are the main ways that misting can be used during a treatment.

   Cooling: Create a misting spray to cool a client during or immediately after a heating treatment, such as a steam or hydrotub treatment. Normally, the face or the back of the neck is misted, but more of the body can be misted if the treatment allows.

   Aromatherapy: Essential oils or hydrosols can be mixed with the water in the spray bottle and misted around the client for aromatherapy.

   Product application: Water-soluble products and small amounts of oils mixed in the water of the spray bottle can be applied to the skin by misting.

   Moistening the skin: For some treatments, misting the skin to make it moist can be of value, for example, when applying certain products to the skin.

Additional Suggestions

- Do not spray directly on the client's face, especially not in the eyes. Spray above the face and let gravity bring the spray down. Most clients know to close their eyes when you spray, but it is good to remind them.

- When natural products are added to the water, add just enough to create a weak solution.

Cryotherapy

CRYOTHERAPY

Cryotherapy is generally associated with the use of ice in the immediate treatment of injuries. Common injuries treated with cryotherapy include sprains, strains, and contusions. These injuries often occur during sports and recreational activities. The main reference source for the use of cryotherapy, including theory and treatment protocols, is taken from the textbook on the subject, *Cryotherapy in Sport Injury Management* by Knight.[2] This authoritative textbook contains references from many scientific studies that deal with the subject of cryotherapy and is referenced by most articles and published papers on cyrotherapy.

Dynamic Water Principles

For ice to transition to the liquid state requires a certain amount of heat. It takes 80 cal of heat to transform 1 g of ice to the liquid state. It takes another 1 cal of heat to raise the temperature of 1 g of liquid water 1°C. See Chapter 1. This makes ice very effective at cooling an injured area of the body for time periods of upto 30 minutes.

Anatomy and Physiology of Cryotherapy

1. Ice—usually crushed ice in a plastic bag—placed on the skin will significantly reduce the temperature of the skin and core body elements, including the cells, blood, and interstitial fluid, and structural elements, such as muscles, ligaments, tendons, and fascia.

2. This reduction in temperature reduces blood flow to the area as blood vessels constrict, which leads to a decrease in edema (swelling).

3. The reduced skin and core temperature reduces the temperature of millions of cells in the area. For every 1°C the temperature of the cells there is a 12% decrease in the metabolic activity.

4. The decrease in temperature reduces cellular damage from secondary hypoxic injury. This means that fewer cells die as a result of the injury due to lack of oxygen, which results in fewer free proteins in the interstitial fluid. This, in turn, reduces the osmotic pull of fluid from the blood plasma to the interstitial fluid, which is a primary cause of edema. Fewer cells dying from the injury also reduces the amount of healing necessary to repair the damaged tissue.

5. After about 15 to 20 minutes of an ice application to the area, there may be a sudden increase in circulation to the area of the body being cooled. This is thought to be the body's protective response, known as **cold induced vasodilatation (VSD)** or **hunting response,** to prevent tissue damage.

Equipment

-   It is recommended to use about 2 lb of crushed ice in a plastic bag. Ice bags created specifically for this purpose can be used. Resealable plastic bags will also work.
-   Caution is recommended when using frozen gel packs, as they can be colder than ice and increase the risk of freezing the skin. When possible, it is recommended to use crushed ice packs for cyrotherapy.

Steps of the Treatment

-   The treatment protocol recommended by Knight is to apply an ice pack (a plastic bag with crushed ice) directly on the site of injury as quickly as possible after the injury. The ice pack should be placed directly on the skin for up to 30 minutes. The ice pack should then be removed for a period of about 2 hours to allow the area to rewarm. The ice pack should then be placed on the injured area again for up to 30 minutes.

NOTE: RECOMMENDATIONS BY OTHER PROFESSIONALS USING ICE THERAPY OFTEN INCLUDE APPLYING THE ICE FOR ONLY 15 TO 20 MINUTES. KNIGHT STATES THAT A PERIOD CLOSER TO 30 MINUTES IS NECESSARY TO DERIVE THE FULL BENEFICIAL EFFECTS OF ICE THERAPY.

-   Cryotherapy should be done for 24 to 72 hours after the time the injury occurred. In general, the greater the injury, the longer the treatment (up to 72 hours).
-   In addition to cryotherapy (ice therapy), it is recommended to use the other well-known treatment modalities of rest, compression, elevation, and stabilization of the injured area.

Safety Considerations

-   Caution! It is very important to avoid freezing the skin of the area being cooled. Once again, according to Knight, using crushed ice is preferable to gel packs, as gel packs are more likely to freeze the skin. The length of time that the ice

Cold induced vasodilatation (VSD)
A protective response in which there is a sudden, dramatic increase in blood flow to a specific tissue area of the body to keep it from being damaged by an extreme drop in temperature. This can happen when applying ice (cryotherapy) after about 20 minutes. Also known as *hunting response*.

Hunting response
See *cold induced vasodilatation (VSD)*.

is placed on the injured area should be limited to reduce the risk of damage to the skin. Once again, the recommendation by Knight is 30 minutes for normal injuries. Whatever protocol is followed, whether it be Knight or another professional, do not exceed the recommended amount of time.

The following are the contraindications for the use of cyrotherapy

- Raynaud's disease: peripheral vascular medical condition
- Cold hypersensitivity
- Cardiac disorder
- Compromised local circulation

NOTE: THE PRIMARY EFFECTS OF CRYOTHERAPY TREATMENTS ARE TAKING PLACE AT THE CELLULAR LEVEL. COLD CAUSES SMOOTH MUSCLE CELLS IN BLOOD VESSELS TO CONTRACT CAUSING CONSTRICTION AND REDUCED BLOOD FLOW. REDUCED METABOLIC RATE OF CELLS DECREASES THE NEED FOR OXYGEN, WHICH DECREASES CIRCULATION TO THE AREA. THE USE OF ICE FOR THERAPY SIGNIFICANTLY REDUCES THE TEMPERATURE OF THE INJURED AREA OF THE BODY. THIS MEANS THAT AT THE CELLULAR LEVEL, MILLIONS OF CELLS ARE BEING AFFECTED. WHEN COLD IS APPLIED, THE BODY PRODUCES SENSATIONS OF DISCOMFORT AND PAIN AS A WARNING OF A THREAT TO THE BODY. REDUCING THE TEMPERATURE OF CELLS CLOSE TO THE LEVEL OF FREEZING CREATES A DRAMATIC CHANGE IN THE PHYSIOLOGY OF THE CELLS AND SHOULD BE DONE WITH GREAT CAUTION SO THAT ADDITIONAL CELLS ARE NOT DAMAGED IN THE PROCESS OF GIVING THE TREATMENT.

Additional Suggestions

- For more in-depth information on the use of cryotherapy in the treatment of injuries, including detailed review of the theory on contrast treatments, cold induced vasodilation, and the use of cyrotherapy in the rehabilitation phase of an injury, please read *Cryotherapy in Sport Injury Management* by Knight.

Hot and Cold Compresses

HOT AND COLD COMPRESSES

Hot and cold compresses, which are created by heating or cooling a cloth compress with hot or cold water, is a form of hydrotherapy that has a long history of traditional use. Compresses, which often include herbs, salts, and oils, have been used in Ayurveda, Thai bodywork, Kneipp, and many other traditions.

Dynamic Water Principles

- Heat exchange occurs between the body and the warmer or cooler water of the compress.
- Products dissolved or mixed in the water of the compress come into contact with the client's skin.

Anatomy and Physiology

- Depending on the temperature of the compress, there will be an increase or decrease in temperature of the area of the body in contact with the compresses. This will, in turn, increase or decrease circulation and cellular metabolism in that part of the body. This can have many therapeutic benefits for the health (healing) and wellness of the skin as well the underlying muscle, ligaments, and fascia.
- Products added to the compress can come into contact with skin. Depending on the product, it may either be absorbed by the skin or have an effect on the surface cells of the skin. Any increase in the temperature of the skin and the product will increase the rate of absorption of the product.

Equipment

Compresses include anything from small towels to special cloth compresses that are specifically designed to allow the addition of products.

Products

Most herbal products, mineral salts, and oils can be used in compresses (usually in hot compresses). This technique is a great way to bring a product into contact with a client's skin (see Figure 7–43). See Appendix C.

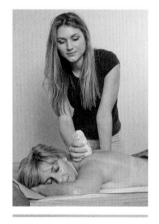

Figure 7–43 Hot compress treatment.

Treatment Suggestions

Hot Compress to Comfort and Heal

It is possible to use a hot compress, with or without products, to increase the speed and degree of healing of an area of the body that has been injured or strained. A hot compress can also be used to stimulated cellar metabolism and circulation as part of a wellness and rejuvenation program.

1. *Pretreatment:* Place a compress in hot water until the compress is heated to the desired temperature range. The temperature of the compress should not be so hot that it causes discomfort to the client's skin. It can be very warm but not too warm. Treatment with a compress is meant to be gentle and soothing. Hot water from a sink is usually hot enough to heat the compress. A hydroculator can also be used if available.

2. *Treatment:* Place the compress on the area of the body to be treated. Depending on the goal of the treatment, pressure can be applied to the compress, or the compress can be used along with massaging the area. The temperature of the compress will decease quickly. Depending on the length of the treatment, it may be necessary to reheat the compress several times or to have several compresses ready for use. A therapist can choose from a wide variety of natural products, including herbs, oils, and mineral salts, with known therapeutic properties, for use in the compress.

Cool Compress

Cool compresses are not used as often as hot compresses. However, there will likely be an increased use of cold compresses as we gain a better understanding of the therapeutic benefits of small decreases in the temperature of the skin and other local deeper areas of the body. A decrease of 1°C of the temperature of a cell decreases its metabolic activity by 12%. It also decreases circulation to that local area of the body. This limited form of **hypothermia** to a local area of the skin and underlying cells is not nearly as dramatic as the application of ice, but it does allow the therapeutic use of hypothermia on a small localized area of the body. This "small" area is actually made up of millions of dynamic metabolically active cells.

The same steps are followed as for a hot compress, except for the cooling of the compress rather than heating it.

- A compress can be cooled by using the coldest water from a sink, which would be in the 50°F (10°C) to 60°F (15.5°C) range.

Hypothermia
The core temperature of the body decreases below its homeostatic set point of 98.6°F, which stimulates a heating response.

- A compress could also be placed in a refrigerator, not the freezer, to bring it to an even cooler temperature of around 40°F (4.4°C).

- When the compress is placed on the client's skin, it should not produce any discomfort due to cold, as this is meant to be a soothing, healing treatment. In general, a cold compress— even one at 40°F (4.4°C)—will not feel uncomfortable and will quickly increase in temperature by absorbing heat from the body. It may be necessary to cool the compress again or have several being cooled in a refrigerator.

- Another use of a cool compress is to soak a small towel in cold water from a sink. This towel is then placed on the head or neck of someone who is getting a heating treatment, such as a steam or hot hydrotub bath. Just as water is being used to heat the body, it can also be used to cool the body. Cooling the head allows a client to be comfortable for a longer period of time while getting a heating treatment.

Dry Hydromassage

SPECIAL DRY HYDROMASSAGE

A new form of hydromassage is the use of a special type of dry hydroballoon massage technology that allows a therapist to massage a client with water without the client or the therapist getting wet. With this hydrotechnology, the therapist controls the pressure, direction, and temperature of the hydromassage on various areas of the client's body. There is a unique synergy between the hydroballoon and the human body as the human body is approximately 80% liquid and made up of 100 trillion cells. The hydroballoon, which is 100% fluid, has a similar shape to many cells in the body. Clients have reported that the pressure from the hydroballoon is very comfortable, even when the pressure is strong. The massage effect is very soothing, relaxing, and therapeutic.

Dynamic Water Principles

- Pressure created by the weight of the water (10–25 lb), the increased pressure created by the therapist, and along with the movement of the hydroballoon, all work together to create a unique massaging effect on the client's body.

- Heat exchange occurs between the hot or cool water in the hydro-balloon and the client's body.

Anatomy and Physiology

- The pressure from the hydroballon will cause increased circulation in the areas of the body receiving the hydromassage due to the pumping effect.

- The heat exchange between hot water in the hyrdoballoon and the body will cause an increase in the circulation and also increase the metabolic activity of the cells.

- The increased heat can also increase the temperature of the underlying muscles and fascial matrix, which can make them easier to stretch and rotate.

- The heat exchange between the cold water in the hyrdoballoon and the body will cause a decrease in circulation and also a decrease in the metabolic activity of the cells.

Equipment

Special equipment and education has been designed for these treatments that include special balloons that will hold sufficient water (10–25 lb). These can be heated or cooled and will allow the therapist to apply additional pressure. The hydroballoons must be strong enough not to break in treatments that may last longer than 45 minutes. For more information about equipment for this treatment, refer to the Hydrotherapy Equipment Resource Guide in Appendix B. The hydroballoon system comes with detailed instructions on performing a wider range of treatments, including the treatments mentioned below.

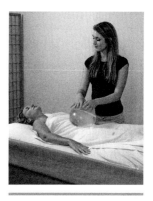

Figure 7–44 Dry hydromassage: Stomach treatment.

Treatment Suggestions

- Hydromassage of the skin, including the epidermis, dermis, and hypodermis: This will produce a massaging effect on the cells, vascular system, and connective tissue matrix of the skin. A light sheet is used to cover the client so that the hydroballoon does not come into direct contact with the clients' skin.
- Cellulite massage
- Hydromassage of the lower back and spine
- Hydromassage of the lymphatic system
- Hydromassage of the vascular system
- Hydromassage of special areas of the body, including the abdomen (see Figure 7–44 and Plate 25), lower back, and solar plexus (see Figure 7–45 and Plate 26)

This form of massage can be gentle yet there can be considerable pressure placed on the surface and deeper layers of the body. This pressure comes from not only the weight of the water in the hydroballoon but also the pressure applied by the massage therapist.

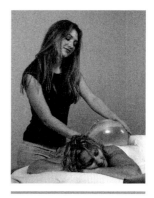

Figure 7–45 Dry hydromassage: Lower back treatment.

 SUMMARY

This chapter provides education on the performance of a wide range of individual hydrotherapy treatments. A number of treatments are given for each main category of hydrotherapy, including hydrotub, steam, shower, underwater hydromassage, hydromassage table, misting, cryotherapy, and hot and cold compresses.

The chapter begins with a discussion of the client evaluation (see Chapter 5) to help a therapist determine each client's unique health and wellness goals as a basis to make recommendations on specific programs, including hydrotherapy, to attain those goals.

For each main category of hydrotherapy treatment, a general overview of common elements is presented, including the principles of the behavior of water, the types of equipment used, natural products that can be incorporated, and the basic principles of the anatomy and physiology. Each discussion also includes a description of contraindications, as well as any special considerations.

The goal of each section, including instructions on specific treatments, is to provide a comprehensive education on how to perform hydrotherapy treatments within a specific category. A therapist should feel competent in providing these types of treatments and he or she should also be able to use this knowledge to create new treatments within each category.

REFERENCE

(1) Bucken H, 2005, *Deutschland: Deine Thermen*. Zeist Geist Media.
(2) Knight, K. (1995). *Cryotherapy in Sport Injury Management*. Champaign, Illinois: Human Kinetics.

SUGGESTED READINGS

Knight, K. (1995). *Cryotherapy in Sport Injury Management*. Champaign, Illinois: Human Kinetics.
Beck, M. (2006). *Theory and Practice of Therapeutic Massage*, (4th ed.). Albany, New York.
Fowlie, L. (2006). *Heat & Cold as Therapy*. Toronto, Ontario: Curties-Overzet Publications.
Dinshah, D. (2001). *Let There Be Light*, (6th ed.). Malaga, New Jersey: Dinshah Health Society.
Weil, A. (AUTHOR ADD YEAR). *Mindbody Tool Kit* (2 CDs). Boulder, Colorado: Sounds True.

REVIEW QUESTIONS

1. List several health and wellness goals of that clients may have.

2. Suggest a hydrotherapy treatment that could help a client to achieve each of these goals.

3. What are some of the main categories of hydrotherapy treatments?

4. What is a key basic behavior of water found in hydrotub treatments?

5. What is a key basic behavior of water found in steam treatments?

6. What is a key basic behavior of water found in shower treatments?

7. List an example of a hydrotherapy treatment in each of the above treatment categories.

8. List a potential safety problem in each of the above treatment categories.

9. List some contraindications for a heating treatment, for example a steam treatment.

10. List some possible combinations of treatments, including a hydrotherapy treatment, as part of a package of treatments.

For additional information on Hydrotherapy, visit our on-line companion at http://www.milady.cengage.com

History of Hydrotherapy— Ancient to Present

KEY TERMS

swedhana   Roman bath
nasya   hypocaust
asclepieion

INTRODUCTION

Traditions of hydrotherapy from around the world can provide us with many ideas about how to incorporate hydrotherapy into our modern spas, wellness, healing, and fitness centers. When we look to the past, we discover the use of hydrotherapy in ancient—as well as more recent—historical traditions of the healing arts and natural approaches to health, wellness, and beauty. See Figure 8–1 for a timeline of hydrotherapy treatments. Many of these traditional uses of hydrotherapy are found today, being used just as they have been for hundreds and even thousands of years.

The same health and wellness goals that people seek today were the main motivating force for the development of the great holistic health and wellness programs of the past. Our modern spa and wellness centers are not new; they are simply modern expressions of health and wellness centers that have been operating since ancient times. Lessons about hydrotherapy can be learned from all cultures and traditions that have developed health and wellness programs based on natural healing modalities. Some of the most interesting and rewarding research into the history of hydrotherapy comes from visiting historical sites in Greece, India, Europe, Japan, and other places

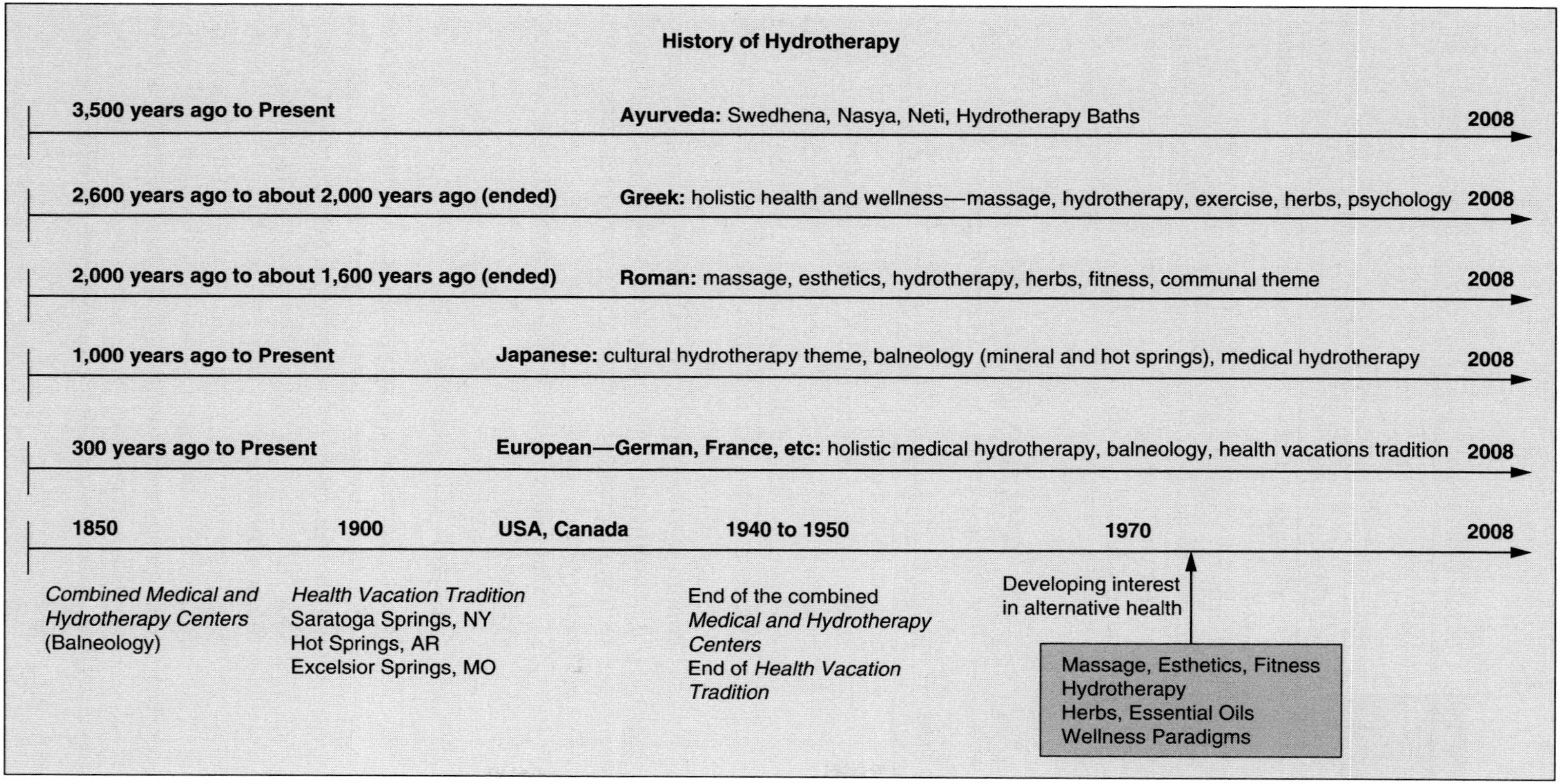

History of Hydrotherapy

3,500 years ago to Present — **Ayurveda:** Swedhena, Nasya, Neti, Hydrotherapy Baths — 2008

2,600 years ago to about 2,000 years ago (ended) — **Greek:** holistic health and wellness—massage, hydrotherapy, exercise, herbs, psychology — 2008

2,000 years ago to about 1,600 years ago (ended) — **Roman:** massage, esthetics, hydrotherapy, herbs, fitness, communal theme — 2008

1,000 years ago to Present — **Japanese:** cultural hydrotherapy theme, balneology (mineral and hot springs), medical hydrotherapy — 2008

300 years ago to Present — **European—German, France, etc:** holistic medical hydrotherapy, balneology, health vacations tradition — 2008

1850 — **1900** — **USA, Canada** — **1940 to 1950** — **1970** — 2008

Combined Medical and Hydrotherapy Centers (Balneology)

Health Vacation Tradition
Saratoga Springs, NY
Hot Springs, AR
Excelsior Springs, MO

End of the combined
*Medical and Hydrotherapy
Centers*
End of *Health Vacation
Tradition*

Developing interest
in alternative health

Massage, Esthetics, Fitness
Hydrotherapy
Herbs, Essential Oils
Wellness Paradigms

Figure 8–1 Hydrotherapy history timeline.

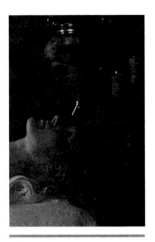

Figure 8–2 Ayurveda shirodhara treatment *(image copyright Alfred Wekelo, 2008. Used under license from Shutterstock .com).*

around the world.* Many of these sites continue to offer the same hydrotherapy experiences that they have offered since ancient times.

The study of the historical use of hydrotherapy reveals that these different traditions share common elements, which can provide insights into understanding the general principles of hydrotherapy. For example, the use of steam therapy in a communal setting is found in the Roman, Middle Eastern (hamam), Russian (banya), German, Mayan, and Native American traditions and have very similar basic approaches. This chapter describes historical uses of hydrotherapy, some of which continue to have a major influence on our modern-day spas, health and wellness, and fitness centers.

AYURVEDA AND HYDROTHERAPY

Ayurveda, which uses hydrotherapy as a component of its holistic programs, is a unique and comprehensive program that offers a wide range of treatments for health, wellness, and beauty using herbs and other natural products. Traditional Ayurveda dates back more than 3,500 years. One of the most ancient archaeological sites that shows evidence of the use of hydrotherapy in India is the Great Bath at Mohenjo-daro, which was built in 2500 B.C.E. Ayurveda, which continues to be popular around the world today, uses a combination of hydrotherapy, massage, yoga, meditation, pranayama (breathing techniques), music, herbs, and other modalities to achieve health and wellness goals.

The following are few examples of the use of hydrotherapy in Ayurveda.

Steam Therapy

Pancha karma is an Ayurvedic balancing and rejuvenation program that involves five different treatment modalities, including the currently popular shirodhara treatment (see Figure 8–2). One hydrotherapy approach included in pancha karma is a steam therapy treatment known as **swedhana.** This treatment begins with a traditional Ayurvedic massage (abyanga), followed by a full-body steam therapy treatment that lasts 20 to 30 minutes. The main purpose of swedhana is to heat the body as comfortably as possible and produce maximum sweating. The combined effect of the massage and the steam treatment produces a significant level

Swedhana
Ayurvedic steam therapy treatments.

---

*While doing hydrotherapy research over many years, the author has visited all the sites that are described below all over the world.

of detoxification. Today, many spa and wellness centers around the world offer this type of Ayurvedic treatment.

Inhalation Therapy

Steam inhalation therapy is part of a total Ayurvedic treatment called **nasya.** This treatment begins with a facial massage with oils and herbs. Drops of an oil herbal mixture are then placed in the nose, followed by steam inhalation. The treatment has a detoxifying, balancing, and enlivening effect on the respiratory system and is particularly beneficial in purifying the system from exposure to high levels of air pollution. Nasya can be found today at many spa and wellness centers offering Ayurvedic treatments.

Nasya
Ayurvedic treatment that uses steam inhalation to detoxify, balance, and enliven the respiratory system.

Home Treatment for Mothers After Childbirth

Another Ayurvedic program involving hydrotherapy that has been used traditionally in India helps mothers recover from childbirth. For several weeks after a mother gives birth, trained therapists come to her home every day to give her a hot bath (more like pouring hot water over the body) until her body is heated. They then wrap her body in warm blankets and have her lie down to rest. Not only is this treatment very relaxing, it also produces purification through sweating. Special oils and herbs, such as ginger, are also used during this treatment.

Usnodaka

Another Ayurvedic therapy is a special program for hydration, called usnodaka, that involves drinking water that has been boiled, sometimes with special herbs added to it. Water is boiled for five minutes, is allowed to cool, and is then used for drinking during the day. The water is never used for more than one day. The purpose of usnodaka is to increase the "intelligence" of the element of fire in the water. Boiled water is thought to enhance the power of *agni,* or the fire of digestion. This procedure is used not only to promote normal daily hydration but also to increase mental and physical stamina, a strong immune system, and healthy, beautiful skin.

JAPANESE HYDROTHERAPY

As with Ayurveda in India, there has been an unbroken tradition of the use of hydrotherapy in Japan for more than a thousand years. Japan has more than 10,000 natural thermal (hot) springs, which have become an essential part of the country's culture, not only for

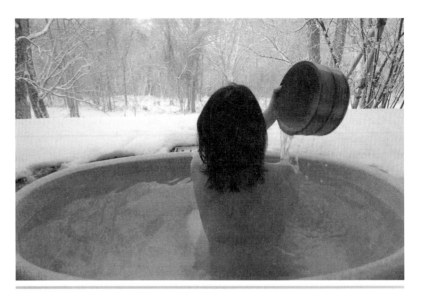

Figure 8–3 Japanese hot springs bath *(image copyright John Leung, 2008. Used under license from Shutterstock.com).*

communal bathing but also for relaxation, rejuvenation, health, wellness, and the treatment of specific medical problems. The Japanese approach includes the healing properties of natural mineral water, herbs, massage, and other natural modalities. Many of Japan's natural hot springs have been developed into modern spas and wellness centers. Some of these sites are well known for their beautiful natural settings and the unique style of the buildings and landscaping. The water, the treatments, the buildings, and the landscaping create a "total experience" that can have a profound healing and restorative effect on a person's physical, mental, emotional, and spiritual levels (see Figure 8–3). The Japanese have developed their hydrotherapy tradition to a very high level of the healing arts, and many spa and wellness centers outside Japan have modeled their programs after this traditional approach to hydrotherapy.

One tradition of hydrotherapy that has been highly developed in Japan is the use of natural mineral waters to produce known therapeutic effects. Every source of natural spring water has its own unique composition of minerals dissolved in the water, as well as its own temperature and pH (see Chapter 2). Mineral waters also have different concentrations of gases—mainly oxygen and carbon dioxide, and possibly radon gas. Over the centuries, the Japanese have found that the proper use of these mineral waters, whether by drinking, bathing, or inhaling, produces specific therapeutic benefits. For example, some mineral waters are used for the treatment and cure of specific medical conditions. Other mineral waters are beneficial for maintaining beautiful skin and healthy joints and muscles and for promoting healthy aging. However, the main therapeutic benefit for most people is the relaxation, rest, and rejuvenation that comes from visits to these special hot springs.

The Japanese have also long used the home bath for hydrotherapy. In Japan, the purpose of the home bath is not for washing the body, which is done before the bath, but for its therapeutic effects, including relaxation. Whether it is a communal bath or a family bath at home, a person washes before getting into the bath. The bath plays an important role in the traditional health and wellness program of the Japanese family; it also has cultural and spiritual significance. Some spa bath treatments around the world are modeled after this famous traditional Japanese home bath tradition.[1]

The Japanese have great respect for their ancient mineral and hot spring traditions. They welcome visitors from around the world to experience this ancient hydrotherapy tradition.[2] It is possible to learn about this great tradition by visiting well-known hot springs, such as famous hot springs at Beppu, or by experiencing a traditional communal bath in any of the Japanese cities, including Tokyo and Kyoto. There is much to learn about hydrotherapy from these ancient and sacred traditions, including elements of medical hydrotherapy; hydrotherapy for general health, wellness, and beauty; and the artistic landscaping found at various sites.

GREEK HYDROTHERAPY

The Asclepieion Tradition

In the ancient Greek healing mythology, Asclepios, the son of Apollo, is the god of healing. Asclepios had two daughters—Panacea, the goddess of healing (her name means "all healing"), and Hygeia, the goddess of the prevention of disease. The **asclepieion** was the physical site (center) in ancient Greece for programs of holistic health, wellness, and medical programs. These healing sanctuaries were built in the tradition of classical Greek architecture and were located in settings of natural beauty with a sacred spring as a source of water. The asclepieion tradition began around the sixth century B.C.E., and by the fourth century B.C.E., most Greek cities had their own asclepieions. The theme of each asclepieion was a holistic, natural approach to wellness, fitness, beauty, prevention, healthy aging,

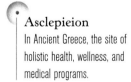
Asclepieion
In Ancient Greece, the site of holistic health, wellness, and medical programs.

and the treatment of medical conditions. The traditional, natural approaches used at the asclepieions included:

- The use of natural herbal remedies
- The use of natural muds and clays
- Nutrition and diet
- The use of natural mineral water from "sacred springs" for therapeutic hydrotherapy treatments, drinking, and bathing
- Massage therapy
- Fitness programs, including physical training and sports programs
- Connection with nature: The asclepieions were developed in areas of natural beauty, including natural sacred springs, with beautiful views and landscaping. The architecture included ornate buildings and statues that complemented the different healing and wellness themes.
- Sleep therapy: The Greeks recognized that normal, healthful sleep patterns contributed to holistic health. Asclepieions also included dream interpretation used to help diagnose health conditions.
- Holistic psychological programs: Attention to mental and emotional health included using the healing value of musical and theatrical performances. Social health and therapy also included the use of the asclepieion as a community center for positive social interaction.
- Spiritual: At the asclepieions, Asclepios, Hygeia, Panacea, and other divinities associated with health and wellness were worshipped, representing a connection with the divine aspect of nature and with a healing power greater than any man-made approaches. It also represented divine models that personified healing and wellness principles and behaviors that were fundamental to the asclepieion tradition.

Aristotle once said, "The whole is greater than the sum of its parts," an expression that captures the essence of the holistic nature of both the Greek and the modern spa, wellness, and fitness center approach to health and wellness. Some modern spa and wellness centers have a remarkable resemblance to the ancient asclepieions of Greece. Today, as in ancient Greece, many spa and wellness centers are developing holistic programs for health, wellness, fitness, and beauty, and are offering programs for weight management, healthy aging, enhancement, and sleep and relaxation therapy. Massage, hydrotherapy, aesthetics, herbs and essential oils, music and light therapy,

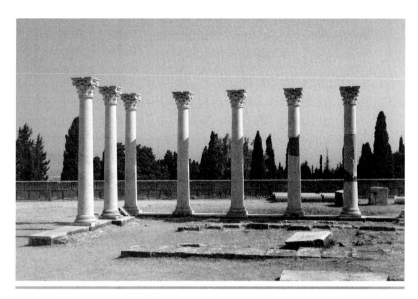

Figure 8–4 Greek healing center of Hippocrates *(image copyright Yan Vugenfirer, 2008. Used under license from Shutterstock.com).*

exercise programs, fitness, and meditation are elements of these programs similar to those found at the asclepieion.

It is possible to visit many of the sites of the ancient Greek asclepieions—sites of natural beauty where one naturally connects with, and can feel transported back to, those ancient times. One such site is the asclepieion on the island of Kos (see Figure 8–4 and Plate 5), the home of Hippocrates (b. 460 B.C.E.). This large asclepieion has a sacred spring, statues, and other architectural remains. From the tree where Hippocrates taught, one can have the same view of the Aegean Sea that Greek citizens saw more than 2,000 years ago. Another site is the Greek city of Loutraki on the Aegean coast, home to a famous thermal spring known for its healing properties. According to Greek legend, when the gods were away from Mount Olympus, they would relax at the hot springs at Loutraki. The protectoress of these mineral springs, the goddess Thermia Artemis, was worshipped there, along with Apollo and Asclepios (see Figure 8–5). History records that the hot mineral waters at Loutraki cured the famous Roman General Sulla in 86 C.E., an event that spread the word of its therapeutic properties throughout the known world. Today, Loutraki has three modern hydrotherapy spa and wellness centers. These centers are fully equipped for thermal mineral water treatments for health, wellness, and aesthetic treatments that are ranked among the finest in the world. Today, you can bathe in the same natural hot springs that centuries ago were used by General Sulla and even possibly by Aristotle and Plato.

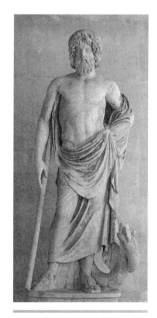

Figure 8–5 Statue of Asclepios.

ROMAN HYDROTHERAPY TRADITIONS

Roman bath
Sophisticated spa, wellness, community, and fitness centers of ancient Rome.

Hypocaust
A system that used advanced plumbing and ventilation systems to produce heated pools and rooms heated with warm or hot air.

The **Roman baths** were actually very sophisticated spa, wellness, community, and fitness centers that are still considered to be architectural marvels. The Romans developed the **hypocaust** system, which used advanced plumbing and ventilation systems to produce heated pools and rooms heated with warm or hot air (see Figure 8–6). The Roman baths also included a pool for a cold plunge, rooms for massage, and instruments for skin exfoliation. The larger facilities had exercise areas, barbers, shops, restaurants, and even libraries. Some offered both fresh and saltwater baths. By 33 B.C.E., there were 170 baths—both public and private—in Rome. Construction of Roman baths continued throughout the Roman Empire. As the Romans continued to develop the hypocaust system, hot or warm water and air could be brought to different areas of the facility, allowing the size of the bath facilities to increase to major proportions. By 305 C.E., the bath of Diocletian could accommodate more than 3,000 bathers.

The Roman baths were obviously far more than a place for bathing. The Romans created a very well-developed and thought-out spa, wellness, and fitness facility that involved heating the body in different stages, including a cold plunge at the end, and then relaxing in a resting area. It also involved immersing one's body in

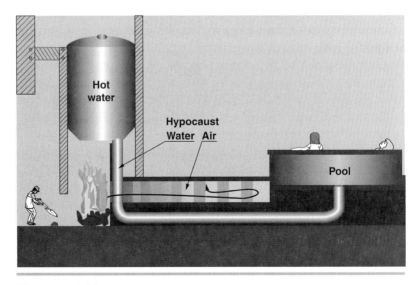

Figure 8–6 Roman hypocaust.

a small pool known as the trepidarium room and swimming in the larger natatio pool. Massage was part of the program, as was skin care using natural products and exfoliation. The Roman baths were also used as a place for social interaction. The relaxed atmosphere made it ideal for discussing business, as well as for spending time with friends and other acquaintances. The architectural beauty of the baths, with their marble floors and walls, paintings, monuments and statues, also contributed to the total wellness experience.

In the Roman baths, we find some of the following fundamental themes, which are shared by many of the spa, wellness, and fitness facilities of today.

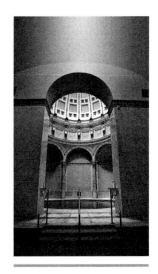

Figure 8–7 Friedrichs-bad classic thermal facility *(courtesy of CAMSAN, Baderbedriebe GmbH).*

- **Architecture and decor:** The Roman baths exemplified the highest level of architectural beauty and decor. This tradition continues today, with spas and wellness centers investing a great deal in their architecture, decor, lighting, fountains, furniture, and so forth. Many spas around the world are modeled after the beauty of the Roman baths. For example, the famous Friedrichsbad Spa in Baden-Baden, Germany (Figure 8–7 and Plate 5), was modeled after the Roman baths and contains similar elements of architectural beauty, rooms, and pools. A detailed description of the experience of visiting the Friedrichsbad Spa is described later in this chapter.

- **Heating the body:** A basic hydrotherapy theme found in most wellness traditions is heating the skin and core body by bathing in natural hot springs or in heated water or by getting a steam or dry hot air (e.g., sauna) treatment.

- **Cold plunge (pool):** A short plunge in a cold pool. This was a small pool with cold water where one could take a short immersion bath, usually following a heating session.

- **Relaxation therapy:** The main theme of the Roman baths was relaxation, rest, and rejuvenation. This is also central to modern health and wellness programs as a natural way to balance the demands and stress of modern life.

- **Rest after treatment:** Sessions that included steam, sauna, baths, and massage ended with a period of rest in a special room, where bathers could lie down, stay warm, and remain quiet.

- **Relaxed social interaction:** One feature of communal bathing is that it helps create a very relaxed social atmosphere, especially at sites of natural hot springs.

GERMANY

Germany has a very impressive and interesting hydrotherapy history that has developed into a highly modern use of hydrotherapy for health and wellness. Today, the hydrotherapy programs in Germany are based on a hydrotherapy tradition several hundred years old, and with connections to the Roman hydrotherapy traditions. Currently, Germany has more than 300 spa and wellness facilities that have hydrotherapy as a main theme.[3] The country has an abundance of thermal mineral springs, and most of its facilities have access to these natural sources of water for pools, hydrotubs, showers, and all other water needs. This abundance of natural hot mineral water, combined with the participation of much of the German population in these facilities, has allowed the development of a wide range of spa and wellness centers. These centers include large specialized swimming pools with hydrojet features, waterfall and exercise pools, multiple steam rooms and saunas, and resting areas. Many also have fitness centers and offer massage, aesthetic, and physical therapy treatments. Some even have water park features, such as slides and wave pools. Most offer hydrotherapy procedures from the Kneipp tradition, including special hot and cold pools for foot bathing and special baths for the arms (see Figure 8–8).

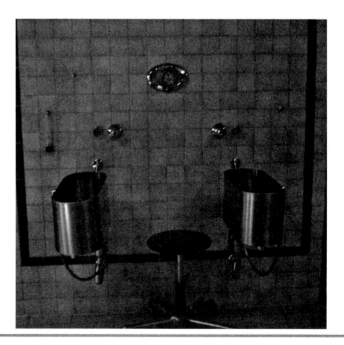

Figure 8–8 Kneipp hydrotherapy foot bath *(compliments of the Edelweiss Hotel, <www.hotel-edelweiss.de>).*

The Kneipp hydrotherapy program was developed by Father Sebastian Kneipp (1832–1897) in Bad Worishofen, and is a total holistic health and wellness program that includes not only hydrotherapy but nutrition, exercise, use of herbs, and connecting with nature. (See Chapter 5 for more detail on the Kneipp Program.)

Wellness centers offering the Kneipp program were established throughout Germany and other European countries, as well as in the eastern part of the United States, in the early part 1900. Today there are more than 40 wellness centers in Bad Worishofen. These centers receive more than 3 million people each year from all over the world, who often stay for one-, two-, three-, or four-week periods. Bad Worishofen is also the home of the Sebastian Kneipp Schule, the educational institute for training on the Kneipp hydrotherapy program, which currently offers a one-week education program in English each year.

Bad Worishofen is a beautiful city with large nature parks and herbal gardens. Walks in these parks are part of the total health program, which is based on specific individual needs. Visiting Bad Worishofen is a great way to learn about the history of a special tradition of hydrotherapy, to see how it continues today, and to receive a total health and wellness program in the Kneipp tradition.

Roman Tradition in Germany

As mentioned earlier, the Roman bath tradition was popular throughout the Roman Empire. Some of the best sites were located where there was a natural supply of thermal hot springs. In Germany, several spa wellness centers are built on the same sites as ancient Roman baths and have programs modeled after the ancient Roman tradition. Perhaps the most famous is the Friedrichsbad Spa in Baden-Baden, Germany. Baden-Baden is world famous for its hot spring mineral wellness centers and its tradition of using hydrotherapy. Baden-Baden has many parks, gardens, and fountains and a classic Hall of Waters, built in 1876. The Hall of Waters is an expression of the appreciation of water for its healing effects and for the essential role it plays in daily health and wellness. Mineral water is available at the Hall of Waters directly from the source and is available to everyone.

The Friedrichsbad Spa, which has the architectural beauty of a traditional Roman bath, was built in 1877 and has been in operation ever since. It includes a program session modeled after the original Roman baths. Mark Twain, after a day at the Friedrichsbad, is quoted as saying, "Here at the Friedrichsbad you lose track of time within 10 minutes and track of the world within 20 minutes." Thermal mineral water from a source near the facility supplies all the water used in the Friedrichsbad Spa, which means that the water

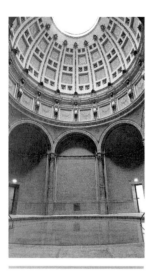

Figure 8–9 Friedrichs-bad temple bathing *(courtesy of CAMSAN, Baderbedriebe GmbH)*.

does not need to be chemically treated. The following is a description of a three-hour session:

The 16 Stages of a Wellness Session at the Friedrichsbad Spa

1. Shower
2. Warm-air bath—129°F (54°C)
3. Hot-air (room) bath—154°F (68°C)
4. Shower
5. Soap and brush massage
6. Shower
7. Thermal steam bath—113°F (45°C)
8. Thermal steam bath—118°F (48°C)
9. Thermal pool—93°F (36°C)
10. Thermal pool with hydrojets—93°F (34°C)
11. Cool thermal pool (under the dome)—82°F (28°C)
12. Shower
13. Cold-water bath—64°F (18°C)
14. Drying off with warm towel
15. Moisturizing cream
16. Resting area

In Baden-Baden, the Friedrichsbad Spa is not referred to as a spa but as a "temple of bathing" (see Figure 8–9).

Another example of the Roman tradition in Germany is the Cassiopeia Therma—a hydrotherapy spa wellness center in Badenweiler, in southwest Germany. The facility is built on the site of a thermal spring, which is the spa's source of water. Like the Friedrichsbad Spa, the Cassiopeia has a complete program modeled after the ancient Roman baths, and session at this spa is very similar to the sessions experienced in the Roman bath that was built at this site hundreds of years ago. After a treatment at this spa, you can visit the well-preserved archaeological site of the original Roman bath just out the door.

 # FRANCE

France, which has a long tradition of hydrotherapy, has many spa and wellness facilities, usually near a thermal hot springs. As in Germany, these facilities are often built on the sites of ancient Roman baths.

There are also many spa and wellness centers along the coast that incorporated the use of natural ocean water, which is known as thallasotherapy, in many different types of hydrotherapy treatments.

One of the most famous centers for hydrotherapy is the town of Vichy in central France. This area is the source of several natural thermal springs and also has a Hall of Waters, where it is possible to drink water from five different mineral springs. Vichy is the source of the famous Celestins mineral water, which is bottled and sold throughout the world. The Hall of Waters is also a museum with descriptions (in French) of the hydrotherapy and cultural history of the town of Vichy, including photos of some of the original Vichy showers.

Each mineral spring at Vichy has a different combination of minerals, and each is known to have specific beneficial and medicinal effects. The natural mineral waters are used for medical, health, and wellness treatments. The amount of water and the timing for drinking the water are prescribed for each type of mineral water depending on the health purpose.

Today, there are three main hydrotherapy facilities in Vichy. The Vichy Les Celestins is the modern, five-star spa wellness facility, offering a variety of hydrotherapy, massage, aesthetics, and fitness programs. The Centre Thermal des Domes offers all the basic hydrotherapy, massages, and aesthetic treatments, but is not as modern and is more moderately priced than Les Celestins. The Thermes de Vichy Callou is a modern, highly developed medical facility that offers programs featuring hydrotherapy to treat various medicinal conditions. These programs combine massage, modern physical therapy, and hydrotherapy, including drinking mineral waters and inhalation therapy. These treatment programs are prescribed by medical doctors and are often paid for by medical insurance. The programs offered at Vichy are similar to programs offered at many locations in France. As with other European spa and wellness centers, the city of Vichy is located on the site of an ancient Roman bath.

The original hydrotherapy programs at Vichy are the source of the Vichy shower, which is one of the best-known and most popular hydrotherapy treatments found at spas around the world. In the original Vichy shower treatment, the client lies on a horizontal wet table. Multiple showerheads spray the client with water as two massage therapists perform a massage. The water flow is generally low pressure with the multiple showerheads keeping a constant flow of warm water over the body. The Vichy shower can be used in combination with other treatments for health, wellness, beauty, and medical benefits. In Vichy, an essential component of the Vichy shower is the use of the mineral waters flowing naturally at the facilities. According to the French Vichy shower tradition, an authentic Vichy shower treatment includes not only the special shower and massage, but also must include the natural Vichy mineral water and its special properties.

OTHER EUROPEAN COUNTRIES

Many other European countries have a historical tradition using hydrotherapy for health, wellness, beauty, and medical purposes. Medical-style facilities have developed over time, mostly at the sites of natural hot springs. Treatments have been developed that have proven to be effective for skin conditions, osteoarthritis, rheumatoid arthritis, kidney problems, and many other conditions. The natural mineral waters are used for hydrotherapy baths and showers, steam treatments, and drinking. Through time, each location has developed its own treatment programs based on the specific qualities of the mineral water at that specific location. Most of these facilities are more medical than other spas, with a staff of doctors, balneologists (those trained in the use of natural mineral water), physical therapists, and massage therapists. Famous centers include those in the Czech Republic, Romania, Hungary, Poland, and Russia. Several scientific studies have been done that demonstrate the effectiveness of these programs in the treatment of various medical conditions.

A well-known form of traditional hydrotherapy from Russia is the banya, a type of Russian communal steam bath. In the banya, steam is created by pouring water over heated stones. There are usually three rooms, including an entry room for leaving one's clothes, a room with hot and cold water for rinsing, and the steam room. The banya has been a very important part of Russian culture and played an important role in communal health and wellness traditions. The banya is another example of the use of heating treatments to produce health and wellness benefits that are also part of the social culture of an entire region.

MIDDLE EAST, SOUTH AMERICA, AND NATIVE AMERICANS

The use of the traditional hamam in the Middle East also has a long cultural history. The hamam has a steam room for heating the body, a massage area, and a resting area, similar to the Roman bath tradition.

In South America, the Mayans developed a tradition of communal steam treatments given in a special room called a *temascal*. They would enter the main room through a very low door. Steam was produced by pouring water on hot stones inside the room. Herbs, spices, and incense were used in addition to prayers. The temascal steam baths were for spiritual, physical, and mental cleansing. This tradition continues even today in some parts of Mexico, where some vacation resorts offer it as an example of a traditional Mayan hydrotherapy treatment.

For centuries before the arrival of Europeans in North America, there was a tradition of the use of water for healing and during communal sweat lodge sessions. In the sweat lodge, water is poured over very hot stones to produce steam. Herbs are also used along with chanting. A sweat lodge session is still a sacred tradition for producing physical, emotional, and spiritual cleansing and for promoting a greater connection (communion) with the creative forces of nature. This sweat lodge tradition continues today and there are some opportunities to experience a sweat lodge session.

It is also possible for spa and wellness centers to incorporate some elements from these ancient traditions in their own hydrotherapy treatments. A theme can be created that includes some kind of sacred intention, combined with the use of special herbs and music that promote a relaxed, spiritual atmosphere. Special steam and hydrotub treatments that combine elements from these mystical traditional treatments can be designed. In developing any hydrotherapy treatment, the intention of the treatment is a key component in its successful outcome (see Chapter 7).

 UNITED STATES

Hydrotherapy, as practiced in Europe, was brought to North America by Europeans who immigrated here during the 1800s. By 1850, there were several hundred "water cure" establishments in the eastern United States. In 1893, Dr. Simon Baruch, professor of balneology at Columbia University, published *The Uses of Water in Modern Medicine*, which supported the use of hydrotherapy in treating specific medical conditions.[4]

Two of the most famous health destinations that emerged with hydrotherapy treatments as a main theme were Saratoga Springs in New York and Hot Springs in Arkansas. By the 1900s, hydrotherapy was considered a mainstream treatment not only for general health and wellness, but also for certain medical conditions, especially orthopedic problems. Hydrotherapy was used at well-known orthopedic hospitals, including the Orthopedic Hospital in Los Angeles and Walter Reid Hospital in Washington, D.C. President Franklin Roosevelt visited Warm Springs, Georgia, for the hydrogymnastics program for polio rehabilitation.

In 1933, the Simon Baruch Institute was founded at Saratoga Springs as the first center for balneology research in the United States. The Government Health Facility, which was developed there in 1935, was the largest health facility in the county. At the facility, which could treat more than 1,000 patients a day, hydrotherapy was an essential component of many of the treatments. In the 1930s and 1940s, more than 750,000 patients a year visited the facilities at Saratoga Springs.[5]

The history of Hot Springs, Arkansas, began in 1832, when Congress designated for protection four sections of land in the area that had natural hot springs. By 1878, more than 50,000 people were coming to health facilities at this location, which featured hydrotherapy programs using water from the hot springs. By 1910, Hot Springs had become a well-developed health and wellness destination. Although most visitors were affluent, even those who could not afford treatments at the bathhouses could bathe for free at the Free Bath House, which saw more than 220,000 visitors in 1911.

Hot Springs included many lavish, highly developed bathhouses that combined a wide range of services, including massage, hydrotherapy, and fitness, as well as medical treatments. As in the European tradition, the bathhouses at Hot Springs were also used for health and wellness vacations. The natural thermal waters were found to have special healing properties for different medical conditions. Dr. Gustav Zander, born in Sweden in 1832, developed physical therapy machines for the bathhouses that are similar to those being used today for fitness and physical therapy. In 1918, the U.S. Public Health Services Division of Venereal Disease established a clinic at Hot Springs. The clinic used treatments combining mineral water, mercury, and arsenic compounds.

On March 4, 1921, the Hot Springs National Park, the smallest national park in the United States, was created. The park includes the historic Bath House Row, natural hot springs, and hiking trails and campsites. It also has a museum with information on the treatments offered at the bathhouses and the fitness equipment designed by Dr. Zander. It is a great national park to visit for those interested in the historical development of hydrotherapy in the United States. It is still possible to get the traditional hydrotherapy and massage treatments in Buckstaff Bath House, one of the original bathhouses

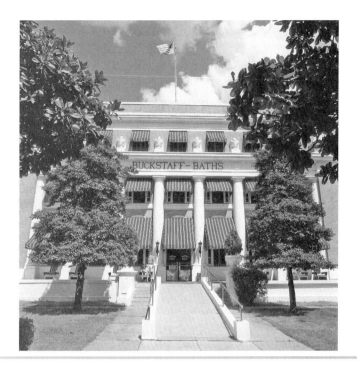

Figure 8–10 Buckstaff Bath House *(courtesy of Buckstaff Hotel, Hot Springs, Arkansas).*

on Bath House Row (see Figure 8–10). The traditional treatment includes a thermal mineral bath, whirlpool, Swedish massage, and loofah mitt exfoliation.

By the end of the 1930s, there was a decline in interest in places like Saratoga Springs, Hot Springs, and other natural hot springs. Not only was the interest in health and wellness vacations decreasing, but also the modern medical approach was developing, with an emphasis on the treatment of medical conditions by more scientific techniques, especially the use of newly developed drugs. For example, after the development of penicillin, which could be used for the treatment of venereal disease, the venereal disease clinic at Hot Springs closed in 1941. As the more modern approaches to the treatment of medical conditions gained in popularity, the former popularity of more natural health facilities declined. By the end of the 1950s, these health facilities were no longer in use, and most closed their doors. Thus, even as the use of hydrotherapy for health, wellness, and medicinal purposes continued in Europe, its use in the United States virtually ended.

In the 1970s, we saw a renewed interest in alternative health and wellness approaches. Even though, the modern medical approach was (and continues to be) the mainstream for the treatment of major medical conditions, it did not offer programs and education that dealt more specifically with such areas as daily wellness, fitness, appearance and beauty, healthy aging, disease prevention, and enhancement of full human potential. More and more people began turning to modern wellness, spa, and fitness centers for education and programs for attaining and maintaining normal, and even optimal levels, of health and wellness. Today's modern holistic spa and wellness centers are able to combine the traditional knowledge of holistic health and wellness, including hydrotherapy, natural products from around the world and the modern scientific understanding of the human body—all to help individuals achieve the health and wellness goals they are seeking.

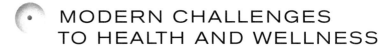

MODERN CHALLENGES TO HEALTH AND WELLNESS

In our modern world, there are also significant new challenges to health and wellness. These challenges will require special programs, including hydrotherapy, to help people manage these problems. Some of these modern-day challenges include:

- Multiple forms of pollution
- Nutrition
- Proper exercise
- Hydration
- Multiple forms of stress
- Disconnect with nature

SUMMARY

The use of hydrotherapy has been found in ancient traditions as an important element of holistic health and wellness programs, including traditions from India, Japan, the ancient Greek, and Roman civilizations, and the past several hundred years in Europe. The use of hydrotherapy in Ayurveda from India is still popular today, both in India and in other countries around the world. The use of natural hot springs and special baths for therapeutic purposes continues today as an essential part of Japanese culture. The hydrotherapy programs of many countries in Europe also continue as they have for several hundred years. All of these programs combined basic approaches to holistic health, including treatments for certain medical conditions as well as time spent at health centers for the beneficial effects of healing, rest, and rejuvenation.

The combined hydrotherapy and medical programs were brought to this country from Europe and were very popular at places like Saratoga Springs, NY and Hot Springs, AR. These centers offered holistic health programs and "health vacations," along with medical treatments. With the development and popularity of the modern medical approach, however, interest in these centers slowly came to an end. By the 1950s, most of these facilities were closed. Many are now museums of the use of hydrotherapy in the United States. With the increased interest in modern medicine and changes in travel trends in the United States, these health and wellness centers lost their former appeal.

Since the 1970s, there have been new developments and an increased interest in hydrotherapy and other forms of alternative health to meet the needs of people wanting to achieve and maintain more developed holistic health and wellness goals. Today, clients have greater expectations for daily wellness, fitness, appearance and beauty, healthful aging, and disease prevention.

Today, our modern life is producing new challenges to health and wellness. For example, there is greater air, water, and soil pollution, which is significantly increasing exposure to toxic levels of various harmful substances. There are also higher personal levels of stress and anxiety. The field of holistic health and wellness is continuing to develop to meet these challenges, offering simpler solutions to these more complex problems. Hydrotherapy has always been an essential element of holistic health and wellness programs, and it will continue to develop as a fundamental treatment modality.

REFERENCES

(1) Altman, N. (2000). *Healing Springs: The Ultimate Guide to Taking the Waters.* Healing Arts Press.

(2) Talmage, E. (2006). *Getting Wet: Adventures in the Japanese Bath.* Kodansha International.

(3) Bucken, H. (2005). *Deutschland: Deine Therman.* Zeist Geist Media.

(4) Baruch, S. (2006; first printing 1892). *The Uses of Water in Modern Medicine.* Kessinger Publishing.

(5) Attman, Healing Springs.

REVIEW QUESTIONS

1. What is a steam treatment used by Ayurveda for detoxification that is still used today?

2. What is an inhalation treatment used by Ayurveda that is still used today?

3. What is meant by the term *holistic health and wellness?*

4. What was holistic about the Greek wellness tradition?

5. What do some of the modern spas and wellness centers have in common with the Roman traditions?

6. What is a famous hydrotherapy treatment from France that is named after the city where the treatment originated?

7. What is the name of the well-known center that was part of the early history of hydrotherapy in the United States, that is now a national park?

8. Discuss why there was such a decline in the popularity and use of hydrotherapy in the United States between 1930 and 1950, when at the same time, hydrotherapy continued to be popular in Europe.

9. Discuss the current increased interest in alternative health approaches and how hydrotherapy, which has long tradition of use for health and wellness, can play a role in the ongoing development of these programs.

The Future of Hydrotherapy

KEY TERM

water isotope

INTRODUCTION

Hydrotherapy has played an essential role in health and wellness programs throughout history and will continue to do so in the future. In the recent past, significant developments have been made in areas connected with hydrotherapy, including a better scientific understanding of the behavior of water, a greater knowledge of the human body's anatomy and physiology, advancements in the technology of hydrotherapy equipment, the availability of more natural products from around the world, and greater sharing of information about hydrotherapy by therapists. We also have a better understanding of the hydrosphere and of the holistic concept of nature. This chapters looks at future trends in each of these areas to provide possible insights into what we can expect from hydrotherapy in the future.

GREATER SCIENTIFIC UNDERSTANDING OF WATER

Currently, much is known about the behavior of water, including the principles of buoyancy, heat capacity, movement, and the solvent nature of water. These scientific principles show that the behavior of water is measurable and predictable. Precise mathematical formulas can be used to calculate changes in temperature, pressure, buoyancy,

317

and flow rates. These formulas are very important because hydrotherapy treatments are done on the human body, which is 60% water. The water inside the human body behaves according to the same principles as the water used in a hydrotherapy treatment. Thus, understanding the behavior of water provides a better knowledge of what is taking place inside the body when water is brought into contact with it during hydrotherapy treatments.

Even though much is known about the behavior of water, there is much that is still being learned. This applies especially to the behavior of water at the molecular level. The interaction between water molecules interacting with other water molecules and molecules of other substances is extremely dynamic and complex. The number of water molecules interacting in even 18.02 g (1 mol) of water is 6.023×10^{23}. And, not all water molecules are exactly the same. There is also a small percentage of water molecules, known as **water isotopes,** that have a slightly different molecular structure. In these isotopes, either the oxygen or the hydrogen molecule that makes up the water molecule will have extra neutrons (see Table 9–1). By measuring the number and combination of water isotopes in a given source of water, hydrologists can determine how long that water has been in a specific location—for example, in a deep water aquifer. For those wishing to study the more complex theories of the behavior of water, please refer to *Water: A Matrix of Life* (see Suggested Readings at the end of this chapter).

Chapter 10 presents the many ways that water is used for healing and wellness that suggest that there is more to the behavior of water than current scientific theories explain. For example, some people speculate that water from certain remote regions in the world is responsible for the exceptional longevity and health of people in that region. They feel that it is the unique behavior of this water at the molecular level that makes it different from "ordinary" water. Other people believe from their experiences that water at certain hot springs has special healing qualities. With a greater scientific knowledge of water in the future, especially at the molecular level,

Water isotope
Water molecule that has a slightly different molecular structure, with either the oxygen or the hydrogen molecule having extra neutrons.

Table 9–1	Isotopes of Water (H_2O)
Isotopes	**Parts per Million (ppm)**
$_1H_2\,_{16}O$ (normal water)	997,280
$_1H_2\,_{18}O$ (isotope)	2,000
$_1H_2\,_{17}O$ (isotope)	400
$_1H_2H\,_{16}O$ (isotope)	320

it may be possible to have a better understanding and application of the full potential of water for healing and wellness.

Greater Understanding of the Behavior of Water in the Human Body

As described in earlier chapters, the human body is approximately 60% water, and all of this water is in a state of constant circulation. Scientific knowledge is continuing to develop regarding the complex nature of the human body as a dynamic, cellular, fluid system. More attention is being placed on the paradigm of the human body as the interaction of trillions of individual cells that function collectively to produce various physiological activities. The activity of all the cells of the body takes place in a fluid environment—the interstitial fluid—through which there is continual circulation of nutrients, oxygen, and other substances. A growing understanding of the body's fluid dynamics and the synergy between water in the body and the water used in hydrotherapy will allow for the further development of the use of hydrotherapy as a treatment modality for influencing the metabolic rate, circulation, cellular alignment, and other cellular functions.

There is also a growing understanding of the structural elements of the body, including the bones, ligaments, tendons, cartilage, and fascia, at the cellular level. Some of these structural systems, especially the fascial matrix, are responsible for much of the alignment of key systems in the body, such as the vascular system, the nervous system, and even the cells. Also, each of these structural systems has its own unique matrix at the cellular level of different protein fibers and ground substance, as well as the crystallized mineral matrix in the bones. We know that hydrotherapy techniques work at the cellular level of these structures. In the future, as our understanding of these elements continues to develop, there will be greater potential to work with and improve the microalignment and integrity of these connective tissue matrixes at the cellular level, to help overcome the effects of traumas, aging, gravity, and daily movement.

Some current special uses of hydrotherapy techniques have been shown to produce dramatic lifesaving benefits. For example, a few hospitals in North America circulate cold water through a special jacketlike system attached to a patient's body immediately following a heart attack. This technique reduces the core body temperature (hypothermia) from 98.6°F to 92°F. This simple and inexpensive procedure increases the survival rate from 10% to 50%. As another example of induced hypothermia, the Children's Pediatrics Hospital in Philadelphia is using a similar procedure immediately after major trauma in children, especially head trauma. The induced hypothermia results in a significant reduction of permanent damage and an improved healing time. There are many implications from these examples for the greater use of cold water (hypothermia) in many other areas of health and wellness in the future.

GREATER USE OF NATURAL PRODUCTS IN HYDROTHERAPY

New levels of global communication and trade have significantly increased the availability of natural products from around the world. Many of these products can be used as a component of hydrotherapy treatments. For example, it is now possible to purchase organic muds from Austria, mineral salts from the Dead Sea, herbs and essential oils from around the world, and seaweed products from different ocean sources. There are likely many other natural products that are yet to be discovered. It is easy to imagine that nature's pharmacy has many secrets to reveal that will aid in achieving all of our complex individual health and wellness needs.

Another future potential development could be the discovery of more effective, unique synergies among the uses of various natural products. The vast number of different products, as well as the ones yet to be discovered, means that we will continuously be finding new ways of combining them, thereby producing new products with unique benefits. Because most hydrotherapy treatments include the use of natural products, these discoveries could enhance the effectiveness of these treatments and also lead to the development of new forms of treatments.

THE FUTURE OF HYDROTHERAPY EQUIPMENT

With hydrotherapy equipment, the therapist brings water into contact with the client's body in a controlled manner to bring about specific therapeutic transformations. Hydrotherapy equipment allows the therapist to adjust the temperature of the water, the pressure of the water, and the exact location of contact with the client's body. Hydrotherapy equipment has improved over the years and will continue to develop with better designs and technological features. The following are some areas in which we can expect to see developments in the design of hydrotherapy equipment.

Improved Control of Water Temperature

Heat exchange, which occurs between water in hydrotubs, showers, or steam equipment and the human body, is one of the most important applied aspects of hydrotherapy. Future developments of hydrotherapy equipment will allow more precise control and measurement of the temperature of the water used in a treatment. There is a very precise relationship between the temperature of the water (liquid, steam, or ice), the specific surface area of the body that the water contacts, and changes in the surface and core temperatures. Being able to more precisely control the water temperature will provide therapists with more control over changes in body temperatures.

Another future development will be more accurate and continual measurements of the surface and/or core temperature of the body. For example, if the goal of the treatment requires the core temperature of the body to be increased by precisely 3°F, then it will be possible to more easily monitor the accuracy of the core temperature during the duration of the treatment.

Improved Control of Water Pressure

When water pressure generated by hydrojets, hydrowands, handheld showers, or other means comes into contact with the client's body, it generates pressure on the surface of the body that, in turn, increases circulation inside the body and also creates a massaging effect on the cells, vascular system, and the structural matrix. Precise control over the water pressure and better control over the exact areas where the water pressure comes into contact with the body will give the therapist more control over changes taking place inside the body.

Improved Comfort

Future developments of hydrotherapy equipment will include designs that are more synergistic with the natural shape and functioning of the human body, which will allow for greater comfort for the client. Other design features for greater client warmth, ease of entering and exiting the equipment system will also add to the quality of the treatment. Currently, much of the hydrotherapy equipment is poorly designed in terms of comfort and other needs of the client.

Multipurpose

Equipment will also become more multipurpose, which will allow a greater variety of treatments to be done with one piece of equipment. There will be a better integration of features for using sound (music) and color light therapy and improved technology for introducing natural products into the water, such as mineral salts and seaweed products.

Another improvement of hydrotherapy equipment will include features that make it easier for therapists to work with the client's body during hydrotherapy treatments. For example, some hydrotubs will be longer, allowing the client to lie in a full horizontal extension in the hydrotub and also will allow the therapist access to all sides the hydrotub.

WISDOM FROM THE PAST

Future developments in hydrotherapy will also come from a better understanding of how it has been used in the past, in such traditions as Ayurveda, Japanese baths, Greek asclepieions, and Roman baths. The European hydrotherapy tradition is rich in special techniques, especially the use of mineral water for medical purposes. It is possible that more can be learned from remote and isolated traditions, such as indigenous cultures in the rainforests of South America and Africa, although there is very limited information currently available.

SHARING KNOWLEDGE AND EXPERIENCE

Hydrotherapy in the future will be further developed by the shared experience of therapists from around the world. Therapists practicing hydrotherapy in different parts of the world will be able to more easily share their knowledge and experiences through the Internet (via Web sites and e-mail), trade magazines and journals, conferences, and health and wellness associations. All therapists, including those using hydrotherapy, share a common goal to promote the health and wellness of their clients, and modern communication technologies can help create a synergy of knowledge and experience between therapists around the world.

GREATER UNDERSTANDING OF CLIENTS' HEALTH AND WELLNESS GOALS

Another area of interest for the future of hydrotherapy is the continuing development of a better understanding of our clients' complex health and wellness goals. Clients are becoming more educated about their own health and wellness and are more motivated to take greater personal responsibility. Clients are seeking programs that are more integrated and holistic and that offer more effective approaches to attaining all of their goals. Also, clients are facing new challenges to health and wellness from increased levels of stress and multiple forms of pollution. These issues will require the development of programs, such as hydrotherapy, that deal with these new and complex challenges of living in our modern world.

 ## GREATER UNDERSTANDING OF THE HYDROSPHERE

Greater knowledge about the hydrosphere (see Chapter 2) can play an important role for hydrotherapy in the future. Recent developments in scientific understanding of the hydrosphere show that there is a fixed amount of water on the planet and that all of this water is interconnected and behaves as one system. This one water system undergoes a dynamic continual process of evaporation, purification, precipitation, and distribution to all regions of the planet (see Figure 9–1). Not only do human beings get water for all their needs, including hydrotherapy, from the hydrosphere, but they are also a part of the hydrosphere, with more than 66 billion gallons of

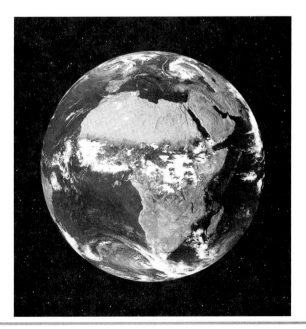

Figure 9–1 Hydrosphere of Africa *(photo courtesy of NASA).*

water in human beings at any given moment. Thus, when we harm the hydrosphere, we harm ourselves.

Much of what has been learned about hydrotherapy throughout history has come from the interaction of people with water in natural settings, such as hot springs, mineral springs, and the oceans. This knowledge and experience has been translated into hydrotherapy treatments and programs, which are usually done at spa, wellness, and health centers or at home. However, as much as we have learned about the hydrosphere, much remains to be discovered.

The hydrosphere is a complex natural system that includes human beings as an element of the system. The relationship of hydrotherapy with the hydrosphere is very important; developing a greater understanding and appreciation of this relationship will benefit the future development of hydrotherapy. In addition, by understanding more about the hydrosphere, its interconnectedness with all living systems, and the fact that all living things depend on the health of the hydrosphere, people will become more aware of behaviors that are harming the hydrosphere, including pollution, overuse, and global warming.

THE NATURE PARADIGM AND HYDROTHERAPY

The hydrosphere, the human body, and products such as herbs and minerals are all natural—they are not man-made. Most therapists integrate natural approaches in their treatments and programs to be more in harmony with the natural behavior of the human body and the healing process, including the use of natural products, light, sounds, and water.

We are continuing to develop a better understanding of what is meant by *nature* and by *natural products* and *therapies*. One source of our understanding of what *nature* is comes from the wisdom of ancient traditions from around the world. Different concepts about nature are also found in different indigenous cultures that continue to live in close harmony with nature. A common theme of these concepts is that nature is a wholeness of all living and non-living natural systems that balance and depend on each other as one unified web of life. These concepts tend to focus more on the sacredness of nature and on being in harmony with the elements of nature, rather than on trying to control nature (see Figure 9–2). The following quote from a member of an indigenous culture in Thailand expresses elements of this vision of nature.

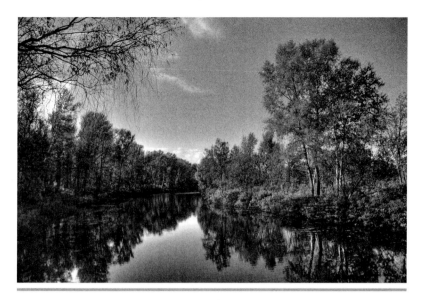

Figure 9–2 Natural water setting *(image copyright Nataliya Peregudova, 2008. Used under license from Shutterstock.com).*

Ancient teachings have been passed down through generations of our people.
These teachings say all life forms are interconnected.
Everything is part of one whole and living organism.
And each part is vital to the survival of the whole.

I believe the Earth is one living being.
The end of any one life form will lead to hardship of another.
And if there are too many hardships
the whole may suffer beyond healing.

I was taught that the most important thing is having a peaceful heart.
When we are content with who we are
we treat other life forms with compassion and kindness.

Nature will always contain mysteries.
We don't need to solve them all.
We just need to open and let it fill us.
The energy of nature moves through the cycle of birth, death, and rebirth.
And it continues on and on
moving from one form of life to another.

—Mae Tui, Hill Tribe, northern Thailand, 2005[1]

Along with ancient wisdom, modern scientific theories and research are also providing insights into a deeper, more complete understanding of the principles of nature. For example, physicists are developing theories, such as the Unified Field Theory and the String Theory, that demonstrate a unity between all the various levels of nature, from the finest levels of matter to the collection of all the galaxies. NASA photos of Earth allow us to see the planet as one natural system that includes the hydrosphere as a key element of the total Earth system.

Other interesting insights about nature come from great writers, such as E. O. Wilson, a famous naturalist and Harvard professor who won two Pulitzer Prizes. The following quote is from *Biophilia* (1984) (See Suggested Readings at the end of this chapter.)

> I have argued . . . that we are human in good part because of the particular way we affiliate with other organisms. They are the matrix in which the human mind originated and is permanently rooted, and they offer the challenge and freedom innately sought. To the extent that each person can feel like a naturalist, the old excitement of the untrammeled world will be regained. I offer this as a formula of re-enchantment to invigorate poetry and myth: mysterious and little known organisms live within walking distance of where you sit. Splendor awaits in minute proportions.

—Edward O. Wilson, *Biophilia,* 1984

The continuing development of our understanding of what we mean by *nature* and of what is natural, from ancient to modern scientific theories, can play an important role in the future development of hydrotherapy. Also, directly working with water to promote healing and wellness can be another dynamic way for us (therapists) to learn more about nature, and our intimate connection with it.

 ## SUMMARY

There are many positive and promising trends for the future development of hydrotherapy. Our clients' desire for more effective, natural ways to attain an increasingly wider range of health and wellness goals will always be a motivating factor for the continued development of hydrotherapy. Likewise, the challenges to health and wellness posed by the stresses of "modern life" will demand better natural technologies to solve these human-made problems. With greater challenges come better solutions, and hydrotherapy will continue to play an important role in health and wellness in the future, just as it has in the past. This chapter described some of the main factors that will contribute to the continued development of hydrotherapy.

Future developments will include a better scientific understanding of the behavior of water at all levels, especially the molecular level, which will provide new insights into the use of water in hydrotherapy treatments. Further developments in the understanding of the anatomy and physiology of the human body, especially its dynamic fluid cellular nature, will provide insights into more effective uses of hydrotherapy. Also important will be a greater understanding of how the behavior of water in the human body is transformed by the behavior of water during hydrotherapy treatments.

More natural products from around the world are now available for use in hydrotherapy, and more are yet to be discovered. The knowledge of how to use these natural products as part of hydrotherapy will continue to develop. It will also be possible to create new synergies by combining different natural products to produce new blends for special uses.

An exciting area for the future of hydrotherapy will be in new technological developments of hydrotherapy equipment. Future equipment will provide more precise control over water temperature, water pressure, and location of water pressure on the body. The design of the equipment will also be in greater harmony with the shape and dynamics of the human body, thereby enhancing relaxation and other hydrotherapy benefits. Future hydrotherapy equipment will also be designed in such a way that allows therapists to work more effectively with clients. Finally, hydrotherapy equipment will continue to be more multipurpose, offering more hydrotherapy modalities in one system.

Modern global communication is making it possible to share information between therapists from around the world. For example, through e-mail, Web sites, and international associations, therapists can share their experiences, insights, scientific research, and enthusiasm, creating a global team of therapists who can more quickly and more effectively develop specialized hydrotherapy treatments to meet any new health and wellness challenges.

The success of the future of hydrotherapy is connected to its successful use for thousands of years. Greater understanding of the use of hydrotherapy from the past will help us continue its development in the future. In addition, learning more about the use of hydrotherapy by remote indigenous cultures can also potentially add to its total understanding.

Clients are becoming more involved in and taking greater personal responsibility for their health and wellness. They also have greater expectations of what they can achieve in areas such as daily wellness, healthy aging, prevention, fitness, and enhancement of full human potential. By better understanding the complex health and wellness goals of clients, hydrotherapy treatments and programs can be developed to support them. Also, modern challenges to health and wellness, including stress and pollution, require special treatment programs. Hydrotherapy will continue to play a key role in facing these challenges.

Today we have a greater understanding of the hydrosphere than ever before, and this understanding will continue to develop. The hydrosphere is not only the source of water for hydrotherapy treatments, it is also the original source of the experiences that led to the development of hydrotherapy. Not only do we get water for all our needs from the hydrosphere, we are also a part of hydrosphere. Because the relationship between the hydrosphere and hydrotherapy is natural and fundamental, future developments in the understanding of the hydrosphere will also lead to the development of hydrotherapy.

There are many new and interesting opportunities available for developing a greater understanding of what we mean by *nature*. Some of this information comes from the wisdom of enlightened people and cultures. Modern science is also contributing to our understanding of nature though theories such as the Unified Field Theory. Because water, the human body and products such as herbs and mineral salts are all natural—having a greater understanding about the total concept of nature can be a positive contribution for the future development of hydrotherapy, which is itself natural approach to health and wellness.

REFERENCE

(1)   From *The Sacred Planet*, Walt Disney Products (2004)—available on DVD (contains beautiful visual expressions of the hydrosphere).

SUGGESTED READINGS

Fothergill, A. (Series producer). (2007). *Planet Earth* [Television series]. Silver Spring, MD: Discovery Communications.

Franks, F. (2000). *Water: A Matrix of Life*. Cambridge, UK: The Royal Society of Chemistry.

Long, J. (Director). (2004). *The Sacred Planet* [Motion picture]. (Available from Living Films, a Walt Disney Company.)

Wilson, E. (1984). *Biophilia*. Cambridge, MA: Harvard University Press.

REVIEW QUESTIONS

1. Discuss how a better scientific understanding of the behavior of water could be of value to the continued development of hydrotherapy.

2. Discuss how a better understanding of the anatomy and physiology of the human body, especially at the cellular fluid level, can be of value to the continued development of hydrotherapy.

3. Discuss how the availability of more natural products and their combined use can be of value to the continued development of hydrotherapy.

4. List some developments in hydrotherapy equipment that can lead to more and better uses of this equipment in the future.

5. Discuss how having a better understanding of the use of hydrotherapy in the past can lead to better use of hydrotherapy in the future.

6. Give some examples of how therapists around the world can share their knowledge and experiences of hydrotherapy and how this can promote the future development of hydrotherapy.

7. Discuss how a better understanding of the hydrosphere as well as the total concept of nature can promote the development of hydrotherapy.

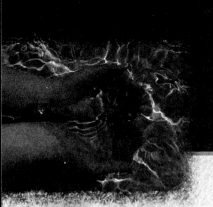

Unique Uses
of Water for Health
and Wellness

INTRODUCTION

Throughout time, people have used water in many special, creative, and unique ways in order to achieve a wide range of wellness goals. In addition to the more traditional uses of water for hydrotherapy, there are other interesting uses of water that may give greater insight and understanding into the total potential of water for its healing and transformational properties. This chapter presents some of the special ways that water has been used, and continues to be used, for health and wellness. The intention of this chapter is not to determine how—or even how well—these special uses work; rather it is to present examples of these interesting approaches.

In each example in this chapter, water plays a primary role in the transformation that takes place. The question is: What is it about the water in each example that allows it to play such a primary role in these special and often mystical transformations? It is also interesting to consider whether there is anything about the special behavior of water that is common to all or some of these phenomena that might provide a greater understanding of these use of water in more traditional hydrotherapy.

These special uses of water are divided into two general categories. The first category lists special uses of water found in more natural settings. The second category deals with special uses of water where the water has been transformed or enhanced by human activity and intention, giving it some special, unique healing and wellness properties.

WATER IN NATURAL SETTINGS

In this category, people benefit in various ways from interacting with water as it is found in natural settings. Nothing is done to the water to change it or try to enhance it. Somehow, the water is already "special" and produces profound health and wellness transformations.

Healing Baths

Many examples of healing baths used to cure major medical conditions—often incurable diseases—are found throughout the world. One of the most famous is in Lourdes, France. The origins of healing pilgrimages to Lourdes began with Bernadette Soubirous, the daughter of a devout Christian peasant. Between February 11 and July 16, 1858, 14-year-old Bernadette saw apparitions of the Virgin Mary in a small grotto called Massabielle, the source of the sacred spring for which Lourdes is now famous. Today, more than 6 million people from all different religious backgrounds visit Lourdes each year to take a healing bath. Water used at the bath flows from the sacred spring into special rooms where any visitor can take a brief cold bath. Nothing is done to change the natural qualities of the water or the natural spring other than having the water flow to man-made bathtubs. At Lourdes, there are many documented cases of cures of major conditions for which there is no medical explanation. It is not understood what role the water plays in the healing transformations, but it is clear that water is an essential element of the process. There are many examples of scared healing baths in different parts of the world, but Lourdes is the most famous modern example and it is possible for anyone to visit and experience this healing bath.

Sacred Baths for Spiritual and Emotional Cleansing, Balancing, and Awakening

Water has played an important role in religious and spiritual rituals that include sacred baths in rivers, lakes, or the ocean. In these cases, water is believed to be an essential element in producing profound physical, emotional, and spiritual transformations. These sacred baths have long traditions and are considered to be both spiritually cleansing and awakening. A well-known example of a river used for sacred baths is the Ganges in India. The Hindus believe that bathing in the Ganges is a sacred experience, especially on specific occasions. One such occasion is during the Kumbha Mela, a pilgrimage every 12 years, when millions of people take a sacred bath, which is actually more a brief, full body immersion, in the Ganges. This special tradition of a sacred bath has a continuous tradition for more than 2,000 years.

Natural Hot Springs, Lakes, the Ocean, and Other Natural Settings

There is an age-old tradition of people going to special locations where water in natural settings, usually hot springs, mineral springs, lakes, or the ocean, is known for producing natural healing effects for medical conditions as well as promoting emotional balance and a sense of well-being. Many people believe, usually from experience, that there is something special about the water at these natural locations that gives it unique transforming powers. Nothing is done to enhance the water, and usually no treatments are given by therapists. A person simply interacts with the water in different ways that produce healing and wellness transformations. For example, there is a long tradition of people in most countries that have natural hot springs of using them not only for their healing benefits but also for the special energy and atmosphere felt at these natural springs. Today, these same hot springs are used for similar purposes by anyone who wishes to visit them.

Some locations have wellness and resort-style facilities built at these sites where people can stay for brief to extended periods of time and receive more complete treatment programs. Many of these locations are famous for the stories of people being healed just by bathing in the waters. For example, in 32 c.e., the famous Roman general Sulla was cured at the hot springs of Loutraki in Greece. The site soon became famous throughout the Roman Empire as being a place of natural healing. The hot springs at Hot Springs, Arkansas, were used for centuries by the local Native Americans and later became a very popular destination for people visiting the numerous wellness clinics and resorts (see Chapter 8). There are many more natural hot springs in the United States, Canada, and around the world that are well known and very popular.

After any form of natural hydrotherapy, people generally feel refreshed, rejuvenated, and balanced. Perhaps it is due to the dynamic energy of water in natural settings, and our natural relationship with water. It may also be related to the fact that water promotes deep relaxation. The special nature of water in these natural settings to promote health and wellness has provided insights into the many uses of water for hydrotherapy that are used today by therapists in the various hydrotherapy treatments and programs.

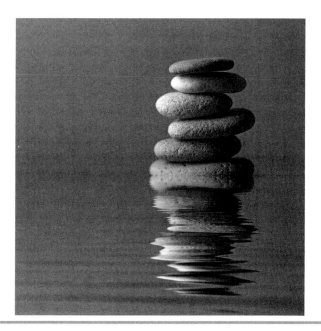

Figure 10–1 Meditative water setting *(image copyright Labetskiy Alexandr Alexandrovich, 2008. Used under license from Shutterstock.com).*

Water in Natural Settings for Contemplation, Meditation, and Creative Insights

Beautiful natural settings that have water as a central theme have long been known as places of mediation, contemplation, and connecting with nature. Feeling the dynamic energy of a waterfall, the serenity of mountain lakes, or the natural rhythm of waves at a beach can have powerful transforming effects on people. Different natural settings with a water theme are some of the most beautiful and inspiring places in the world (see Figure 10–1). For ages, people have spent time at these places for creative, artistic, and spiritual inspiration. The dynamic movement of water, combined with other natural rhythms and energy at these locations, produces very special experiences. In fact, many spa and wellness centers in urban settings attempt to re-create in their facilities some of the natural beauty and energy of water found in natural settings.

Water has also inspired many beautiful poetic and philosophical expressions, including the following quote from the *Tao Teh Ching:*

Nothing in the world is softer or more yielding than water

But, for wearing down the hard and strong, there is nothing like it

The yielding overcomes the strong and softness overcomes the hard

Is something that is known by all, but practiced by few

—Lao Tzu, *Tao Teh Ching*, Verse 78[1]

Communal Uses of Water in Natural Settings

When water is used in a communal setting, especially in natural settings, it appears to enliven a special connection between people. For example, the Roman baths, which were often built at the sites of hot springs, were places that provided an opportunity for relaxed social interaction. In North America, different Native American tribes would often gather peacefully and interact at natural hot springs, even if they were in a state of conflict. Even today, at natural hot springs and hot springs resorts, people seem more naturally relaxed, promoting a greater ease of social interaction (see Figure 10–2).

Likewise, therapists who work with clients in water—especially in such traditions as WATSU®, where relaxation is a theme—report a special connection to their clients that appears to be enhanced by working directly with them in water. This phenomenon of water creating a special connection with the client has also been experienced by therapists during other types of hydrotherapy treatments.

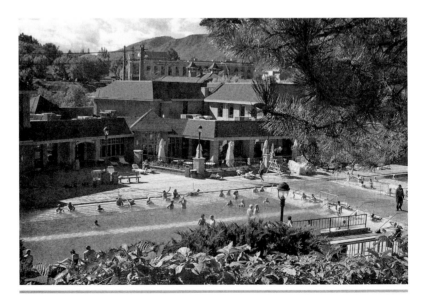

Figure 10–2 Glenwood Springs, Colorado *(compliments of Glenwood Hot Springs Pool, Glenwood Springs, Colorado).*

Perhaps it is because all living systems are connected by the same one water system (hydrosphere) or that the human body is 60% water, but there is something unique about the use of water in communal settings, especially natural settings, that enhances a greater sense of connectedness.

Recreational Use of Water in Natural Settings

Some great experiences come from recreational activities involving water in natural settings. There is the exhilarating feeling of riding a wave, of skiing down a snow-covered mountain, or of rafting through white water rapids. Just swimming in an ocean, lake, or river or skating on a frozen lake can be very refreshing, relaxing, and enlivening. There are many options for dynamic interaction with water in natural settings, and each of these forms of hydro-recreation is an expression of natural hydrotherapy and another way of interacting with water to produce positive wellness benefits. Recreational use of water is probably the way that most people have a dynamic interaction with water other than in a home setting. See Plate 3.

Natural Water for Health and Longevity

In a few locations around the world, the people who live there enjoy exceptional health and longevity. One possible explanation put forth is that the natural water found in these regions possesses special properties that contribute to the remarkable health and longevity of the people. The Hunza people, who live high in the Karakorum Mountains in northern Pakistan, are one such group of people. Research done on the water from those mountains indicates that the water may have special properties that contribute to their longevity. Attempts have been made to replicate the properties of water in these locations, but this is still something that is being developed and tested.

WATER ENHANCED BY MAN-MADE TECHNOLOGIES AND INTENTION

In this category, different technologies are used to transform and enhance ordinary, natural water. This water is then used to create health and wellness transformations in people who drink or otherwise come into contact with it. The idea is that naturally occurring water can be transformed by specific actions, technologies, or conscious intentions to gain a unique vibrational energy that can change the vibrational energy of a person who drinks or comes into contact with it.

Similar to the way therapists transform water by adding mineral salts, herbs, or oils to create a special mixture with certain benefits, water in the following examples is thought to be transformed at a subtler vibrational level. The special vibrational energy of the water then resonates with the water and energy in the person, transferring that special influence to the person. Perhaps from the following examples, insights can be gained in ways that a therapist can transform the water used in a hydrotherapy treatment that in turn will produce various transformational effects on their clients.

Crystals and Other Gemstones

A well-known technique for transforming the vibrational energy of water is to bring the water into contact with natural quartz crystals. Either the crystal is placed in the water or the water flows over the crystals. This water is then brought into contact with a person's body with the intention of transferring the special crystal energy to the person by the process of resonance. Massage and other therapists doing energy work with the intention of creating special positive benefits sometimes use this technique, and many massage schools teach energy work as part of their curriculum. For example, Chapter 7 presents a hydrotub treatment in which natural quartz crystal clusters are used as a key element.

Crystals are visually beautiful, especially when combined with water. It is also interesting to note that quartz crystals have a natural hexagonal structure, similar to the hexagonal structure of frozen water and the shape of snowflakes. Although other types of gemstones are used in a similar way, quartz crystals are most commonly used for energy treatments with water (see Figure 10–3).

Color Light Therapy

The natural colors of light have been used in many ways for healing and for enhancing a person's state of well-being. Each color of light has a specific wave frequency and energy. A rainbow is one of the most beautiful natural phenomenon of light, created when sunlight passes through raindrops (water) at specific angles.

In some special hydrotherapy treatments, specific colors of light are used to change the energy of the water. This, in turn, changes the

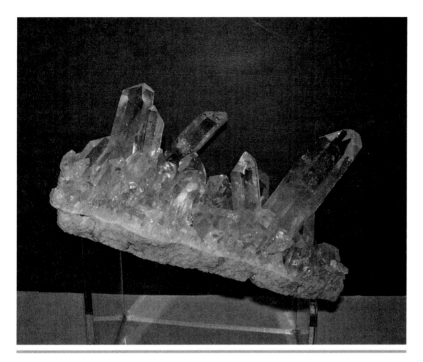

Figure 10–3 Crystal for hydrotherapy treatments.

energy of a person who comes into contact with the water. Another theory regarding color light is that the light energy is enhanced and magnified as it passes through the water to a person's body. Color light therapy is currently used in some hydrotherapy treatments in spas and wellness centers, but its use is very limited. With the development of better color light therapy equipment as well as more hydrotherapy treatments using color light therapy, the therapeutic use of color light with hydrotherapy should continue to evolve.

Natural Sounds, Music, and Water

Because sound travels through water and can be easily heard underwater, it can be combined with hydrotherapy treatments. Natural and primordial sounds, such as dolphin and whale sounds, chanting, and special sounds played on certain instruments, resonate and change the vibration not only of the water used in a hydrotherapy treatment but also the water inside the person being treated. Because water may also enhance the sound waves as they travel through water, listening to music while relaxing underwater, as in a hydrotub or flotation treatment, can produce a unique and wonderful experiences.

Communal Steam Treatments for Spiritual Cleansing

Many cultures use communal steam baths for not only relaxation, cleansing, and social bonding, but also for spiritual awakening. Examples of this are the banya in Russia, the hamam in Turkey, and the Native American sweat lodges. A sweat lodge, for example, is an intense steam session that includes the use of herbs and chanting, and is used not only for spiritual cleansing but also as a connection with nature and as preparation for special ceremonies. The ancient Mayans performed similar steam session rituals, but instead of a temporary sweat lodge, they used a more permanent structure called the temescal.

By studying the use of water and other elements in these traditions, we may be able to gain greater insights into ways to develop treatments that produce similar experiences of spiritual awakening and greater connection with nature. Even in current spas and wellness centers, it is possible to create similar experience by combining special music, herbs, and aromatherapy during a steam treatment along with an intention to produce a level of spiritual enlivenment and greater awareness. As mentioned in Chapter 7, the intention of a hydrotherapy treatment is a key element of the treatment and can influence its outcome.

Blessing Water: Hydrotherapy by Intention

People who are considered to be spiritually developed or in certain religious positions will often bless water with the intention of transforming ordinary water into water with special properties. This blessed water is then shared with others, with the idea that the special, positive qualities of the water can be transferred to the people who drink it, bless themselves with it, or keep it in their homes. As in the other examples in this section, ordinary water is transformed by contact with the higher intentions of a spiritually developed or religious person. It may be possible that therapists—most of whom have naturally developed healing skills and energy—are transforming water used in hydrotherapy treatments by their positive intentions for greater healing.

Water Responding to Thoughts, Intentions, and the Environment

Dr. Masaru Emoto's popular book *The Hidden Messages in Water* describes his research of using a special technology to freeze samples of water that had been subjected to various influences, including peoples' negative and positive thoughts.[2] He also tested samples of water from pure, pristine sources as well as water from polluted sources. Using the special freezing techniques on these different samples of water, he was able to produce different hexagonal crystal patterns, similar to snowflakes. Photographs of these crystals showed that samples from sources exposed to positive thoughts and feelings as well as those from pure water sources, produced beautiful patterns. Water crystals exposed to negative thoughts or feelings and from polluted sources, on the other hand, produced deformed crystals.

Dr. Emoto believed that he was able to objectively demonstrate that normal water absorbs and is transformed by the positive and negative influences to which it is exposed. It is another example of the theory that water can be transformed in positive or negative ways by subtle influences and that the water can then transfer those positive or negative influences to people or the environment. According to this theory, therapists are able to have a transforming effect on the water they use for hydrotherapy simply with their own positive thoughts, feelings, and intentions. This water then has a greater positive effect on their clients during a hydrotherapy treatment.

Feng Shui, Sthapatya Veda, and the Power of Flowing Water

Feng shui is the well-known tradition from China in which the architectural design of buildings and the directional orientation of buildings and landscaping, including flowing water, should follow specific guidelines that bring the structure and its surroundings into harmony with nature. The results of good feng shui are health, prosperity, and success for the people living or working in the building.

Feng shui offers specific rules for flowing water, one of which is that water should flow naturally, as a natural stream does; water should not flow in straight lines or through square (90°) angles. Properly flowing water is felt to contain an abundance of chi, or life force energy, which is essential to the total health of the building, of the people dwelling in the building, and of the land surrounding the building.

Traditional Chinese medicine also states that there is a similar flow of chi in the human body that must remain balanced and healthy as a basis for individual health. The flow of chi in the body appears to follow similar principles as the flow of water—that is, chi should flow in a continual, unobstructed manner, without any excess or restricted flow. The correlation between the healthy flow of chi and the healthy flow of water in the body is interesting to consider, especially now that we have greater understanding of the complex nature of the circulation of water in the human body (see Chapter 3). Chapter 7 describes a hydrotherapy treatment that combines underwater hydromassage with the practice of shiatsu massage. The hydromassage is done along the client's energy lines and points in a similar way that hands are used on a client during a shiatsu treatment on a massage table.

Sthapatya Veda, from the Vedic tradition of India, is similar to feng shui. Like feng shui, it is thousands of years old and deals with similar principles of architecture and landscaping to bring a building into harmony with nature. This, in turn, brings happiness, health, and prosperity to those who dwell in the building. The flow and location of any water in relationship to the building, and in the streams, ponds, and lakes, must be according to specific rules to ensure maximum healthy prana, or life force. These guidelines are very detailed and are fundamental to Vedic architecture and landscaping. Sthapatya Veda, as a form of architecture that is in harmony with the natural environment, is becoming popular in other countries outside of India, similar to the way Ayurvedic health treatments and yoga have become popular. Figure 10–4 shows a modern Sthapatya home in the United States that is located facing east with a lake (not shown) in the correct location to the north side of building.

In the Ayurveda health tradition, properly flowing water in the body's circulatory system is seen as being essential for a healthy flow of prana in the body. Because hydrotherapy promotes healthy

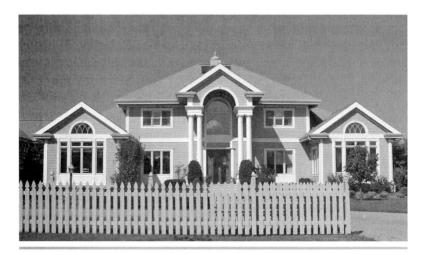

Figure 10–4 Sthapatya Vedic home, Fairfield, Iowa *(courtesy of Sthapatya Vedic Home, Fairfield, Iowa).*

circulation of water in the body, it may also at the same time be improving the flow of prana.

These ancient traditions help us see that there may be much more to what makes water "healthy" than just what we know from a scientific perspective. These special traditions of the application of water to enhance the health of buildings and the landscaping that surrounds them, and the people in them, is another interesting use of the full potential of water in areas related to health and wellness.

Special Technologies to Make Drinking Water "Healthier"

Some different approaches are now being used to modify the behavior of water, usually at the molecular level, to make it healthier for various metabolic activities at the cellular level in the human body. The general idea is that "normal" water has lost much of its natural essential qualities due to the addition of chemicals, such as chlorine to drinking water, as well as pollution from industry, agriculture, and other sources. It is also thought that artificially changing the natural flow of water, as occurs in the process of municipal treatment plants, water storage towers, city water lines, and bottled water, disturbs the natural energy of the water.

Attempts are being made to use special technologies, such as magnetic fields, to restore or even enhance the health benefits of the water. Some brands of water that have been "enhanced" at the molecular level are available at health and natural food stores. Each of these brands has different claims as to how their enhanced water provides special health benefits. There are also some special technologies that take water that has "lost" its natural energy as a result of flowing though straight lines and angles and creates ways by which the water flows in unique vortex patterns. This is believed to restore and enhance the natural energy of the water.

Many of the claims by the companies who are attempting to improve the quality of water are difficult to prove, but some of the "enhanced" waters are popular and those interested in possibly using or recommending them to clients should carefully research them to understand the theory behind what makes the water special for greater health and wellness.

Hydrotherapy and the Treatment of Major Medical Conditions

Historically, hydrotherapy has been used in conjunction with traditional medical approaches in the treatment of serious medical conditions including infectious diseases, cancer, auto-immune disorders, and skin and mental health problems. As we saw in Chapter 8, natural mineral water is currently being used as part of treatments, mainly in Europe and Japan, to treat a wide range of medical problems. These treatments are usually combined with some form of massage, physical therapy, exercise, herbs, and even prescription drugs. In Europe, these techniques have been used for several hundred years and in Japan for more than a thousand years. There is considerable scientific research that has been done to verify the effectiveness of these approaches, which include hydrotherapy as a major component, for treatments in many areas including:

- Asthma
- Diabetes
- Essential hypertension
- Cardiac arrhythmias
- Hepatitis
- Osteoarthritis
- Rheumatoid arthritis
- Psoriasis
- Depression

For more detailed information on the use of hydrotherapy at medical facilities located at the sites of natural mineral springs, including references to scientific studies, please refer to *Healing Springs* by Nathaniel Altman.[3]

Even in the United States, there are historical examples of the use of hydrotherapy as part of a treatment program in Saratoga Springs, NY and also Hot Springs, AR. In 1911 at Hot Springs, the U.S. government founded a clinic for the treatment of venereal diseases that used bathing in the natural mineral waters as part of the treatment, even though the clinic closed in 1948 with the introduction of penicillin. Today, except for some countries in Europe and Japan, hydrotherapy is not commonly used in the treatment of major medical conditions. It is more often used by physical therapists, occupational therapists, and massage therapists in rehabilitation treatments and programs.

Because this hydrotherapy textbook has been developed for massage therapists, aestheticians, body workers, and other alternative therapists that are not trained nor licensed to treat major medical conditions, hydrotherapy treatments for specific major medical conditions are not covered in this textbook. However, the same basic hydrotherapy skills that a therapist learns in this textbook and that are used in the various treatments presented in Chapter 7, are the same skills that therapists use in special hydrotherapy treatments for major medical conditions, for example, hyperthermia treatments (steam, hydrotub) that heat the core temperature of the body. The basic hydrotherapy principles are the same, however, the use of hydrotherapy to treat major medical conditions must be done under the supervision of medical personnel who are also trained in the use of hydrotherapy techniques.

There is also a growing positive trend in the use of integrative medicine that includes the use of alternative health programs, including hydrotherapy, along with traditional medicine as a total treatment program for many major medical conditions. For example, a physician may find that a client with cancer would benefit from the deep relaxation and comfort that clients experience with certain hydrotherapy treatments, which could help them in dealing with the anxiety and emotional discomfort that clients experience with such conditions.

 ## SUMMARY

This chapter presents an overview of some of the special and unique approaches in the use of water for achieving a wide variety of health and wellness goals. By considering certain common elements found in the different examples presented in this chapter, we may gain deeper insights into the full potential of the behavior of water as a therapeutic modality. This chapter looks at two general categories of the special use of water: the use of water as it naturally occurs without any modifications, usually in natural settings, and the use of water that has been modified or enhanced by man-made technologies and intentions.

The following are the different types of the use of water, usually found in natural settings.

- Healing baths: used naturally heal major medical conditions. The example used was the famous healing baths at Lourdes, France.
- Sacred baths: used to awaken greater spiritual consciousness. An example was a sacred bath in the Ganges.
- Time spent for healing and relaxation at natural hot springs, lakes, rivers, and oceans.

- Time spent in meditation and contemplation in beautiful natural settings with a water theme, for example, a waterfall.

- Benefits from interacting with water for recreational purposes, for example, swimming, skiing, skating, surfing, and rafting.

The following are ways that people modify, or "enhance" ordinary water that give it added power to produce health and wellness transformations:

- Use of quartz crystals and water to enhance the effects of hydrotherapy treatments.

- Use of color light therapy and water to transform the water used during a hydrotherapy treatment or to enhance the power of the color light as it comes into contact with the body.

- Use of natural sounds, primordial sounds, and music during hydrotherapy treatments.

- The use of sacred communal steam treatments to enliven spiritual awareness and greater connection with nature.

- Transforming water in positive ways by blessing it.

- Water being automatically influenced by the thoughts and feelings of people, and also by the quality of the environment in which the water is found.

- Ancient traditions of feng shui and Sthapatya Veda enhance the natural life force in buildings and their surroundings by the proper placement and flow of water.

- Enhancing normal water used for drinking by the use of special technologies to increase its health potential, especially at the cellular level.

- The use of hydrotherapy programs in the treatment of major medical conditions.

REFERENCES

(1) Ni, Hua-Ching. (1995). *The Complete Works of Lao Tzu.* Los Angeles, California: Seven Star Communications.

(2) Emoto, M. (2004). *The Hidden Messages in Water.* Hillsboro, Oregons: Beyond Words Publishing.

(3) Altman, N. (2000). *Healing Springs.* Rochester, Vermont: Healing Arts Press.

SUGGESTED READING

Thrash, A., & Thrash, C. (2006). *Home Remedies: Hydrotherapy, Massage, Charcoal, and Other Simple Treatments.* A New Lifestyle Book.

REVIEW QUESTIONS

1. Describe some of your own experiences of water in natural settings that produced some special, notable experience, healing, or awakening.

2. What are two of the basic principles of the behavior of water found at hot springs that people using the hot springs experience? What are two of the basic principles of the behavior of water found in oceans that people experience?

3. Describe how it is possible to transform water for a hydrotherapy treatment using natural products such as herbs or mineral salts. Describe how it might be possible to transform water using crystals, color light, music, or intention?

4. Describe any experiences you have had using crystals, color light, sound, intention, or any other subtle effects to transform water used for a hydrotherapy treatment.

Marketing Hydrotherapy Programs

11

INTRODUCTION

This chapter looks at how to successfully market hydrotherapy treatments to current and potential clients as part of your spa or wellness programs. As many therapists and spa owners are not as familiar with hydrotherapy programs and themes as they are with other programs, such as massage and aesthetic treatments, this chapter will present creative ways to promote hydrotherapy treatments and programs.

MARKETING HYDROTHERAPY TREATMENTS AND PROGRAMS

Hydrotherapy programs have been an essential part of the most successful holistic health and wellness traditions. In fact, as has been mentioned, two of the oldest traditions—Ayurveda from India and Japanese hydrotherapy programs, which both date back thousands of years—continue to be popular today in spa and wellness centers around the world. In addition, Germany has many technologically advanced and esthetically beautiful spa and wellness complexes that use water from natural mineral and hot springs. Many of these German spas are modeled after the Roman bath complexes that were once located on the same sites as the modern facilities.

The reason for the success of hydrotherapy treatments, programs, and themes is that they work on many different levels. Human beings have a natural relationship with water (our bodies are 60% water), and 70% of Earth's surface is covered by water (100% when you include water in the atmosphere). Hydrotherapy treatments and programs

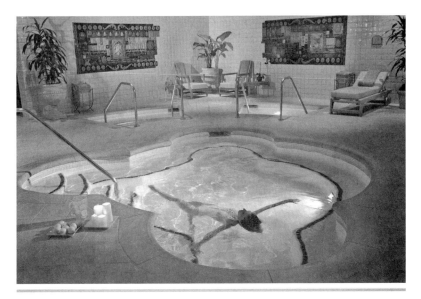

Figure 11–1 Resort hydrotherapy program *(courtesy of Marriott Hotels).*

allow us to further develop our natural relationship with water by using it as a therapeutic modality for producing multiple health and wellness benefits. The creative challenge now becomes how to successfully communicate and promote these hydrotherapy programs to current and potential clients (see Figure 11–1 and Plate 7).

The following are the goals of a hydrotherapy marketing program:

- To increase the number of new clients to the facility getting hydrotherapy treatments
- To increase the number of current clients at the facility getting hydrotherapy treatments
- To increase client retention by offering a broader spa menu that includes hydrotherapy treatments

PROMOTIONAL MATERIALS AND HYDROTHERAPY PROGRAMS

Clients are not always aware of the many benefits of hydrotherapy treatments and how these benefits can help them achieve their personal health and wellness goals. Thus, it is necessary to use creative, engaging marketing materials to communicate how they can enjoy and benefit from hydrotherapy treatments and how wonderful those treatments can be.

Spa Menu and Brochure

Create descriptive explanations of your hydrotherapy programs can be included that capture the interest of those reading the spa menu or brochure. Because only limited information can be included on spa menus and brochures, descriptions need to be brief but enticing. Include photographs of water in natural settings, such as a beach on a tropical island, a lake, or a waterfall. There are now several quality stock photography sites that provide beautiful photos of spa and water themes. There are hundreds of photos to choose from and these photos can be used for your brochures, Web site, printed materials, and DVD presentations. One example of a stock photography Web site is Shutterstock at www.shutterstock.com (see Figure 11–2). Search for photographs using key words, such as "waterfall," "tropical beach," and "spa relaxation."

Special Printed Descriptions

In addition to menus and brochures, you may want to provide special printed descriptions (leaflets) about the hydrotherapy programs

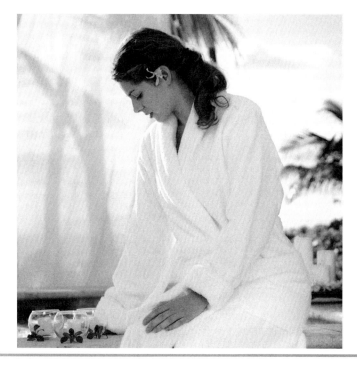

Figure 11–2 Web site spa photograph *(image copyright iofoto, 2008. Used under license from Shutterstock.com).*

and treatments. These may be one-page, front-and-back leaflets that provide more detailed explanations of the benefits of each treatment. You may also want to include color photos of the actual treatments. These leaflets can easily be printed from a computer onsite.

DVD Presentation

Another great way to market hydrotherapy programs is with a DVD presentation. It is now possible for anyone with creative computer skills to create a DVD presentation on a home computer. A DVD presentation can include any number of color photographs as well as video clips of not only water and spa themes but photos of hydrotherapy treatments being offered at the spa or wellness center. A DVD presentation can also include audio descriptions and soothing music. These DVD presentations can be played in the reception area and copies can also be sent to potential clients as part of a total marketing program.

Web Site

Web sites are now as fundamental to marketing as brochures once were. Unlike brochures, Web sites offer unlimited space for written descriptions, photos, and even video/audio clips. They provide you with a cost-effective way to communicate directly with potential or existing clients. In any advertisements, brochures, or leaflets, be sure to include and emphasize your Web address (URL) so that people can visit your Web site.

When looking for a Web site designer, shop around until you find the right source at a reasonable cost. Another option is to have someone who has good computer skills who is connected with your business learn the basic skills of Web site design. With some basic training, just about anyone can use Web site design software programs to create a professional Web site.

Spa Magazines in the Reception Area

Spa trade magazines often include beautiful presentations of spas from around the world that feature hydrotherapy programs and themes. These magazines could be placed in the reception or resting area for clients to read. The following are suggested resources for spa magazines:

American Spa Magazine: www.americanspamag.com

Skin Inc.: www.skininc.com

Day Spa Magazine: www.dayspamagazine.com

Les Nouvelles Esthétiques: www.nouvelles-esthetiques.com

Spa Finder: www.spafinder.com

Some of these magazines also contain excellent articles on managing a spa and wellness center.

CLIENT INTERVIEW: KEY TO SUCCESS

A key aspect of any spa and wellness program is attention to the personal needs of the client. Therefore, it is important for a current or potential client to have a personal interview with a therapist or trained staff member. At the interview, any questions the client has can be answered. In addition, you can determine what the client is interested in and recommend a personalized program that suits him or her best. Most clients are seeking knowledgeable advice on different treatments and programs. Although they may have a general idea of what they are looking for, they often find it very helpful to speak with someone who understands the available programs and who can make a personal recommendation suited to the client's specific needs. Thus, based on the interview, it should be possible to determine what health and wellness benefits the client is seeking and make recommendations that include the appropriate hydrotherapy treatments.

COMBINATION TREATMENT PACKAGES AND A SERIES OF TREATMENTS

A good way to introduce clients to the wonderful experiences and benefits of hydrotherapy treatments is to offer packages that combine hydrotherapy with other treatments. For example, hydrotherapy works very well in combination with massage, esthetic treatments, and fitness programs. The profound relaxation of hydrotherapy, in addition to its other benefits, can enhance the effect of the total combination. See Chapters 5 and 7 for suggestions on the many combination packages that can include hydrotherapy.

Special packages generally have specific goals, such as skin care, weight management, stress management, and general wellness. For a client to realistically attain these goals, it is often necessary to offer a series of treatment sessions at regular intervals over a specified period of time. At a minimum, clients should receive maintenance and tune-up programs on a regular basis as part of their own health and wellness program. Some very successful holistic health and wellness programs, such as Ayurveda or the Kneipp program, include not only a daily home health and wellness routine but also a regular program of treatments from a professional therapist. For example, in the Ayurvedic tradition, a person receives a special balancing and renewal treatments four times each year. Such programs are similar to regular maintenance program for your car. Of course, the human body is far more complex than the best luxury car and greatly benefits from regular care and rejuvenation programs.

 ## SPA TEAM

Another approach that has proven successful at spa and wellness centers is to involve all the therapists, staff, management, and anyone else who has direct contact with clients as part of an integrated "spa team," so that from the time a client arrives until he or she leaves, every experience contributes toward a completely rewarding and satisfying session. As part of this team approach, every person who interacts with a client should be educated about the different hydrotherapy treatments and their benefits. In addition, everyone involved should also have the experience of receiving the different hydrotherapy treatments, which will make them more enthusiastic in promoting those treatments to clients. Although brochures, Web sites, and other promotional materials can be effective, a well-educated, knowledgeable, enthusiastic spa team will have perhaps the greatest influence in inspiring and motivating clients about taking advantage of the special hydrotherapy programs being offered.

 ## HYDROTHERAPY SPA THEMES

Another way to promote hydrotherapy is to create a theme within the facility that expresses all of the healing, rejuvenating, relaxing, mystical and magical qualities of water as found in various beautiful, natural settings. Some of the best spas in the world, in places like Bali, Hawaii, Thailand, Japan, France, and Germany, have water themes along with offering quality hydrotherapy programs. Developing this theme can be as simple as placing photographs of beautiful water settings or of treatments with water themes in the facility (see Figure 11–3). Music can also be played that includes the natural soothing sounds of water

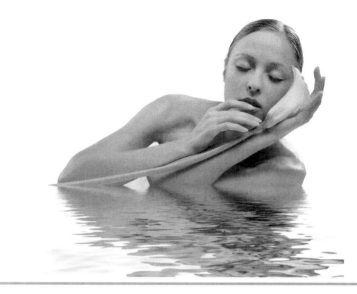

Figure 11–3 Hydrotherapy spa theme *(image copyright Solovieva Ekaterina, 2008. Used under license from Shutterstock.com).*

flowing, either in the reception area or during a hydrotherapy treatment. Another option is to include water fountains to create the sounds and the vision of flowing water.

 ## CLIENT RETENTION

Adding hydrotherapy treatments to your total treatment menu can improve client retention. Not only are the number of treatment options available greater, but also total client satisfaction and motivation to continue to get treatments on a regular basis can be increased. Great treatments produce great word-of-mouth advertising, making your clients one of your best marketing resources.

After all the effort, time, and expense of persuading clients to get a hydrotherapy treatment, the experience should be such that clients not only want to get the treatment again but will also share with others how great it was. When you talk to someone who has been to many spas, that person will have stories about the best treatments (often a hydrotherapy treatment) and the worst treatments (also often a hydrotherapy treatment). The following are some of the basic mistakes that can ruin what should have been a great experience:

- The most common complaint by clients during hydrotherapy treatments is that they got cold or overheated. You cannot tell by looking at a client what he or she is experiencing;

you must ask for feedback. Some clients will suffer in silence unless you ask them for feedback. Sometimes, those clients will not come back.

- Don't start a hydrotherapy treatment, especially a heating treatment, and then leave the client alone until the end of the treatment. Give the client as much personal attention as possible at regular intervals and get enough feedback to know that the treatment is going well and if any adjustments need to be made.

- Make sure therapists are properly trained in the steps of the treatment as well as in the use of the equipment. Even the best hydrotherapy equipment will produce limited results if not used properly.

The following is an inspirational message from Monica Tuma Brown to those who are planning to offer and promote hydrotherapy in their business.

Water is Nature's wonder drug . . . it soothes, it nourishes, cleanses, and restores. It is the "source" of "Spa," be it ancient springs, the oceans, a simple bath, modern hydrotherapy, a steam, shower, or even a moist, warm towel. Water adapts beautifully to all health, wellness, and relaxation needs. Heat it, cool it, and add to it, it can be a most efficacious compliment to natural therapies, enhancing holistic benefits and outcomes.

Historical wisdom is now a scientific fact. We possess a better understanding of the action and benefits of hydrotherapy as it relates to human physiology. We have access to advanced research, technological developments, and availability of unique spa products and equipment to enhance the spa experience. This has fostered a keen desire to again seek the "source" from the simplest of applications, such as a footbath, to a sophisticated, computerized hydrotub or shower treatment. The beauty of hydrotherapy is the ability to incorporate water into your own healing philosophy via a vast array of forms, treatments, products, and equipment.

Water's precious position in spa therapies and experiences is back. Recognized and esteemed as a vital, natural resource around the globe, the spa industry is enjoying the homecoming of one of nature's most fundamental and enjoyable, natural healing elements.

—Monica Tuma Brown

Monica possesses more than 35 years of health and spa experience, spanning international health care, wellness, and spa positions in management, development, and consulting. She is known for her creative concepts and solutions to spa operations and signature experiences. Monica has specialized in integrating hydrotherapy programs into modern spa and health and wellness programs.

The following are suggestions by Monica about marketing hydrotherapy:

- Power up the Purpose: Highlight the benefits of each treatment and promote the holistic experience.
- Romance the History: The stories of hydrotherapy are intriguing and generate interest.
- Live It in Your Menu: Create and promote hydrotherapy treatments that become a "have to" in your spa menu.
- Be a Hydro Host: Offer tours, insight, information, and promotions; host hydrotherapy lectures and information; do special mineral water tasting. Be creative and have fun!

 ## SUMMARY

The purpose of marketing a hydrotherapy program is to increase the number of new clients getting hydrotherapy treatments, to increase the number of current clients getting hydrotherapy treatments, and to increase client retention. Developing marketing materials for hydrotherapy can be a very creative and enjoyable process. Use beautiful photographs and other multimedia options to promote a hydrotherapy theme in your brochures, Web site, DVD presentations, and advertisements to create an interest in hydrotherapy treatments and programs.

Another effective way to motivate clients to choose hydrotherapy is through the personal client interview. From the interview, a knowledgeable therapist or staff person can learn about the client's health and wellness goals and then make recommendations about a personalized treatment program, which includes hydrotherapy. It also provides them with a personalized program designed to meet their special personal needs.

Hydrotherapy treatments are great as part of a package of treatments. By having a hydrotherapy treatment as part of a package of treatments, clients can be introduced to the wonderful experience and benefits of hydrotherapy. To achieve the full benefits of a treatment program, such as weight or stress management, it is also a good idea to offer a program as part of a series of sessions. Ongoing programs for regular maintenance should also be part of a client's total holistic health and wellness program for maintenance and rejuvenation of body, mind, emotions, and spirit.

Many of the top spas around the world include a water theme as part of their total spa and wellness theme. This can include beautiful photos of natural water settings and other spa themes. Sounds of ocean waves, waterfalls, and rain can add to the effect. Water fountains and pools can also produce special healing and soothing effects. This can be another option in promoting hydrotherapy programs.

Hydrotherapy treatments produce some of the most relaxing, healing experiences of any types of spa and wellness treatments. However, they must be done properly. Clients who get cold or overheated during a hydrotherapy treatment can become very uncomfortable. Clients should not be left alone during a hydrotherapy treatment for long periods of time, especially a heating treatment. By attention to simple details, clients will have a positive experience with every hydrotherapy treatment.

REVIEW QUESTIONS

1. What are the three key goals of a successful marketing program?

2. What are some different approaches to market a hydrotherapy program?

3. What advantages does a Web site offer in marketing hydrotherapy programs.

4. What advantage does an interview with a client offer in determining what treatments he or she wants compared to simply providing the client a spa menu?

5. Discuss how including hydrotherapy treatments as part of a "special package" of treatments can help promote a hydrotherapy program.

6. Discuss some ways a hydrotherapy theme could be added to a facility to enhance a hydrotherapy program.

7. What are some guidelines to follow to help decrease the chance of a client having an unfavorable hydrotherapy treatment?

Appendix A

Fahrenheit to Celsius Conversion Chart	
Fahrenheit	**Celsius**
32	0
60	15.5
65	18.3
70	21.1
75	23.9
85	29.4
86	30.0
87	30.5
88	31.1
89	31.6
90	32.2
91	32.8
92	33.2
93	33.9
94	34.4
95	35.0
96	35.5
97	36.1
98	36.6

continues

Fahrenheit to Celsius Conversion Chart *(continued)*

Fahrenheit	Celsius
98.6	37.0
99	37.2
100	37.7
101	38.3
102	38.8
103	39.4
104	40.0
105	40.5
106	41.1
107	41.7
108	42.2
109	42.7
110	43.3
111	43.9
112	44.4
113	45.0
114	45.5
115	46.1
116	46.7
117	47.2
118	47.7
119	48.3
120	48.9
121	49.4
122	50.0
123	50.6
124	51.1
125	51.7
130	54.4
212	100.0

Appendix B

Trade Magazines and Trade Shows

(Current listing of trade shows can be found on some of the trade magazine Web sites listed below)

- *American Spa Magazine:* www.americanspamag.com
- *Skin Inc.:* www.skininc.com
- *Day Spa Magazine:* www.dayspamagazine.com
- *Les Nouvelles Esthétiques:* www.nouvelles-esthetiques.com
- *Dermascope Magazine:* www.dermascope.com
- *Spa Finder Magazine:* www.spafinder.com

Internet Keywords for Hydrotherapy Equipment

Hydrotub Equipment
- spa hydrotub, therapeutic hydrotub, wellnesshydrotub

Steam Equipment
- steam canopy, steam cabinet, steam room, steammassagetable
- steam inhalation equipment, mabis steam inhaler

Shower Equipment
- Vichy shower, Swiss shower

Hydromassage Table
Most hydromassage tables on the Internet are mainly robotic in nature and are not designed for use on a client by a therapist. The following key words are more likely to locate a manual hydromassage table for use on a client by a therapist.
- manualwatertherapy, manualhydromassage, hydromassage table

continues

359

Hydrotherapy Equipment Resource Guide *(continued)*

Hot and Cold Herbal Compresses
- make herbal compresses, herbal compresses

Hydroballoon Equipment
- hydroballoon massage, hydroballoon massage, hydrosphere massage

Appendix C

Hydrotherapy Product Resource Guide

Trade Magazines and Trade Shows

(Current listing of trade shows can be found on some of the trade magazine Web sites listed below)

- *American Spa Magazine:* www.americanspamag.com
- *Skin Inc.:* www.skininc.com
- *Day Spa Magazine:* www.dayspamagazine.com
- *Les Nouvelles Esthétiques:* www.nouvelles-esthetiques.com
- *Dermascope Magazine:* www.dermascope.com
- *Spa Finder Magazine:* www.spafinder.com

Internet Keywords for Hydrotherapy Products

Herbs and Seaweed
- herbal baths, herbs spa treatments, herbal spa bath
- seaweed spa treatments, seaweed bath treatments

Essential Oils
- spa bath essential oils, bath essential oils, therapeutic essential bath oils

Hydrosols
- organic hydrosols, hydrosols, bath hydrosols

Minerals
- therapeutic mineral salts, therapeutic sea salts, spa mineral baths

Moor Mud
- Moor mud, Moor mud spa, therapeutic Moor mud, Moor spa mud

Clays and Mud
- mud spa treatments, therapeutic mud treatments, clay spa treatments, therapeutic clay treatments

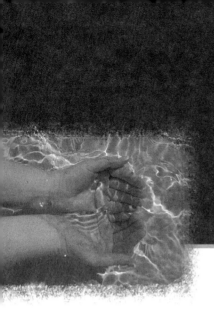

Glossary

A

Adhesion The behavior of water that allows water molecules to be attracted to other types of molecules on the surface of other substances.

Aquatic therapy pool Modern, smaller therapy pool specifically designed for clients and allows for exercise in water and other hydrotherapy features.

Asclepieion In ancient Greece, the site of holistic health, wellness, and medical programs.

Ayurveda A holistic form of health and wellness that originated in India thousands of years ago and that uses hydrotherapy as a key element.

B

Bacteria Single-cell, plantlike microorganisms, some of which cause disease.

Balanced Hydration Program A systematic, personalized hydration treatment.

Balneotherapy The study and use of natural mineral water for improving health and wellness.

Baroreceptor Neurons that are sensitive to changes in blood pressure.

Blood plasma The liquid that remains after red and white blood cells and platelets have been separated from the blood.

Broad-spectrum disinfectant A high-grade disinfectant that kills the normal range of germs. Recommended for use in hydrotherapy rooms and equipment.

Buoyancy The upward pressure exerted by the fluid in which a body is immersed.

C

Cell The basic structural and functional unit of the body capable of performing all the activities vital to life.

Cohesion The attraction between water molecules that allows water to behave as a liquid between temperatures of 32°F (0°C) and 212°F (100°C).

Cold induced vasodilatation (VSD) A protective response in which there is a sudden, dramatic increase in blood flow to a specific tissue of the body to keep it from being damaged by an extreme drop in temperature. This can happen when applying ice (cryotherapy) after about 20 minutes. Also known as *hunting response*.

Colon therapy A form of therapy that uses specially designed equipment for the purpose of colon cleaning.

Contact time (dwell time) The time required to leave a disinfectant on a surface in order to be effective.

Crystal therapy Natural quartz crystals that have a hexagonal shape, the same as the structure as water. Used in hydrotherapy to energetically transform the water.

D

Diffusion The movement of a substance from an area of high concentration to an area of lower concentration.

E

Evaporation The transformation of water from the liquid or frozen state to the gas (vapor) state.

G

Gravity The natural force of attraction exerted by a celestial body, such as Earth, upon objects at or near its surface, tending to draw them toward the center of the body.

H

Handheld shower The use of a single shower head connected to a flexible hose that allows a therapist to rinse product off the client.

Heat capacity The ability of a substance to absorb and release heat. Water has a high heat capacity.

Humidity A measure of the amount of water vapor in the air.

Hunting response See *cold induced vasodilatation (CIVSD).*

Hydrogen bond The term used to describe the cohesive attraction between water molecules.

Hydrologic cycle The dynamic movement by which water is constantly evaporating and becoming part of the atmosphere, condensing, and then precipitating back to the ground, flowing from higher to lower elevations, and then evaporating to begin the cycle again.

Hydrology The study of the behavior of water, especially as it occurs in the hydrosphere.

Hydrophilic Substances that dissolve naturally in water (*hydro* means "water," *phyllic* means "love").

Hydrophobic Substances that do not dissolve in water, such as oils (*phobic* means "fear").

Hydrosol Water-soluble essence of plants (as compared with essential oils, which are the oil essence of the plant).

Hydrosphere All the water on Earth (which is generally a fixed amount) and its behavior as one integrated system.

Hydrotherapy The use of water to produce a therapeutic transformation in a person (client).

Hydrotub A bathtub used for hydrotherapy treatments that can range from a simple bathtub to a more complex hydrotub with hydrojets, hydrowands, and/or music and color therapy.

Hydrowand An underwater hose that allows a therapist to direct a stream of water under pressure to very specific areas of the client's body.

Hypocaust A system in ancient Rome that used advanced plumbing and ventilation systems to produce heated pools and rooms.

Hypothermia The core temperature of the body decreases below its homeostatic set point of 98.6°F, which stimulates a heating response.

I

Infiltration The process by which some of the water that falls on land is absorbed by the soil to become groundwater.

Integrative medicine Combination of the use of alternative health programs, including hydrotherapy, with traditional medicine for the treatment of major medical conditions.

K

Kinetic energy The mechanical energy that a body has by virtue of its motion.

Kneipp therapy A holistic program of health and wellness that includes hydrotherapy, founded by Sebastian Kneipp around 1875. A foundation for modern hydrotherapy programs in Germany.

L

Lubricant A substance that lessens friction, such as water on a hard, smooth surface.

Lymphatic vascular system A system that helps drain and purify the interstitial fluid surrounding the cells of the body returning back into the cardiovascular system.

M

Methicillin-resistant *Staphylococcus aureus* (MRSA) A strain of staphylococcus that has developed a resistance to modern antibiotics.

Mineral salts Natural occurring substances that dissolve easily in water, for example, sea salt (mainly sodium chloride), calcium, and magnesium.

Mold Microfungus that grows in warm, moist conditions and that can produce respiratory irritation and allergies.

Mole A combination of the atomic weights of the atoms that make up a substance.

Moor mud A rare form of nutrient-rich peat that has been created by the gradual transformation of herbs, plants, and flowers that have been permanently submerged underwater or underground.

N

Nasya Ayurvedic treatment that uses steam inhalation and certain herbs to detoxify, balance, and enliven the respiratory system.

Negative ions Molecules that have gained an extra electron.

O

Osmolarity The measure of osmoles of solute per liter of solution.

Osmoreceptor Neuron in the hypothalamus that is sensitive to changes in the blood's osmolarity.

Osmosis The flow of water molecules through a semipermeable membrane from the side of a higher concentration of water molecules to the side of a lower concentration of water molecules.

P

pH level A measure of the acidity or alkalinity of a specific solution.

Pressure balance A feature on some hydrotherapy equipment that prevents fluctuations in water temperature when water is being used elsewhere.

Pumping Applying pressure, or force, to water to cause water flow.

R

Roman bath Sophisticated spa, wellness, community, and fitness centers of ancient Rome.

S

Scald protection A feature on some hydrotherapy equipment that prevents the temperature of the water from becoming excessively hot or scalding hot and possibly injuring the client.

Solute The substance dissolved in a given solution, for example, salt in water.

Solvent A substance that dissolves another to form a solution. Water is a solvent.

Specific gravity The weight in grams of 1 cm^3 of a substance. The specific gravity of water is 1 g.

Surface tension Water molecules on the surface of water have a greater attraction to each other than to the water molecules below the surface.

Suspension The mixing of a substance in water. When the mixing ceases, the substance will separate from the water.

Swedhana A steam treatment in Ayurveda that induces sweating for detoxification.

Swiss shower A vertical shower system with multiple showerheads (approximately ten) that showers a client on all sides, including the head, as the client stands.

T

Thallasotherapy The use of seawater for hydrotherapy; generally limited to facilities located very close to the ocean.

Thirst center The portion of the brain, found in the hypothalamus, that governs the urge to drink.

W

Water isotope Water molecule that has a slightly different molecular structure, with either the oxygen or the hydrogen molecule having extra neutron(s).

WATSU Form of hydrotherapy in which the therapist works with the client in a special pool, taking the client through a series of passive flowing motions.

Wet room Special hydrotherapy treatment room that allows water to flow from a wet table onto the floor and drain to a central floor drain.

V

Vichy shower A horizontal shower with multiple showerheads (approximately seven) that showers a client lying on a wet table, often as the client is being massaged. The origin of the treatment is from Vichy, France.

Virus Smallest disease-causing microorganism.

Y

Yeast Microfungus that produce diseases such as ringworm, nail fungus, and athlete's foot.

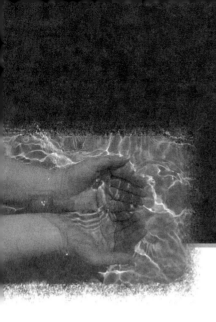

Index